Chinese
Medical
Obstetrics

Chinese Medical Obstetrics

Bob Flaws

Blue Poppy Press

Published by:
BLUE POPPY PRESS
A Division of Blue Poppy Enterprises, Inc.
1990 N 57th Court, Unit A
BOULDER, CO 80301

FIRST EDITION, JULY, 2005
SECOND PRINTING, JULY, 2009
THIRD PRINTING, JANUARY, 2013

ISBN 1-891845-30-6
ISBN 978-1-891845-30-7
LOC #2006273082

COMP **Designation:** Original work using a standard translational terminology

Cover design by Eric Brearton
Interior design by Debra Topping

Printed at Edwards Brothers Malloy, Ann Arbor, MI

10 9 8 7 6 5 4 3

Contents

Book Two   Postpartum Diseases

Preface

Path of Pregnancy was the first book I wrote on Chinese medicine, now 23 or more years ago. Since then, this book has gone through four incarnations. If one where to compare the evolution of these four editions, one would get not only a good impression of my development as a Chinese doctor but also, I think, of the development of the profession as a whole in the West. This current edition is a combination of the previous *Path of Pregnancy, Volumes 1 & 2*, in a single volume. It is meant as a textbook and clinical manual of Chinese medical obstetrics.

Some of the changes in this fourth edition include up-dating the terminology to more closely agree with that found in Nigel Wiseman and Feng Ye's *A Practical Dictionary of Chinese Medicine* as well as other, newer Blue Poppy Press books. I have corrected a number of inconsistencies and errors in the Latinate pharmacological identification of medicinals. In addition, I have standardized the Pinyin identifications of all the medicinals so that a given medicinal is always referred to by its full standard Chinese name, and I have added English language translations of all Chinese formula names. Other additions consist of more lengthy and up-to-date Western medical introductions of each disease category, abstracts of representative Chinese research, representative case histories (whenever I could find these), and acupuncture and moxibustion formulas for each pattern of most, if not all, diseases. I have changed the table of contents so that it is more congruent with modern Western medicine, for instance, talking about such things as postpartum infection instead of postpartum fever and postpartum depression instead of postpartum palpitations and abstraction. Hopefully, I have also improved the quality of the Chinese medical theory.

In preparing this edition, one of my goals was to make the book easier to use for Western students and practitioners alike. Therefore, I have included standard daily doses under each of the guiding formulas. These doses are for use in bulk-dispensed, water-based decoction. They are congruent with contemporary standards of care in the People's Republic of China. However, they are only meant as a rough guide. Depending on the situation, most of these doses may be increased or decreased beyond the range of textbook standards. However, it is still my opinion that, unlike many other conditions, gestation and postpartum (gestation especially) are not times to be trying to teach oneself how to do Chinese medicine out of a book. Before attempting to use any of the protocols described in this book, I would expect all practitioners to have completed certain basic, entry-level requirements, such as Chinese medical theory, the four examination, pattern discrimination, and the treatment of internal disease in general before going on to gynecology in particular. Especially when it comes to the internal administration of Chinese medicinals, I would expect all practitioners to have completed their entry-level study of materia medica, formulas and prescriptions, and how to write and modify a prescription. While Chinese medicinals are relatively benign, the uninformed practice of Chinese medical obstetrics can have severe, irremedial consequences.

As an extension of the above, some students and practitioners may ask why I have given so many different formulas under many of the patterns in this book. Many individuals simply want to know which formula is the right or best one. However, in presenting a number of different formulas, I am hoping that the reader becomes better able to see and understand the underlying methodology of Chinese medicine. If one understands this methodology, then there is no one right or best formula. Rather, there are a large number of possible combinations which may all adequately deal with the situation at hand. Textbook formulas typically have to be modified to fit the needs of individual patients. Hopefully, by seeing the range of possibilities of formulas for a particular pattern of a particular disease, one will be more confident in writing their own formulas for their own patients, albeit, perhaps, based on the examples given in this book.

In terms of acupuncture nomenclature, Lu = lung, LI = large intestine, St = stomach, Sp = spleen, Ht = heart, SI = small intestine, Bl = bladder, Ki = kidney, Per = pericardium, TB = triple burner, GB = gallbladder, and Liv = liver. In addition, CV = conception vessel, and GV = governing vessel. Extra-channel points are identified by Bensky and O'connor's numerical system as it appears in *Acupuncture: A Comprehensive Text* (Eastland Press, Seattle, 1981).

I hope readers find this new edition an improvement over the old. For readers interested in going further in Chinese medical gynecology, Blue Poppy Institute offers an 18-month, Distance Learning, postgraduate program. To find out more about this program, go to the Blue Poppy Institute subsite at www.bluepoppy.com.

Bob Flaws
Boulder, CO
Mar. 2005

BOOK ONE

Gestational & Birthing Diseases

1
Introduction

Western medicine & pregnancy

Development & growth of the embryo

After fertilization in the fallopian tube, the zygote divides repeatedly to form a solid sphere of cells referred to as the morula. This morula reaches the uterine cavity by the seventh day after ovulation and is fully embedded by the 14th day after ovulation. During the first 14 days of pregnancy, the growth of the uterus and the decidua or endometrium of pregnancy is maintained by the corpus luteum under the influence of luteinizing hormone secreted from the hypophysis. After 14 days, the primitive chorion secretes a luteinizing hormone (chorionic gonadotrophin) which assumes control of the corpus luteum and inhibits pituitary gonadotrophic activity. Under the influence of the placental luteinizing hormone, the corpus luteum continues to grow and secrete steroids in order to maintain the growth of the uterine decidua. Around weeks 10-12, chorionic gonadotrophin out-put reaches its peak and then declines to an almost constant level until term. The activity of the corpus luteum fails along with this decline. However, production of steroids by the placenta replaces it so that the estrogen and progesterone out-put rises steadily to term.

When the morula reaches the uterine cavity, an eccentric space appears resulting in the formation of a hollow sphere or blastocyst with a mound of cells on one side of the inner surface. This mound is the inner cell mass. The outer shell of the blastocyst becomes the trophoblast responsible for the nutrition of the embryo. Up until this point, the zygote has relied on the secretions within the fallopian tube and uterus for nutrition which has been sufficient for the initial growth of the zygote. However, further growth demands an increased supply of food and oxygen. Therefore, the zygote embeds in the decidua in order to gain access to the maternal blood supply. The inner cell mass differentiates and forms two distinct masses, the outer or ecto-

3

dermal layer and the inner or endodermal layer. A further differentiation produces a third layer—the mesoderm—between these two. This grows outward and eventually lines the blastocyst. Two small cavities appear, one in the ectoderm forming the amniotic sac, the other in the endoderm forming the yolk sac. These two small spheres, covered by mesoderm, then move into the middle of the blastocyst cavity, the mesoderm forming the connecting stalk and expansion of the amniotic sac takes place. It is the two opposing layers of the ectoderm and endoderm together with the interposing mesoderm which form the actual embryo.

Blood vessels develop in the embryonic mesoderm and in the mesoderm of the trophoblast which eventually result in the formation of the umbilical arteries and vein. Within the embryo, the vessels at the cephalic end differentiate and form the heart, with fetal blood formation occurring within the primitive blood vessels of the trophoblast and fetus. Interchange between mother and fetus is facilitated by the formation of this feto-trophoblastic circulation. The formation and differentiation of the hemopoietic vascular system occurs between the third and fourth week of pregnancy. From then on, full development of the fetus can take place.[1]

TIME-TABLE FOR ORGAN DEVELOPMENT

Organ	Differentiation	Complete formation
Spinal cord	3-4 weeks	20 weeks
Brain	3 weeks	28 weeks
Eyes	3 weeks	20-24 weeks
Olfactory apparatus	4-5 weeks	8 weeks
Auditory apparatus	3-4 weeks	24-28 weeks
Respiratory system	5 weeks	24-28 weeks
Heart	3 weeks	6 weeks
Gastrointestinal system	3 weeks	12 weeks
Liver	3-4 weeks	12 weeks
Renal system	4-5 weeks	12 weeks
Genital system	5 weeks	7 weeks
Face	3-4 weeks	8 weeks
Limbs	4-5 weeks	8 weeks

Functions of the placenta

The functions of the placenta include respiration, nutrition, and secretion. Although some authorities also include excretion as a function of the placenta, little is known about this activity. Due to the fact that maternal blood is relatively high in oxygen and low in carbon dioxide, oxygen is passed from maternal to fetal blood and carbon dioxide flows from fetal to maternal blood. Nutritional substances are exchanged between mother and fetus via the placenta by active transport mechanisms. The hormones secreted by the placenta include estrogens, progesterone, chorionic gonadotrophin, placental lactogen, corticosteroids, and probably ACTH and TSH substances.[2]

Amniotic fluids

The amniotic fluid is derived directly from maternal circulation, by diffusion through the umbilical cord, and by secretion by the amnion. It consists of a number of substances, including protein, creatinine, urea, uric acid, glucose, lipids, and electrolytes. It also includes a number of hormones, such as chorionic gonadotrophin, placental somatotrophic hormone, estrogens, progesterone, and corticosteroids. Likewise, there are a wide variety of enzymes. The amniotic fluid increases up to the 38th week of pregnancy, falls slightly up to term, and then falls more rapidly after that. Amniocentesis, *i.e.*, withdrawal of a small amount of amniotic fluid allows for prognostication in cases of rhesus incompatibility, antenatal sex determination, detection of chromosomal abnormalities, diagnosis of fetal storage disorders, and diagnosis of fetal enzyme deficiencies.[3]

Maternal adaptations to pregnancy

Due to rising levels of hormones secreted first by the corpus luteum and later by the placenta, women experience a number of physiologic and psychologic changes during pregnancy. As a functioning gland, the placenta produces large quantities of both peptide and steroid hormones. Serum progesterone and estradiol levels rise by six or seven times during pregnancy, deoxycorticosterone rises 20-fold, and plasma levels of human chorionic somatomammotropin (hCS) quadruples. Rises in progesterone result in relaxation of the vascular, gastrointestinal, and genitourinary smooth muscle, reduction in uterine motility, and modulation of the immune system. Rises in deoxycorticosterone result in salt and water retention. Rises in estrone and estradiol result in increased blood flow in the uterus, promote salt and water retention, and increase production of binding proteins by the liver, and rises in human chorionic somatomammotropin mobilize free fatty acids, inhibit the effects of insulin on glucose uptake, and promote nitrogen retention. By 32 weeks of pregnancy, blood and plasma volume has increased as much as 40% and there is typically a net fluid gain of 6-8L. In response, maternal heart rate increases by 15-20% during pregnancy and the kidneys must work 40% harder. In addition, there is vasodilation in the skin to allow for more efficient heat radiation and there is development of the mammary glands within the breasts.

Due to the effects of progesterone on smooth muscle activity, esophageal reflux and heartburn are common. Due to progesterone's effects on the biliary system, there is the possibility of cholestatic jaundice during pregnancy. Estrogen-induced increases in clotting factors cause an increased risk of thrombosis. Due to estrogen's effect on the liver, cholesterol and triglyceride concentrations are elevated. Low back pain during pregnancy is due to changes in posture in response to the growing fetus as well as increased pliability and mobility of the sacroiliac and pubic symphysis joints. Striae gravidarum (*i.e.*, stretch marks) are most likely due to changes in hormones, not actually the stretching of the skin. Because melanocyte activity is increased, there is typically darkening of the areola, the skin of the midline from umbilicus to pubis, and melasma of the face and neck, the so-called mask of pregnancy. Superficial varicosities occur in 40% of women. These mostly occur in the lower extremities but may also result in hemorrhoids. Increases in estrogen are also thought to be responsible for the occurrence of spider angiomata distributed over the upper chest, extensor surfaces of the hands and arms, and on the face. And finally, many women experience increased hair growth during pregnancy.[4]

Most women experience an increase of weight during pregnancy equivalent to 25% of their non-pregnant weight. This averages 12.5kg, with the main increase occurring in the second half of pregnancy. In terms of distribution, 1-1.5kg of this weight is added to the breasts, 0.5-1.0kg is added to the uterus, water and electrolytes

SIGNS & SYMPTOMS OF PREGNANCY

4 weeks	Amenorrhea, morning sickness
6 weeks	Increased urination, cervical softening
7 weeks	Palpable uterine enlargement (the size of a large hen's egg)
8 weeks	Increased pulsation in lateral fornices (Osiander's sign) Darkening of vaginal mucus membrane (Jacquemier's sign) Sensation of fingers almost meeting during bimanual examination (Heigar's sign)
6-8 weeks	Increased breast heaviness Increased pigmentation of primary areola Increased prominence of Montgomery's tubercles
10 weeks	Vulval varicosities (Kluge's sign)
14 weeks	Internal ballotment can be felt, *i.e.*, rise and fall of fetus in response to a tap on the cervix
15 weeks	Increase in abdominal size apparent
16 weeks	Colostrum secreted and able to be manually expressed
16-18 weeks	Quickening, the sensation of fetal movement
20 weeks	Palpable uterine contractions (Braxton Hicks' sign) Palpable fetal movements
24 weeks	External ballotment can be felt, *i.e.*, side to side movement of fetus felt by tapping abdomen Auscultation of the fetal heartbeat
26 weeks	Palpable fetal parts[6]

account for 1-1.5kg, increases in subcutaneous fat account for 4-4.5kg, and the fetus and placenta add 5kg. Weight gain should not exceed 2.25kg per month or 0.9kg per week and should not be less than 0.22kg per week.[5]

Length of gestation

Normal gestation lasts from 38 to 42 weeks. This period is divided into three three-month sections referred to as the first, second, and third trimesters respectively. Pregnancy is considered prolonged if it exceeds 294 days or 42 weeks, after which perinatal morbidity begins to climb.[6]

Western medical gestational conditions

The main Western medical gestational conditions are: nausea and vomiting of pregnancy(NVP), hyperemesis gravidarum, spontaneous abortion, rhesus incompatibility, ectopic pregnancy, gestational trophoblastic disease (GTD), including hydatidiform mole, diabetes mellitus, incompetent cervix, placenta previa, hypertension/pre-eclampsia, eclampsia, fetal growth disorders, preterm labor and delivery, and prolonged pregnancy.

Stages of labor

Delivery, or labor, is divided into three stages: first, second, and third, with the first stage being subdivided into early, active, and transition phases. In addition, some authorities also describe a prelabor stage. In that case, prelabor refers to the last five weeks of gestation, during which time there may be some thinning, ripening, and dilation of the cervix. The mother-to-be may lose her mucus plug as a result of this dilation. Typically, during prelabor, Braxton Hicks contractions become more frequent and the fetus's head turns downward and engages in the pelvis.

First stage

During the first stage of labor, the cervix thins, ripens, and fully dilates as a result of the mother's uterine contractions. It is during this stage that the amniotic sac typically ruptures. This is the longest of the three stages of labor. In early first stage labor, contractions occur every 10 minutes or so and last approximately 30 seconds. The cervix dilates 3-5cm and this stage of labor commonly lasts 12-14 hours. During active early stage labor, contractions occur every 4-5 minutes and last approximately 60 seconds. This stage of labor commonly last six hours or so. In the transition stage (meaning the transition from first to second stage labor), contractions come every 2-3 minutes and last up to 90 seconds each. By the time this phase is over, the cervix is fully dilated and the fetus is ready to be born. During the transition phase, women may experience fluctuations in body temperature, pressure against the rectum, nausea or vomiting, an urge to push, cramps in the legs, and/or sensitivity to touch. In some women, the transition phase is followed by 20 minutes or so of weak contractions. This is referred to as the interval. In general, how long any of these stages last is variable from expectant mother to expectant mother. However, these phases tend to be shorter in women who have given birth vaginally before and longer in primiparas.

Second stage

During the second stage there is an intense urge to push. This is the stage during which the fetus is forced out of the birth canal, ending with the birth of the baby. The second stage may last anywhere from 20 minutes to an hour or more for primiparas.

Third stage

The third stage refers to the explusion of the placenta. This usually occurs 5-30 minutes after birth and is accompanied by mild contractions.

LONGITUDINAL DIAGRAM OF WESTERN GESTATIONAL & BIRTHING DISORDERS

First trimester
   Morning sickness
   Miscarriage
   Large for dates

Second trimester

Third trimester
   Pre-eclampsia-eclampsia
   Antepartum hemorrhage
   Abruptio placentae
   Placenta previae

First stage of labor
   Dystocia
   Disproportion
   Malposition of the fetus
   Malpresentation
   Multiple pregnancy

Second stage of labor
   Dystocia
   Disproportion
   Malposition of the fetus
   Malpresentation
   Multiple pregnancy

Third stage of labor
   Retained placenta
   Postpartum hemorrhage

Chinese medicine & pregnancy

According to Chinese medical theory, conception takes place when the white reproductive essence of the male unites with the red reproductive essence of the female. This then forms the *tai* or fetus which grows and takes shape within the *bao gong* or uterus. The uterus is connected via the *bao luo* or wrapper network vessels to the kidneys from which it receives nourishment in the form of essence. The uterus is also attached to the heart via the *bao mai* (wrapper vessel)/*chong mai* (thoroughfare vessel) and is nourished by blood sent down by the heart. The latter heaven root of blood engenderment is the spleen and stomach which are also the latter heaven root of qi engenderment and transformation. Spleen or central qi helps to lift and contain the abdominal contents, including the uterus and the fetus it contains. The thoroughfare vessel is called the sea of blood and arises from the uterus. Conception can only take place if the sea of blood is full and the conception vessel is freely flowing and uninhibited. The liver stores the blood and so there is a close connection between the uterus, the thoroughfare vessel, and the liver. In addition, the course of the liver channel traverses the lower abdomen and genitalia.

For the fetus to grow, it must receive essence from the kidneys as well as qi and blood engendered by the five viscera but sent downward by the heart. Therefore, the mother's qi, blood, and essence must not only be sufficient in amount but must be able to flow freely to the uterus. It is said that blood and essence have a common source. That common source is the kidneys. It is also said that blood and fluids have a common source since both are part of systemic yin fluids. If either latter heaven or original qi are insufficient or likewise yin blood and fluids and humors, problems may arise with the growth and development of the fetus and the successful completion of gestation. Therefore, Chinese medical obstetrics addresses many seemingly minor complaints during pregnancy in an effort to maintain the best and balanced engenderment and free flow of qi, blood, fluids, and essence.

Ye Heng-yin's description of conception

Ye Heng-yin was a gynecological specialist who wrote a pithy little obstetrics and gynecology text in the Qing dynasty titled, *Nu Ke Zhi Nan (A Guide to Gynecology)*. The following is Ye Heng-yin's description of the origin of the fetus.

> The *tian gui* is the endowment of the father and mother, the former heaven true qi which engenders the body. The essence and blood which are transformed from water and grains are the root of the latter heaven's production of the form. In males, the *tian gui* arrives at two [times] eight [years of age], since men are categorized as yang and correspond to the sun. Therefore, their essence daily becomes [more and more] exuberant. In women, the *tian gui* arrives at two [times] seven [years of age]. This is because women are categorized as yin and correspond to the moon. Therefore, their blood flows freely once each month. At the time when men and women unite, their former heaven true qi, latter heaven essence and blood, and yin and yang come together and unite, thus enabling the getting of children. At this time, if the *qian*[7] *dao* is exuberant, this produces a male. If the *kun*[8] *dao* is exuberant, this produces a female.[9]

Ye Heng-yin on the proper timing of conception

> The *dao* of a male's gathering of essence must be to decrease [sexual] desire, and intercourse should occur at the proper time. It is not ok to be too early or too late [literally, slow]. It should occur after the menstrual movement when the influence that brings lovers together arrives [to such an extent that the couple] have difficulty bearing their joyous desire. This is the true occasion for producing the fetus's engenderment and transformation.[10]

Ye Heng-yin on the determination of sex

Former sages held that essence and blood, former and latter could divide male from female. If blood arrives first to envelope the essence, this will produce a boy. If essence arrives first to envelope the blood, this produces a girl. It is also possible that the profuse [*i.e.*, odd] or scanty [*i.e.*, even, number on which intercourse occurred] can divide male from female. [If pregnancy occurs] on the first, third, or fifth [day of the lunar month], this produces a male. [If it occurs on] the second, fourth, or sixth, this produces a female. [Another theory has it that] males are formed on the first and second days, while females are produced on the fourth and fifth days. It is also possible [to determine] male from female according to the fixing [of the fetus] on the left or right [side] of the uterus. If the qi is received on the left [side of] the uterus, this makes for males. If the qi is received on the right [side of] the uterus, this makes for females. All [the various past masters who proposed the above] each stuck to their own view; so one cannot know among which of these is [the real] factor. However, if one wants to obtain from among these the truth, it is that only [when] the *qian dao* yang is exuberant are males produced and [only when] the *kun dao* yin qi is exuberant are females produced.[11]

Ye Heng-yin on the conception of twins

The ancients had it that twin fetuses were due to essence qi exuberance. This causes the blood to divide and gather [into two]. There are other [situations] where it is possible not to produce [either] a male or a female, [and yet other cases where] the male [child] cannot make a father, while the female [child] cannot make a mother.[12] It is also possible for [the child] to have male and female forms simultaneously.[13] All [these are due to] abnormalities in yin and yang and the contraction of contradictory qi. Although such affairs have their reasons, these are hard to fully clarify. No one can verify these.[14]

Ren shen bing or *Tai qian bing*

Diseases or pathoconditions occurring from conception to delivery are called either *ren shen bing*, "diseases of pregnancy," or *tai qian bing*, literally, "before birth diseases." The causes of gestational complaints may be due to former heaven natural endowment insufficiency, the seven affects, the six external evils, irregularities in diet, stirring (*i.e.*, activity), stillness (or rest), sex, and traumatic injury. In addition, during pregnancy, blood accumulates in the *chong* and *ren* in order to nourish the fetus. Depending upon the mother's constitution and condition, this may lead to a yin blood vacuity in the rest of the body and hyperactivity of yang. Further, as the fetus grows physically, distending the abdomen and putting pressure on the abdominal contents, the qi mechanism may be disturbed, thus negatively affecting the upbearing and downbearing, floating and sinking of qi and fluids.

Complaints encountered during pregnancy should be corrected as soon as possible so that viscera and bowel function is not compromised resulting in either diminished engenderment of qi and blood or their impaired flow. Thus both the mother's and the fetus's health and survival are guaranteed. The safest method for prescription during pregnancy is treating on the basis of pattern discrimination since this takes the individual's total condition into account. Thus side effects are avoided or minimized.

The traditional *tai qian bing* or gestational diseases include nausea and vomiting, abdominal pain, fetal stirring restlessly, vaginal bleeding, miscarriage, habitual miscarriage, edema, diarrhea, dysentery, cough, loss of voice, urinary problems, malaria-like disease, so-called epilepsy while with child, dizziness, insanity, vexation, and dysphoria. To these, modern Chinese medicine has added hypertension, pre-eclampsia, eclampsia, ectopic pregnancy, hydatidiform mole, and chorioadenoma. However, these are but modern names which cover aspects of traditional Chinese diseases. For instance, ectopic pregnancy as a modern disease category is associated with abdominal pain, and so-called epilepsy while with child is eclampsia.

Diagnosing pregnancy

In Chinese medicine, early diagnosis of pregnancy is important for at least two reasons. First, it is important so that the woman does not eat or do anything that might negatively affect fetal development or jeopardize the pregnancy. Secondly, it is important that the doctor know if their patient is pregnant so as to avoid certain potentially dangerous or contraindicated treatments. In traditional Chinese medicine, diagnosis of early pregnancy is accomplished by three of the four examinations.

Inspection

Inspection is always the first part of a Chinese medical examination, and the first thing the Chinese doctor inspects is the facial color or complexion. During early pregnancy, most women's complexion is normal. However, it may also be pale or sallow. Secondly, the doctor should inspect the patient's carriage. Pregnant women may often appear more tired than usual and may change their position frequently. Closer inspection typically reveals enlargement of the breasts and darkening of the areola of the nipples after two months of pregnancy. During early pregnancy, the tongue color may remain unchanged but typically there will be white, possibly slimy fur.

Questioning

Questioning is the next method of examination employed by the Chinese doctor. One may question specifically about the menses and one can also question concerning the patient's general signs and symptoms. In terms of the menstruation, if a woman is of child-bearing age, is sexually active without the use of birth control, has had a regular menstrual cycle for some time, and her menses are currently 10 days overdue, pregnancy should be suspected. Although some women may continue menstruating for several months after conception, cessation of menstruation is the single most important indicator of possible pregnancy.

In terms of general signs and symptoms, if the woman reports nausea and vomiting, lack of appetite, increased saliva, cravings for sour or other peculiar foods, and a dislike of fatty foods or certain smells, fatigue, weakness of the four limbs, dizziness, or breast distention, any or all of these may help confirm that a woman is pregnant. A woman may or may not experience any of these signs and symptoms and there are other disease mechanisms which may account for any of these other than pregnancy.

Palpation

Most women's pulses are fine compared to men's. The pulse of pregnancy tends to be slightly rapid and slippery compared to usual. During early pregnancy, the pulse may be floating and slippery and either fine or wide. Often the slippery quality denoting pregnancy is mostly felt in the bar and cubit positions. However, it may also be felt at the inch position instead or as well.

Nowadays in the West, women can buy home pregnancy testing kits over the counter at their pharmacists. These test kits are quite reliable and are able to detect pregnancy quite early on. Although the Chinese medical practitioner may want to note any changes in the pulse or other corroborating signs and symptoms of early pregnancy, if pregnancy is suspected, they should immediately advise their patient to use such an early pregnancy, home testing kit.

Prohibitions during pregnancy

Since Chao Yuan-fang and Sun Si-miao in the Tang dynasty, it has been traditionally believed that certain channels or organs develop or are nourished during each month of gestation. For a millennia or more, Chinese doctors used this idea to guide their diagnosis and treatment during pregnancy. Although this idea is not used much in contemporary Chinese medicine, some practitioners may want to consider it. According to Sun Si-miao, during the first month the foot jue yin is being nourished and, therefore, no acupuncture or moxibustion should be used on this channel. During the second month, the foot shao yang is being nourished and, therefore, no acupuncture or moxibustion should be used on it. Likewise, during the third month one should avoid needling or moxaing the hand shao yin channel; the fourth month, the hand shao yang; the fifth month, the foot tai yin; the sixth month, the foot yang ming; the seventh month, the hand tai yin; the eighth month, the hand yang ming; and the ninth month, the foot shao yin. By the tenth month, the viscera and bowels are complete and, therefore, delivery occurs.

In terms of treatment methods, forceful exterior-resolving is prohibited during pregnancy for fear of consuming yang and damaging yin by profuse perspiration. Purgation is also prohibited for fear it may also injure yin and, therefore, damage the blood. In addition, attacking and precipitation may dislodge the fetus and result in miscarriage if the fetal ligation is tenuous to begin with. And excessive seeping water or dispelling dampness is prohibited also for fear of consuming and damaging yin fluids.

THE "THREE PROHIBITIONS" DURING PREGNANCY

1. Unwarranted or excessively forceful exterior-resolving
2. Unwarranted or excessively forceful attacking and precipitation
3. Unwarranted or excessively forceful seeping water

Based on the above general prohibitions, it is traditionally advised to avoid certain medicinals which quicken the blood too forcefully, move the qi and body fluids downward too forcefully, or are too toxic. These may cause miscarriage or injury to the fetus. They include:

Dan Pi (Cortex Moutan)
Ma Chi Xian (Herba Portulacae)
She Gan (Rhizoma Belamcandae)
Huai Niu Xi (Radix Achyranthis Bidentatae)
Mang Xiao (Mirabilitum)
Fan Xie Ye (Folium Sennae)
Lu Hui (Herba Aloes)
Qian Niu Zi (Semen Pharbitidis)
Gan Sui (Radix Euphorbiae Kansui)
Yuan Hua (Flos Daphnis Genkwae)
Jing Da Ji (Radix Euphorbiae Seu Knoxiae)
Shang Lu (Radix Phytolaccae)
Mu Tong (Caulis Akebiae)
Qu Mai (Herba Dianthi)
Che Qian Zi (Semen Plantaginis)
She Tui (Periostracum Serpentis)
Kuan Jin Teng (Ramus Tinosporae Sinensis)
Tian Hua Fen (Radix Trichosanthis)
Tian Nan Xing (Rhizoma Arisaematis)
Zhi Bai Fu Zi (Rhizoma Praeparata Typhonii)
Zao Jiao (Fructus Gleditschiae Chinensis)
Zao Jiao Ci (Spina Gleditschiae Chinensis)
San Qi (Radix Notoginseng)
Qian Cao (Radix Rubiae)
Hua Rui Shi (Ophicalcitum)
Yan Hu Suo (Rhizoma Corydalis)

Yi Mu Cao (Herba Leonuri)

Yue Ji Hua (Flos Et Fructus Rosae Chinensis)

Hong Hua (Flos Carthami)

Tao Ren(Semen Persicae)

E Zhu (Rhizoma Curcumae)

San Leng (Rhizoma Sparganii)

Ru Xiang (Resina Olibani)

Mo Yao (Resina Myrrhae)

Chuan Niu Xi (Radix Cyathulae)

Wang Bu Liu Xing (Semen Vaccariae)

Lu Lu Tong (Fructus Liquidambaris Taiwaniae)

Xue Jie (Sanguis Draconis)

Su Mu (Lignum Sappanis)

Shui Zhi (Hirudo)

Tu Bie Chong (Eupolyphaga Seu Opisthoplatia)

Zhi Fu Zi (Radix Praeparatus Aconiti Carmichaeli)

Hai Long (Syngnathus)

Hai Ma (Hippocampus)

Gui Ban (Plastrum Testudinis)

She Xiang (Secretio Moschi Moschiferi)

Niu Huang (Calculus Bovis)

Wu Gong (Scolopendra)

Dong Bei Guan Zhong (Rhizoma Dryopteridis Crassirhizomae)

Qing Fen (Calomelas)

Xiong Huang (Realgar)

Liu Huang (Sulphur)

Ma Qian Zi (Semen Strychnotis)

Mu Bie Zi (Semen Momordicae Cochinensis)

Zhang Nao (Camphora)

Ban Mao (Mylabris)

Chan Su (Secretio Bufonis)

However, some of these medicinals are found in the formulas contained in this book. Although they are listed as prohibited during pregnancy, in some cases they are used depending upon the circumstances. They should not be used, however, without good and sufficient cause or if some other medicinal will achieve the same result just as effectively. In other words, these prohibitions are not absolute. They are mostly meant for those specifically untrained in Chinese obstetrics. In many cases, if these medicinals are warranted by the patient's pattern discrimination and disease diagnosis, they not only can be used but must or should be used. As an example of this principle, blood stasis is one of the disease mechanisms which may cause or contribute to fetal stirring restlessly or threatened miscarriage. In that case, one must use one or more of the above "prohibited" blood-quickening medicinals in order to quiet the fetus and prevent the abortion. Failure to do so out of untutored fear may very well fail to eliminate the disease mechanism causing the miscarriage and, hence, fail to prevent the miscarriage itself.

Other ingredients are not prohibited but care is cautioned in their use during pregnancy. These include:

Chan Tui (Periostracum Cicadae)
Mu Zei (Herba Equiseti Hiemalis)
Dan Zhu Ye (Herba Lophatheri)
Ye Ming Sha (Feces Vespertilii)
Xi Jiao(Cornu Rhinocerotis)
Bai Hua She She Cao (Herba Hedotis Diffusae)
Ya Dan Zi (Fructus Bruceae)
Da Huang (Radix Et Rhizoma Rhei)
Yu Li Ren (Semen Pruni)
Hua Shi (Talcum)
Yi Yi Ren (Semen Coicis)
Tong Cao (Medulla Tetrapanacis)
Dong Kui Zi (Fructus Malvae)
Hou Po (Cortex Magnoliae Officinalis)
Shen Qu (Massa Medica Fermentata)
Zhi Ke (Fructus Aurantii)
Pu Huang (Pollen Typhae)
Yu Jin (Tuber Curcumae)
Ze Lan (Herba Lycopi)
Wu Ling Zhi (Feces Trogopterori Seu Pteromi)
Gan Jiang (dry Rhizoma Zingiberis)
Rou Gui (Cortex Cinnamomi)
Chuan Jiao (Fructus Zanthoxyli)
Bie Jia (Carapax Amydae Chinensis)
Chi Shi Zhi (Hallyositum Rubrum)
Dai Zhe Shi (Haematitium)
Bing Pian (Borneolum)
Ci Ji Li(Fructus Tribuli)

Should any of the above medicinals be warranted and, therefore, used to remedially treat a specific disease or pathocondition, as soon as that condition is relieved, their use should be suspended. As Ye Heng-yin says, "[Although] one should treat following the pattern, [whether] exterior or interior, vacuity or repletion, cold or hot, it is not ok to [use] excessively harsh [methods]."[15]

Endnotes:

[1]   Garrey, Matthew M. *et al.*, *Obstetrics Illustrated*, Churchill Livingstone, Edinburgh, 1980, p. 5-12

[2]   *Ibid.*, p. 17-18

[3]   *Ibid.*, p. 20-21

[4]   Moore, Thomas R., "Maternal Adaptation to Pregnancy," *Gynecology & Obstetrics: A Longitudinal Approach*, ed. by Thomas R. Moore *et al.*, Churchill Livingstone, NY, 1993, p. 223-233

[5]   Garrey, *op. cit.*, p. 25

[6]   *Ibid.*, p. 73-78

[7]   *Qian* is the name of the heavenly or creative trigram and signifies yang and male.

[8]   *Kun* is the name of the earthly or receptive trigram which signifies yin and female.

[9]   In other words, the offspring are sterile.

[10] *Ie.*, hermaphroditism

[11] Ye Heng-yin, *A Guide to Gynecology*, trans. by Bob Flaws & Shuai Xue-zhong, Blue Poppy Press, Boulder, CO, 2001, p. 45

[12] *Ibid.*, p. 46

[13] *Ibid.*, p. 46-47

[14] *Ibid.*, p. 47

[15] *Ibid.*, p. 51

2

Nausea & Vomiting
of Pregnancy

The first and most common complaint associated with pregnancy is both a traditional Chinese and modern Western medical disease—nausea and vomiting of pregnancy. Nausea and vomiting of pregnancy, referred to by the acronym NVP in Western medical obstetrics, affects 50-80% of pregnant women.[1] Of those women who experience NVP, a third only experience nausea, while 2/3 experience some vomiting.[2] Such nausea and vomiting typically begin between the 4-6th weeks of gestation, with 60% of affected women better by the 12th week and 90% better by the 16th week.[3] In a small number of cases, nausea and vomiting may persist through the entire pregnancy. Half of all women with NVP feel that it is uncomfortable enough to adversely affect their work, and 25% actually require time off from work.[4] One out of 20 women are affected so severely that they experience weight loss, dehydration, and electrolyte disturbances which may require hospitalization.[5] Such severe, intractable nausea and vomiting during pregnancy is referred to as hyperemesis gravidarum. In English, nausea and vomiting of pregnancy are colloquially called morning sickness. This is because, in some women, their nausea and vomiting are worse in the morning and improve as the day wears on. However, many women experience nausea all day long, and, in others, their nausea worsens during the latter part of the day and evening.

The Western medical causes of NVP are not fully understood. It is probable that they are multifactorial and include some combination of increased hormone levels (possibly estrogen and/or human chorionic gonadotropin [hCG]), physiologic changes, such as excess stomach acid, increased sense of smell, emotional stress, and fatigue. The Western medical treatment of NVP consists mainly of dietary recommendations, for instance, eating many small meals consisting of bland foods, and maintaining adequate hydration. Vitamin B_6 (pyridoxine) has been used at doses of 20-50mg three times per day. If the discomfort is severe and intractable, antiemetics may be prescribed. Such anti-emetics falls into several different categories. There are the antihistimines such as Antivert (meclizine), the phenothiazines such as Thorazine (chlorpromazine), the dopamine antagonists such as Reglan (meto-clopramide), and the apomorphine antagonist Inapsine (droperidol). For the treatment of hyperemesis gravidarum, treatment typically consists of intravenous fluids and parenteral antiemetics. In addition, the patient is commonly placed on enteric rest, with nothing *per os* (PNO) for 24-48 hours.

Chinese medical disease categorization

In Chinese medicine, nausea and vomiting of pregnancy are referred to as *ren shen e zu*. *Ren shen* means pregnancy, and *e zu* means malign obstruction.

Disease causes & disease mechanisms

No matter what the cause, nausea *per se* has to do with disharmony of the stomach. This means that stomach qi which should normally flow down, counterflows upward. If this upward counterflow is strong enough, it may even result in vomiting. There are three basic mechanisms that lead to upward counterflow of the stomach qi after conceiving. The first has to do with the spleen-stomach alone, the second has to do with the stomach and liver, and the third involves the kidneys. Based on these three scenarios, a number of other disease mechanisms may also complicate the situation.

When conception occurs, the menses cease. The fetus blocks the *bao men* or uterine gate. The *chong* which sends blood down to the uterus continues to do so, but this blood has nowhere to go. As yet the fetus is not sufficiently developed to make full use of all the blood accumulating in the *bao gong*. The *chong* is connected to the *yang ming*. It is *yang ming* qi which helps descend the thoroughfare vessel qi. The *chong mai* and *yang ming* intersect at *Qi Chong* (St 30). If the stomach and spleen are vacuous and weak to begin with, the qi associated with the blood accumulating in the *bao gong/chong mai* may counterflow upward by flowing into the *yang ming*, overwhelming the *yang ming* qi. This then results in nausea and even vomiting.

Since the spleen engenders and transforms the blood, the increased demand for blood after conception to nourish the fetus may result in the spleen's function of promoting transportation and transformation declining and becoming weak. The spleen governs upbearing and the stomach governs downbearing. Upbearing and downbearing are mutually reflexive. One cannot occur without the other. Therefore, uninhibited upbearing promotes proper downbearing and *vice versa*. Hence spleen vacuity weakness resulting in non-upbearing of the clear can aggravate the upward counterflow of stomach qi due to excessive and counterflowing thoroughfare qi. In other words, if the spleen does not properly upbear, the stomach cannot properly downbear. Faulty diet, worry, and taxation and fatigue may all weaken the spleen and can, therefore, aggravate this condition.

As the fetus grows, it begins to make full use of the qi and blood sent down to it via the *chong mai/bao mai* and thus the thoroughfare qi no longer accumulates and counterflows upward. Therefore, this nausea and vomiting cease spontaneously sometime around the end of the first trimester. Obviously, in the majority of women, morning sickness has to do with a temporary readjustment in the flows and uses of certain qi and body fluids. Otherwise the condition would persist throughout gestation.

Secondly, the liver is the viscus that treasures the blood and its function of controlling coursing and discharge is dependent on the liver obtaining sufficient blood to nourish it. If the blood being sent down to and accumulating in the uterus fails to also adequately nourish the liver, the liver may fail to control coursing and discharge. Instead, the liver may become depressed and the qi stagnant. Liver depression is a species of repletion. Because of the relationship of the liver and stomach described by five phase theory, a replete liver may counterflow horizontally to attack the stomach. Because the liver also governs upbearing, if the liver assails the stomach, the stomach may lose its downbearing and harmony and its qi may counterflow upward. Women with a tendency to liver depression and/or blood vacuity are prone to this scenario.

Fu Qing-zhu, arguably the most famous premodern Chinese gynecological specialist, especially emphasized this mechanism of nausea and vomiting of pregnancy. Since it is my experience that this is the single most common pattern of nausea and vomiting of pregnancy in Western women, I believe it is appropriate to quote Fu Qing-zhu at length on this issue:

> [Some] pregnant women suffer from nausea, retching, and vomiting with a desire for sour [foods] to quench their thirst but an aversion to any food in sight, fatigue, and somnolence. People call this pregnancy malign obstruction. Who would suspect extreme dryness of liver blood? Conception in women is based on effulgent kidney qi. Only when the kidneys are effulgent can the essence be contained. However, once the kidneys have received the essence [from the male] and engendered pregnancy, kidney water begins to grow the fetus [and thus becomes] too busy to moisten the five viscera.

> The liver is the child of the kidneys and has to live on the qi of its mother every day to be soothed. Whenever it is in need of nourishing fluids, its qi will be pressing for them. As now kidney water is unable to meet this demand, the liver becomes more impetuous or temperamental. When the liver becomes impetuous, fire stirs and [live qi] counterflows. Once live qi counterflow occurs, problems such as retching, vomiting, and nausea arise.[6]

However, the disease mechanism of liver depression causing counterflow may also arise due to emotional stress during the first trimester. Because of conflicting emotions, desires may be unfulfilled and the coursing and discharge may become inhibited. This is yet another cause of liver attacking the stomach.

The third basic mechanism associated with nausea during pregnancy has to do with the kidneys. As Fu Qing-zhu points out, after conception, it is the kidneys which nourish the fetus with essence. In addition, it is said the blood and essence share a common source, and that source is the kidneys. With so much essence and blood focused on nourishing the fetus, kidney yin may become vacuous and depleted. In that case, vacuous and insufficient yin may fail to enrich and moisten the liver. Similar to blood vacuity, if the liver does not obtain sufficient yin to enrich and moisten it, it cannot control its function of coursing and discharge. This then leads to liver depression with the liver's attacking the stomach and the stomach's loss of downbearing and harmony. This is simply a further extension of the disease mechanism described above by Fu Qing-zhu. This scenario is most often encountered in women who are constitutionally weak, women in their mid 30s to early 40s, drug abusers, those who are overtaxed physically, emotionally, and sexually, or those who have suffered a long time from chronic disease.

As to the complications derived from these three basic mechanisms, if the spleen and stomach lose their ability to promote the movement and transformation of water fluids, dampness may accumulate internally. If this dampness accumulates past a certain point, it may also congeal and turn into phlegm and turbidity. Likewise, if the stomach qi fails to downbear and descend, untransformed food may accumulate and stagnate in the stomach. Or, if the spleen and stomach are further weakened by the upward counterflow of stomach qi and, therefore, lack of proper dispersion and transformation and thus the engenderment of qi, they may exhibit signs of yang vacuity-vacuity cold, remembering that yang is only a sufficient quantity of qi to experience the qi's intrinsic warmth besides its function.

Further, if liver qi stagnates and becomes depressed, this depression may transform into fire. In this case, the fire may steam body fluids congealing them into phlegm. It may also cause the stomach to exhibit signs of evil heat or fire, and this heat may ascend to harass the heart spirit above. If this heat endures, it may consume and damage yin fluids within the stomach itself and eventually kidney yin below, aggravating any tendency to yin vacuity in any of the viscera and bowels of the body.

Conversely, if kidney water is insufficient to both nourish the fetus and moisten and emolliate the liver, such yin vacuity itself can cause the liver to become anxious, worried, and irritated. This worry and anxiety lead to stirring of liver fire and counterflow of liver qi.

Therefore, as one can see from the above disease mechanisms and their ramifications as described by Chinese medical theory, nausea and vomiting in pregnancy can be a somewhat complicated affair. However, I believe that the three main viscera involved with counterflow of stomach qi during pregnancy are the spleen, liver, and kidneys.

Patterns common to this condition

Spleen-stomach vacuity weakness
Phlegm dampness obstruction & stagnation
Liver assailing the stomach
Liver depression transforming heat
Qi & yin dual vacuity

Treatment based on pattern discrimination

Spleen-stomach vacuity weakness

Main symptoms: Nausea and vomiting during pregnancy, hunger but no desire to eat, vomiting clear water, a bland taste in the mouth, lassitude of the spirit, fatigue, desire to sleep, superficial edema of the face and eyes, a lusterless facial complexion, lack of strength of the four limbs, a fat, swollen tongue with thin, white or white, slimy fur, and a slippery, soggy, fine, and/or forceless, possibly moderate (*i.e.*, slightly slow) pulse

Note: In my experience, this pattern in its pure form is not very common in Western women. However, spleen vacuity does complicate many cases of NVP. This is reflected in the fact that most of the formulas suggested below under this pattern contain one or more medicinals which also rectify the qi, eliminate dampness, or transform phlegm. Simply fortifying the spleen and boosting the qi is rarely a sufficient treatment plan for treating NVP.

Treatment principles: Fortify the spleen and boost the qi, harmonize the stomach and downbear counterflow

Guiding formulas:

Ren Shen Ban Xia Wan (Ginseng & Pinellia Pills)
Ban Xia (Rhizoma Pinelliae), 9g
Ren Shen (Radix Ginseng), 3-9g
Gan Sheng Jiang (dry and uncooked Rhizoma Zingiberis),
   3-6g each

This formula is for the treatment of spleen-stomach vacuity weakness with cold fluids obstructing the stomach.

Ren Shen Ju Pi Tang (Ginseng & Orange Peel Decoction)
Ren Shen (Radix Ginseng), 3-9g
Ju Hong (Pericarpium Citri Erythrocarpae), 6-9g
Bai Zhu (Rhizoma Atractylodis Macrocephalae), 9g
Fu Ling (Poria), 12g
Hou Po (Cortex Magnoliae Officinalis), 9g
mix-fried *Gan Cao* (Radix Glycyrrhizae), 3-6g

E Zu Xiao Fang (Malign Obstruction Effective Formula)
Ju Hong (Pericarpium Citri Erythrocarpae), 9g
Ren Shen (Radix Ginseng),[7] 3-9g
Bai Zhu (Rhizoma Atractylodis Macrocephalae), 9g
Hou Po (Cortex Magnoliae Officinalis), 9g
Mai Men Dong (Tuber Ophiopogonis), 12g
Sheng Jiang (uncooked Rhizoma Zingiberis), 6g
Zhu Ru (Caulis Bambusae In Taeniis), 6-9g

Xiang Sha Liu Jun Zi Tang (Auklandia & Amomum Six Gentlemen Decoction)
Ren Shen (Radix Ginseng), 3-9g
Bai Zhu (Rhizoma Atractylodis Macrocephalae), 9g
Fu Ling (Poria), 12g
mix-fried *Gan Cao* (Radix Glycyrrhizae), 3-9g
Chen Pi (Pericarpium Citri Reticulatae), 3-9g
processed *Ban Xia* (Rhizoma Pinelliae), 9g
Mu Xiang (Radix Auklandiae), 6-9g
Sha Ren (Fructus Amomi), 3-4.5g

This formula treats spleen qi vacuity complicated by dampness and qi stagnation. Han Bai-ling suggests deleting *Ban Xia* since it may damage the fetus. However, it is commonly used to treat nausea and vomiting in pregnancy since at least Zhang Zhong-jing in the *Jin Gui Yao Lue (Essentials from the Golden Cabinet)*.

Zhu Ru Tang (Caulis Bambusae Decoction)
Zhu Ru (Caulis Bambusae In Taeniis), 9g
Chen Pi (Pericarpium Citri Reticulatae), 6-9g
Ban Xia (Rhizoma Pinelliae), 9g
Fu Ling (Poria), 12g
Sheng Jiang (uncooked Rhizoma Zingiberis), 6g

Bao Sheng Tang Er Hao (Protect Engenderment Decoction #2)
Bai Zhu (Rhizoma Atractylodis Macrocephalae), 9g
Sha Ren (Fructus Amomi), 3-4.5g
Xiang Fu (Rhizoma Cyperi), 9g
Wu Yao (Radix Linderae), 9g
Chen Pi (Pericarpium Citri Reticulatae), 6-9g
Gan Cao (Radix Glycyrrhizae), 3-6g
Sheng Jiang (uncooked Rhizoma Zingiberis), 6g
Da Zao (Fructus Jujubae), 2-3 pieces

Wu Qian gives this version of the above formula for habitual stomach weakness without phlegm fluids. If the qi is vacuous, add *Ren Shen* (Radix Ginseng). If the qi is replete, *i.e.*, stagnant, add *Zhi Ke* (Fructus Aurantii).

Phlegm dampness obstruction & stagnation

Main symptoms: Vomiting of phlegm and saliva, stomach duct glomus or fullness, possible heart palpitations, difficulty swallowing, a bland taste in the mouth, a cold body, fatigue and weakness of the four limbs, a fat, swollen tongue with white, glossy, slimy fur, and a slippery pulse

Treatment principles: Transform phlegm and downbear counterflow, harmonize the spleen and transform dampness

Guiding formulas:

Ban Xia Fu Ling Wan Jia Jian
(Pinellia & Poria Pills with Additions & Subtractions)
Zi Su Ye (Folium Perillae Frutescentis), 9-12g
Chen Pi (Pericarpium Citri Reticulatae), 6-9g
ginger-processed *Ban Xia* (Rhizoma Pinelliae), 9g
Sheng Jiang (uncooked Rhizoma Zingiberis), 6g
Mei Gui Hua (Flos Rosae Rugosae), 9g
stir-fried *Gu Ya* (Fructus Germinatus Oryzae), 9-15g
Sha Ren (Fructus Amomi), 3-4.5g
Fu Ling (Poria), 12g

Xiao Ban Xia Fu Ling Tang Jia Wei
(Minor Pinellia & Poria Decoction with Added Flavors)
Ban Xia (Rhizoma Pinelliae), 9g
Sheng Jiang (uncooked Rhizoma Zingiberis), 6g
Fu Ling (Poria), 12g
Chen Pi (Pericarpium Citri Reticulatae), 6-9g
Huo Xiang (Herba Pogostemous), 9g

Er Chen Tang (Two Aged [Ingredients] Decoction)
Fu Ling (Poria), 12g
Chen Pi (Pericarpium Citri Reticulatae), 6-9g
Qing Ban Xia (Rhizoma Pinelliae), 9g
Gan Cao (Radix Glycyrrhizae), 3-6g

If there is heat, add *Zhi Zi* (Fructus Gardeniae) and *Zhu Ru* (Caulis Bambusae In Taeniis) to clear heat, downbear counterflow, and stop vomiting. If heat is prominent and phlegm is less so, delete *Qing Ban Xia* which may damage the fetus. If there is vexation within the chest and vexatious stuffiness, add *Gua Lou* (Fructus Trichosanthis) and *Zhi Zi* (Fructus Gardeniae) to move phlegm stagnation within the chest.

Si Qi Tang (Four [Times] Seven Decoction)
Ban Xia (Rhizoma Pinelliae), 9g
Hou Po (Cortex Magnoliae Officinalis), 9g
Zi Su Ye (Folium Perillae Frutescentis), 9-12g
Fu Ling (Poria), 12g
Sheng Jiang (uncooked Rhizoma Zingiberis), 6g

Liver assailing the stomach

Main symptoms: Nausea and vomiting during pregnancy, easy anger, tendency to sigh, chest oppression and stuffiness, a darkish tongue with normal or white fur, and a slippery, bowstring[8] pulse

Treatment principles: Regulate and harmonize the liver and stomach

Guiding formulas:

Bao Sheng Tang **(Protect Engenderments Decoction; see above)**
Because of the inclusion of *Xiang Fu* (Rhizoma Cyperi) and *Wu Mei* (Fructus Mume), this formula can be seen as a harmonizing formula, even though some Chinese doctors have recommended this formula under spleen qi vacuity.

An Wei Yin **(Quiet the Stomach Pills)**
Ban Xia (Rhizoma Pinelliae), 9g
Huo Xiang (Herba Pogostemonis), 9g
Fu Ling (Poria), 12g
Chen Pi (Pericarpium Citri Reticulatae), 6-9g
Shen Qu (Massa Medica Fermentata), 6-9g
Bai Zhu (Rhizoma Atractylodis Macrocephalae), 9g
stir-fried *Xiang Fu* (Rhizoma Cyperi), 9g
Dang Gui (Radix Angelicae Sinensis), 9g
Bai Shao (Radix Albus Paeoniae Lactiflorae), 9g
Sha Ren (Fructus Amomi), 3-4.5g

Shun Gan Yi Qi Tang **(Normalize the Liver & Boost the Qi Decoction)**
Ren Shen (Radix Ginseng), 3-9g
Bai Zhu (Rhizoma Atractylodis Macrocephalae), 9g
Bai Shao (Radix Albus Paeoniae Lactiflorae), 9g
Dang Gui (Radix Angelicae Sinensis), 9g
Fu Ling (Poria), 12g
Zi Su Zi (Fructus Perillae Frutescentis), 9-12g
Shu Di (cooked Radix Rehmanniae), 12-15g
Mai Men Dong (Tuber Ophiopogonis), 9-12g
Chen Pi (Pericarpium Citri Reticulatae), 6-9g
Sha Ren (Fructus Amomi), 3-4.5g
Shen Qu (Massa Medica Fermentata), 6-9g

This formula harmonizes both the liver and spleen and liver and stomach.

Liver depression transforming heat

Main symptoms: Nausea and vomiting during pregnancy, heart vexation, vomiting of bitter water, dizziness, chest oppression, a tendency to sighing, vexatious thirst for cold drinks, dry, bound stools or difficult, reddish urination, a feverish feeling in the hands and feet, a red facial complexion, chapped lips, a red tongue with dry, yellow fur, and a bowstring, slippery, rapid pulse

Treatment principles: Level the liver and clear heat, harmonize the stomach and stop vomiting

Guiding formulas:

Qing Re Zhi Ou Tang (Clear Heat & Stop Vomiting Decoction)
Zhu Ru (Caulis Bambusae In Taeniis), 9-12g
Chen Pi (Pericarpium Citri Reticulatae), 6-9g
Zhi Shi (Fructus Immaturus Aurantii), 3-9g
Fu Ling (Poria), 12g
Mai Men Dong (Tuber Ophiopogonis), 9-12g
Lu Geng (Rhizoma Phragmitis), 9g
Huang Qin (Radix Scutellariae), 9-12g

If there is constipation, add a small amount of *Da Huang* (Radix Et Rhizoma Rhei) to clear heat, downbear counterflow, and stop vomiting. In this case, do not use *Gan Cao* which warms the middle and aids evils.

Wen Dan Tang Jia Wei
(Warm the Gallbladder Decoction with Added Flavors)
Chen Pi (Pericarpium Citri Reticulatae), 6-9g
Ban Xia (Rhizoma Pinelliae), 9g
Fu Ling (Poria), 12g
Gan Cao (Radix Glycyrrhizae), 3-6g
Zhi Ke (Fructus Aurantii), 3-9g
Zhu Ru (Caulis Bambusae In Taeniis), 9g
Huang Qin (Radix Scutellariae), 9-12g
Huang Lian (Rhizoma Coptidis), 3-6g
Lu Geng (Rhizoma Phragmitis), 9g
Mai Men Dong (Tuber Ophiopogonis), 9-12g
Sheng Jiang (uncooked Rhizoma Zingiberis), 6g
Da Zao (Fructus Jujubae), 2-3 pieces

Ren Shen Ju Pi Tang Jia Wei
(Ginseng & Orange Peel Decoction with Added Flavors)
Ren Shen (Radix Ginseng), 3-9g
Chen Pi (Pericarpium Citri Reticulatae), 6-9g
Bai Zhu (Rhizoma Atractylodis Macrocephalae), 9g
Mai Men Dong (Tuber Ophiopogonis), 9-12g
Gan Cao (Radix Glycyrrhizae), 3-6g
ginger stir-fried *Hou Po* (Cortex Magnoliae Officinalis), 9g
Fu Ling (Poria), 12g
Zhu Ru (Caulis Bambusae In Taeniis), 9g
Huang Qin (Radix Scutellariae), 9-12g

Wan Mi-zhai recommends this formula for thin women with both phlegm and heat.

Xiao Chai Hu Tang (Minor Bupleurum Decoction)
Chai Hu (Radix Bupleuri), 9g

Ren Shen (Radix Ginseng), 3-9g
mix-fried *Gan Cao* (Radix Glycyrrhizae), 3-9g
Huang Qin (Radix Scutellariae), 9-12g
Ban Xia (Rhizoma Pinelliae), 9g
Da Zao (Fructus Jujubae), 2-3 pieces
Sheng Jiang (uncooked Rhizoma Zingiberis), 6g

This formula treats a liver-stomach, liver-spleen disharmony with depressive heat and even some phlegm turbidity. Therefore, it is an extremely useful, commonly used guiding or base formula for the treatment of many women's NVP. If liver depression is more pronounced, *Zhu Ru* (Caulis Bambusae In Taeniis), *Zi Su Ye* (Folium Perillae Frutescentis), and/or *Wu Mei* (Fructus Mume) may be added.

Qi & yin dual vacuity

Main symptoms: Severe, violent vomiting during pregnancy, recurrent vomiting, dry heaves or bringing up matter from the stomach mixed with streaks of blood, lassitude of the spirit, fatigue, lack of strength, a thin body, dry skin, deep, possible deep, sunken eye sockets, dizziness, thirst, scanty urination, generalized heat, a red tongue with no moisture and thin, yellow or smooth, bare, peeled fur, and a fine, rapid, forceless pulse

Treatment principles: Boost the qi and nourish yin, harmonize the stomach and stop vomiting

Guiding formulas:

Zeng Ye Tang (Increase Fluids Decoction) plus *Sheng Mai San* (Engender the Pulse Powder) with Added Flavors #1
Ren Shen (Radix Ginseng), 3-9g
Mai Men Dong (Tuber Ophiopogonis), 9-12g
Wu Wei Zi (Fructus Schisandrae), 9g
Sheng Di (uncooked Radix Rehmanniae), 9-15g
Xuan Shen (Radix Scrophulariae), 9-15g
Chen Pi (Pericarpium Citri Reticulatae), 6-9g
Zhu Ru (Caulis Bambusae In Taeniis), 9g

Zeng Ye Tang (Increase Fluids Decoction) plus *Sheng Mai San* (Engender the Pulse Powder) with Added Flavors #2
Tai Zi Shen (Radix Pseudostellariae), 9-15g
stir-fried *Mai Men Dong* (Tuber Ophiopogonis), 9-12g
Wu Wei Zi (Fructus Schisandrae), 9g
Sheng Di (uncooked Radix Rehmanniae), 9-15g
Xuan Shen (Radix Scrophulariae), 9-15g
Bai Shao (Radix Albus Paeoniae Lactiflorae), 9g
stir-fried *Wu Mei* (Fructus Mume), 9g
Chen Pi (Pericarpium Citri Reticulatae), 6-9g
ginger stir-fried *Zhu Ru* (Caulis Bambusae In Taeniis), 9g

Gou Teng (Ramulus Uncariae Cum Uncis), 9-15g
mix-fried *Gan Cao* (Radix Glycyrrhizae), 3-9g

Because qi and yin vacuity leads to liver fire effulgence, *Bai Shao* and *Wu Mei* have been added to restrain the liver.

Acupuncture & moxibustion: Although acupuncture is generally considered prohibited or contraindicated during pregnancy, as with the use of "prohibited" medicinals, it is really the unwarranted use of acupuncture that is prohibited. In fact, acupuncture may be quiet useful in the treatment of a number of gestational disorders, NVP being one of them. Often nausea during pregnancy is so bad that the thought of drinking a foul or strange-tasting, bitter decoction is more than the patient can bear. In that case, or if internal medicine is insufficient, one can do acupuncture.

Main points: *Nei Guan* (Per 6), *Zhong Wan* (CV 12), *Zu San Li* (St 36)[9]

Needles may be left in place for up to an hour if necessary and two or more treatments can be given per day. For liver invading the spleen and stomach, add *Tai Chong* (Liv 3) and/or *Zhang Men* (Liv 13). For depressive liver heat, add *Xing Jian* (Liv 2). For excessive phlegm, add *Feng Long* (St 40). For stomach heat, add *Nei Ting* (St 44). For spleen vacuity, add *Pi Shu* (Bl 20) and *Wei Shu* (Bl 21). For yin vacuity, add *Zhao Hai* (Ki 6) and *Nei Ting* (St 44).

Abstracts of representative Chinese research:

From "The Treatment of 155 Cases of Severe Nausea During Pregnancy Based on Chinese Medical Pattern Discrimination" by Jiang Xi-ping & Wu Xiang-hong, *Zhong Yi Za Zhi (Journal of Chinese Medicine)*, #4, 1994, p. 225

Cohort description:

From 1982-1992, the authors treated 115 women with severe nausea during pregnancy based on pattern discrimination. Of these 115 women, 50 were between 22-25 years of age, 49 were between 26-29, and 16 were 30 years old or older. The onset of this disease during pregnancy occurred between days 40-59 of gestation in 63 cases, between days 60-89 of gestation in 37 cases, and on days 90 or more in 15 cases. There were 75 primiparas and 40 multigravidas.

Treatment method:

1. Liver-stomach disharmony

After becoming pregnant, the women exhibiting this pattern tended to vomit after eating. The vomitus consisted of a sour or bitter water. They also had dizziness and vertigo, chest and rib-side distention and pain, hiccup, a bitter taste in the mouth, heart vexation, insomnia, a red tongue with thin, white or thin, yellow fur, and a slippery, bowstring pulse. The treatment principles consisted of repressing the liver and harmonizing the stomach, downbearing counterflow and stopping vomiting. Therefore, these patients were given self-composed *Su Lian Hu Qin Tang* (Perilla, Coptis, Bupleurum & Scutellaria Decoction): *Huang Lian* (Rhizoma Coptidis), 3g,

Su Ye (Folium Perillae Frutescentis), 6g, *Chai Hu* (Radix Bupleuri), 6g, *Huang Qin* (Radix Scutellariae), 9g, *Zhu Ru* (Caulis Bambusae In Taeniis), 6g, *Lu O Mei* (Flos Mume), 9g, *Ju Pi* (Pericarpium Citri Reticulatae), 9g, ginger-processed *Ban Xia* (Rhizoma Pinelliae), 9g.

2. Spleen-stomach vacuity weakness

After becoming pregnant, these women experienced vomiting and inability to eat. There was a bland, tasteless feeling in their mouths. They vomited clear water, had epigastric distention and fullness, lassitude of the spirit, and lack of strength. Their tongues were pale with white fur, and their pulses were fine, slippery, and force-less. The treatment principles were to fortify the spleen and boost the qi, harmonize the center and downbear counterflow. Therefore, they were given *Ju Pi Zhu Ru Tang Jia Jian* (Orange Peel & Caulis Bambusae Decoction with Additions & Subtractions): *Ju Pi* (Pericarpium Citri Reticulatae), 10g, *Zhu Ru* (Caulis Bambusae In Taeniis), 10g, *Tai Zi Shen* (Radix Pseudostellariae), 10g, *Ban Xia* (Rhizoma Pinelliae), 10g, *Fu Ling* (Poria), 10g, *Bai Zhu* (stir-fried Rhizoma Atractylodis Macrocephalae), 12g, *Pi Pa Ye* (mix-fried Folium Eriobotryae), 9g, *Sheng Jiang* (uncooked Rhizoma Zingiberis), 3 slices, *Da Zao* (Fructus Jujubae), 5 pieces.

3. Phlegm dampness internally obstructing

These women began vomiting after conceiving and the vomitus was phlegmy, oily, and slimy looking. They were fatigued and were addicted to sleeping. Their tongues were fat and enlarged with white, slimy fur, and their pulses were fine and slippery. The treatment principles were to eliminate dampness and transform phlegm, down-bear counterflow and stop vomiting. Therefore, they were given *Huo Po Er Chen Tang Jia Jian* (Agastaches & Magnolia Two Aged [Ingredients] Decoction with Additions & Subtractions): *Huo Xiang* (Herba Pogostemonis), 10g, *Hou Po* (Cortex Magnoliae Officinalis), 9g, *Chen Pi* (Pericarpium Citri Reticulatae), 10g, *Fu Ling* (Poria), 12g, *Ban Xia* (Rhizoma Pinelliae), 9g, *Bai Bian Dou* (Semen Dolichorisis), 30g, stir-fried *Bai Zhu* (Rhizoma Atractylodis Macrocephalae), 12g, *Zhi Ke* (Fructus Aurantii), 10g, *Zhu Ru* (Caulis Bambusae In Taeniis), 6g.

4. Qi & yin dual vacuity

After conceiving, these women experienced incessant, enduring vomiting. When severe, no water would even come out (*i.e.*, they had dry heaves). Their bodies were emaciated, their eyelids fell downward, both eyes lacked spirit, their mouths were dry, and they had vexatious thirst. Their urination was scanty and their stools were bound. They had red tongues with scanty fur and fine, slippery, rapid pulses. The treatment principles were to boost the qi and nourish yin, engender fluids and stop vomiting. Therefore, they were given self-composed *Yi Qi Yang Yin Tang* (Boost the Qi & Nourish Yin Decoction): *Sheng Di* (uncooked Radix Rehmanniae), 20g, *Mai Men Dong* (Tuber Ophiopogonis), 10g, *Wu Wei Zi* (Fructus Schisandrae), 10g, *Xuan Shen* (Radix Scrophulariae), 15g, *Bai Shao* (Radix Albus Paeoniae Lactiflorae), 15g, *Shi Hu* (Herba Dendrobii), 9g, mix-fried *Pi Pa Ye* (Folium Eriobotryae), 9g, *Zhu Ru* (Caulis Bambusae In Taeniis), 6g, *Wu Mei* (Fructus Mume), 10g, and *Fo*

Shou (Fructus Citri Sacrodactylis), 9g.

Patients were administered one packet per day decocted down to 200ml of liquid. This was given in many small doses.

Treatment outcomes:

Cure was defined as cessation of vomiting and nausea after taking the medicinals, disappearance of the clinical signs and symptoms, three negative urine analyses for protein, and, eventually, a normal birth. Marked improvement meant that, after taking the medicinals and intravenous fluid replacement, the clinical signs and symptoms disappeared, there were three negative urine analyses, and, eventually, there was a normal birth. Some improvement meant that, after taking the Chinese medicinals and intravenous fluid replacement and Western antiemetic medicinals, the signs and symptoms were reduced, urine analysis was negative, and, eventually, there was a normal birth. No results would have meant that after combined treatment, the vomiting did not stop and the pregnancy eventually had to be terminated due to damage and detriment to liver and kidney function.

Based on the above criteria, 78 cases or 67.8% were cured after 2-3 weeks of treatment. Thirty cases or 26.1% experienced marked improvement. Seven cases or 6.1% got some results. Thus the total amelioration rate was 100%. However, the cure rate was highest (88.5%) for the patients in the liver-stomach disharmony pattern group and lowest (20.0%) in the yin and qi dual vacuity pattern group.

From "The Treatment of 47 Cases of Gestational Malign Obstruction with *Wen Dan Tang Jia Jian* (Warm the Gallbladder Decoction with Additions & Subtractions)" by Huang Jian, *Fu Jian Zhong Yi Yao (Fujian Chinese Medicine & Medicinals)*, #6, 2000, p. 40

Cohort description:

All 47 patients in this study were seen as outpatients. Forty-one were primiparas, while for six, this was a second pregnancy. The youngest patient was 25 and the oldest was 31 years old. All met the criteria for gestational malign obstruction appearing in *Zhong Yi Bing Zheng Zhen Duan Liao Xiao Biao Zhun (Chinese Medicine Diseases, Patterns, Diagnosis, Treatment & Outcomes Criteria)*. The symptoms seen were recurrent nausea and vomiting, vomiting of sour or bitter water, chest oppression, dizziness, heart vexation, insomnia, a red tongue with slimy, yellow fur, and a slippery or slippery, rapid pulse. The Chinese medical pattern discrimination was phlegm heat internally obstructing with stomach loss of harmony and downbearing.

Treatment method:

Wen Dan Tang consisted of: *Ban Xia* (Rhizoma Pinelliae), 9g, *Chen Pi* (Pericarpium Citri Reticulatae), 6g, *Fu Ling* (Poria), 9g, *Zhi Ke* (Fructus Aurantii), 5g, *Zhu Ru* (Caulis Bambusae In Taeniis), 10g, *Gan Cao* (Radix Glycyrrhizae).

Additions and subtractions consisted of the following:

For dry mouth, red tongue with yellow fur, and heart vexation, *Huang Qin* (Radix Scutellariae), 9g, was added. For enduring, incessant vomiting and chest oppression, *Fu Long Gan* (Terra Flava Usta), 10g, *Huang Lian* (Rhizoma Coptidis), 6g, and *Zi Su Ye* (Folium Perillae Frutescentis), 6g, were added. For heart vexation, poor sleep, and a dry mouth, *Huang Lian* (Rhizoma Coptidis), *Mai Men Dong* (Tuber Ophiopogonis), and *Yu Zhu* (Rhizoma Polygonati Odorati), 10g, were added. For lower abdominal aching and pain, *Bai Shao* (Radix Albus Paeoniae Lactiflorae), 20g, was added. For central qi insufficiency with heart fluster and shortness of breath, *Dang Shen* (Radix Codonopsitis), 12g, was added. For low back soreness and pain, *Xu Duan* (Radix Dipsaci), 15g, and *Sang Ji Sheng* (Herba Taxilli), 12g, were added.

Treatment outcomes:

Cure was defined as disappearance of vomiting, normalization of eating, and no recurrence of symptoms on follow-up. Improvement meant that the number of times of vomiting was markedly reduced, the patient was able to eat a little more, and other symptoms had lessened. No effect meant that food taken in was vomited back out and there was no obvious lessening of accompanying symptoms. Based on these criteria, 33 cases (70.2%) were judged cured, 12 cases (25.5%) were judged improved, and two cases (4.3%) got no effect. Therefore, the total amelioration rate was 95.7%.

From "The Treatment of 86 Cases of Severe Vomiting During Pregnancy by the Methods of Acridly Opening & Bitterly Downbearing" by Ye Wu-rong, *He Nan Zhong Yi (Henan Chinese Medicine)*, #3, 2001, p. 48-49

Cohort description:

All 86 women in this study were between 24-37 years of age and all had been confirmed to be pregnant by urine analysis or ultrasound. The course of disease had lasted in all these cases from 0.5-3 months. There was severe vomiting of whatever was eaten, phlegmy drool, clear water, bile, or even bloody fluids.

Treatment method:

The basic formula was *Ban Xia Xie Xin Tang* (Pinelliae Drain the Heart Decoction): *Ban Xia* (Rhizoma Pinelliae), 10g, *Dang Shen* (Radix Codonopsitis), 10g, *Huang Qin* (Radix Scutellariae), 6g, *Huang Lian* (Rhizoma Coptidis), 3g, *Gan Jiang* (dry Rhizoma Zingiberis), 3g, mix-fried *Gan Cao* (Radix Glycyrrhizae), 3g, *Da Zao* (Fructus Jujubae), 5 pieces.

If there was heart vexation, *Dan Dou Chi* (Semen Praeparatus Sojae), 10g, stir-fried *Zhi Zi* (Fructus Gardeniae), 6g, and *Zhu Ru* (Caulis Bambusae In Taeniis), 6g, were added. If there was phlegm heat, *Zhu Ru* (Caulis Bambusae In Taeniis), 6g, *Chen Pi* (Pericarpium Citri Reticulatae), 6g, and *Pi Pa Ye* (Folium Eriobotryae), 6g, were added and *Dang Shen* was removed. If there was hematemsis, *Xian He Cao* (Herba Agrimoniae), 10g, *He Ye* (Folium Nelumbinis), 10g, carbonized *Wu Mei* (Fructus Mume), 10g, *Lu Ge* (Rhizoma Phragmitis), 10g, *Dai Zhe Shi* (Haemititum), 10g, and *Zhe Bei Mu* (Bulbus Frtillariae Thunbergii), 10g, were added. If there was spleen vacuity and cold, *Dang Shen* was replaced by *Ren Shen* (Radix Ginseng), 6g, and *Sha Ren* (Fructus Amomi), 3g, *Pei Lan* (Herba Eupatorii), 10g, *He Ye* (Folium Nelumbinis), 10g, and *Huo Xiang* (Herba Pogostemonis) were added. If there was stomach yin vacuity, *Shi Hu* (Herba Dendrobii), 10g, *Bai Hu* (Bulbus Lilii), 10g, and *Sha Shen* (Radix Glehniae), 10g, were added. If there was low back pain, *Du Zhong* (Cortex Eucommiae), 10g, *Tu Si Zi* (Semen Cuscutae), 10g, and *Xu Duan* (Radix Dipsaci), 10g, were added. If there was dizziness, *Mu Li* (Concha Ostreae), 15g, was added. These medicinals were combined with the following ear points: Spleen, Stomach, Triple Burner, Uterus, Liver, Gallbladder, and Internal Secretion.

Treatment outcomes:

Fifty of the 86 patients were cured in six packets of the above medicinals, Twenty-seven were cured after taking nine packets. Seven were cured after 12 packets, and only two cases got no effect and had to have their pregnancies terminated. Therefore, the total amelioration rate was 97.7%.

From "The Treatment of 28 Cases of Severe Vomiting during Pregnancy Accompanied by Liver Function Abnormality with *Jue Ming Gua Lou Tang* (Abalone Shell & Trichosanthes Decoction)" by De Ping, *Jiang Xi Zhong Yi Yao (Jiangxi Chinese Medicine & Medicinals)*, #6, 2000, p. 31

Cohort description:

Of the 28 patients in this study, the youngest was 24 and the oldest was 31 years old, with an average age of 27.1 years. All these patients experienced the onset of this condition between days 36-102 of their pregnancy. Eight cases had begun vomiting within 49 days, 12 had begun vomiting between 50-84 days, and eight cases had begun vomiting between 85-102 days. This was a first pregnancy for 10 cases and a second pregnancy for 18 cases. All the patients were positive for urine ketones. Two cases were ++, 12 cases were +++, and 14 cases were ++++. All cases had high ALT between 50-192 U/L. Twenty cases had a U/L of 50-100, and eight cases had a U/L of 101-192. In two cases, bilirubin was high, but albumin was normal in all cases. Four cases had ST-T abnormalities on their EKG. One case was seen to have gallstones on ultrasound, and three cases had accompanying threatened abortion.

Treatment method:

The basic formula consisted of: *Shi Jue Ming* (calcined Concha Haliotidis), 24g, *Gua Lou Ren* (Semen Trichosanthis), 12g, *Bai Shao* (stir-fried Radix Albus Paeoniae Lactiflorae), 10g, *Dang Gui* (Radix Angelicae Sinensis), 10g, *Sang Ye* (Folium Mori), 12g, *Huang Qin* (Radix Scutellariae), 10g, *Zi Su Ye* (Folium Perillae Frutescentis), 6g, *Zi Su Gen* (Caulis Perillae Frutescentis), 6g, *Lu Mei Hua* (Flos Mume), 5g, ginger-processed *Ban Xia* (Rhizoma Pinelliae), 9g, mix-fried *Gan Cao* (Radix Glycyrrhizae), 5g.

If dry mouth and parched throat were marked, 12 grams of *Shi Hu* (Herba Dendrobii) and 10 grams of *Mai Men Dong* (Tuber Ophiopogonis) were added. If there was scanty qi and disinclination to speak, 12 grams of *Tai Zi Shen* (Radix Pseudostellariae) were added. If the tongue fur was thick and slimy, six grams of *Hou Po* (Cortex

Magnoliae Officinalis) was added. If the tongue was red with scanty fur, two grams of *Xi Yang Shen* (Radix Panacis Quinquefolii) was added. If there was low back soreness, abdominal pain, and vaginal bleeding, 24 grams of *Zhu Ma Gen* (Radix Boehmeriae Niveae) and 15 grams of *Sang Ji Sheng* (Herba Taxilli) were added. One packet of these medicinals was decocted in water per day and administered in many small doses.

Treatment outcomes:

Cure was defined as cessation of the nausea and vomiting with urine ketones testing negative three successive times, ALT normal, and normal fetal growth and development. Some effect was defined as cessation of the nausea and vomiting, but urine ketones not testing negative three successive times, and abnormal ALT. No effect meant that the nausea and vomiting did not stop, ketones tested positive, liver function did not improve, and the pregnancy had to be terminated. Based on these criteria, 23 cases were judged cured and five got some effect. Therefore, the total amelioration rate was 100%. The shortest number of days in the hospital was six and the longest was 39, with an average stay of 14.64 days.

Representative case histories:

Case 1: The patient was a 32 year-old female married worker who had given birth once in four pregnancies. At the time she was examined, it was 26 days since her last menstruation and urine examination for pregnancy was positive. The patient's main complaints were severe nausea and vomiting. The vomitus consisted of phlegmy drool and clear water. The patient had no thought for eating or drinking. Previously, she had liked to eat a lot of enriching, slimy foods. There was also chest and stomach duct distention and pain, loose stools and increased number of bowel movements, dizziness, thin, slimy tongue fur, and a slippery pulse.

Based on these signs and symptoms, the patient's Chinese medical pattern was categorized as spleen vacuity mixed with phlegm, and she was prescribed four packets of the following medicinals: stir-fried *Dang Shen* (Radix Codonopsitis), scorched *Bai Zhu* (Rhizoma Atractylodis Macrocephalae), and *Fu Ling* (Poria), 12g each, ginger-processed *Ban Xia* (Rhizoma Pinelliae), 9g, *Gan Jiang* (dry Rhizoma Zingiberis), *Mei Gui Hua* (Flos Rosae Rugosae), mix-fried *Gan Cao* (Radix Glycyrrhizae), and *Zhi Ke* (Fructus Aurantii), 3g each, *Chen Pi* (Pericarpium Citri Reticulatae), 5g, and *Zi Su Gen* (Caulis Perillae Frutescentis), 6g.

At the second examination, the patient reported that the previous medicinals had decreased her vomiting and that she had more appetite. However, her stools were still loose, she was fatigued, and there was lack of strength. Therefore, she was prescribed another four packets of the following medicinals: stir-fried *Dang Shen* (Radix Codonopsitis), scorched *Bai Zhu* (Rhizoma Atractylodis Macrocephalae), and *Shan Yao* (Radix Dioscoreae), 15g each, *Fu Ling* (Poria), 9g, stir-fried *Bai Shao* (Radix Albus Paeoniae Lactiflorae) and *Zhu Ma Gen* (Radix Boehmeriae Niveae), 12g each, and *Mei Gui Hua* (Flos Rosae Rugosae), *Chen Pi* (Pericarpium

Citri Reticulatae), *Gan Jiang* (dry Rhizoma Zingiberis), and mix-fried *Gan Cao* (Radix Glycyrrhizae), 3g each.

At the third examination, the patient reported that now her stools were formed and she had a bowel movement only 1-2 per day. All her other symptoms were cured. In order to consolidate the treatment effect, the woman was prescribed an undisclosed number of packets of: stir-fried *Dang Shen* (Radix Codonopsitis), scorched *Bai Zhu* (Rhizoma Atractylodis Macrocephalae), and *Shan Yao* (Radix Dioscoreae),15g each, *Zhu Ma Gen* (Radix Boehmeriae Niveae) and *Xu Duan* (Radix Dipsaci), 12g each, mix-fried *Huang Qi* (Radix Astragali), 9g, and *Mei Gui Hua* (Flos Rosae Rugosae) and mix-fried *Gan Cao* (Radix Glycyrrhizae), 3g each.

Case 2: The patient was a 26 year-old female teacher who was first examined on Nov. 6, 1978. This woman's menstruation had stopped two months before and she had had recurrent nausea and vomiting for 40 days. Gynecological examination showed that she was in early pregnancy. Because of the vomiting, she was not able to eat. Because her urine contained ketones, the patient was hospitalized. After two days, her vomiting was brought under control and she was discharged from the hospital. However, in the last half month, she had become nauseous again and vomited whenever she ate. The vomitus consisted of sour, bitter water. This was accompanied by fatigue and somnolence, scanty urination and constipation, a red,tongue with scanty fluids and thin, white fur, and a deep, weak pulse.

Based on these signs and symptoms, the patient's Chinese medical pattern was categorized as spleen vacuity-stomach heat with enduring vomiting having damaged yin. Based on the treatment principles of fortifying the spleen, harmonizing the stomach, and nourishing yin, the woman was prescribed *Yi Gong San Jia Wei* (Strangely Effective Powder with Added Flavors): *Ren Shen* (Radix Ginseng), 6g, *Bai Zhu* (Rhizoma Atractylodis Macrocephalae), 9g, *Fu Ling* (Poria), 10g, *Chen Pi* (Pericarpium Citri Reticulatae), 6g, *Huo Xiang* (Herba Pogostemonis), 9g, *Zhu Ru* (Caulis Bambusae In Taeniis), 12g, *Huang Qin* (Radix Scutellariae), 10g, *Wu Mei* (Fructus Mume), 9g, *Lu Gen* (Rhizoma Phragmitis), 15g, *Shi Hu* (Herba Dendrobii), 15g, and *Sheng Jiang* (uncooked Rhizoma Zingiberis), 8 slices.

The patient was re-examined on Dec. 10 when she reported that, after taking two packets of the above medicinals, the vomiting had stopped and she was able to eat and drink normally again. In addition, her affect had improved.

Case 3: The patient was 28 years old. Her initial examination occurred on Nov. 29, 1978. She was 50 days pregnant and nausea and vomiting were especially severe. There was dizziness and lack of strength, low back soreness and lower leg weakness, a cold body, and hard stools. The pulse was fine and slippery and the tongue fur was thin. Treatment, therefore, was in order to boost the qi and fortify the spleen, harmonize the stomach and downbear counterflow. The formula used was *Huo Xiang Er Chen Tang Jia Wei* (Agastaches Two Aged [Ingredients] Decoction with Added Flavors): *Huo Xiang Gen* (Caulis Pogostemonis), 9g, *Chen Pi* (Pericarpium Citri Reticulatae), *Ban Xia* (Rhizoma Pinelliae), and *Zi Su Gen* (Caulis Perillae Frutescentis), 6g each, *Sha Ren* (Fructus Amomi), 8g, added later, *Dang Shen* (Radix Codonopsitis), *Bai Zhu* (Rhizoma Atractylodis Macrocephalae), *Xu Duan* (Radix Dipsaci), and *Sang Ji Sheng* (Herba Taxilli), 9g each, and ginger-processed *Huang Lian* (Rhizoma Coptidis), 1.5g. Five packets were administered.

After taking these medicinals, the patient's nausea and vomiting diminished and her low back soreness and lower leg weakness were relieved. Intake was improved, but the bowel qi was still stagnant. The pulse was fine and slippery and the tongue fur was thin and yellow. Therefore, *Huo Xiang, Ban Xia,* and *Chen Pi* were removed from the original formula and *Sheng Di* (uncooked Radix Rehmanniae) and *Gua Lou Ren* (Semen Trichosanthis), 12g each, were added in order to enrich fluids and moisten the intestines. After continuing another five packets, the patient was cured.

Case 4: The patient was a 27 year-old female who was first examined on Apr. 20, 1993. The patient was three months pregnant and had no desire to eat. When she ate, this led to oppression in the space between the chest and diaphragm and a desire to vomit. Her mouth was dry but she did not desire to drink much. The woman's tongue was red with thin, slightly yellow fur, and her pulse was slippery and rapid. Therefore, her pattern was categorized as stomach heat with qi stagnation, and she was prescribed the following medicinals: *Bai Bian Dou* (Semen Dolichoris), 30g, *Bai Zhu* (Rhizoma Atractylodis Macrocephalae), 10g, *Sha Shen* (Radix Glehniae), 12g, *Shi Hu* (Herba Dendrobii), 15g, *Huang Qin* (Radix Scutellariae), 10g, *Zhu Ru* (Caulis Bambusae In Taeniis), 10g, *Sha Ren* (Fructus Amomi), 10g, *Bai Dou Kou* (Fructus Cardamomi), 10g, *Sheng Di* (uncooked Radix Rehmanniae), 10g, and *Zi Su Ye* (Folium Perillae Frutescentis), 6g. One packet of these medicinals was decocted in water per day and administered orally. After taking 10 packets of this formula, all the symptoms were eliminated and the patient's eating and drinking had returned to normal.

Remarks

1. Some Chinese doctors do not consider simple nausea during pregnancy a disease or pathocondition. They regard it as a normal symptom of pregnancy which itself is also not a disease. Therefore, these doctors simply advise their patients to be patient and the nausea will clear up on its own. However, nausea is a species of pain and suffering and a doctor's duty is to relieve such suffering if possible. In addition, nausea, no matter what its disease mechanism, involves disharmony of the stomach, and the spleen

and stomach are the root of latter heaven qi and blood engenderment and transformation. Therefore, if one is nauseous, it is reasonable to surmise that their qi and blood engenderment and transformation are impaired. Since it is the mother's qi and blood which nourish the developing fetus, it is also only reasonable to think that treating nausea during pregnancy does have a systemic salutary effect on both the mother and fetus. In my opinion, whether or not to treat simple nausea during pregnancy should depend on the severity of the condition and the wishes of the patient. However, practitioners would do well to remember that Fu Qing-zhu believed that, "Retching and vomiting may not be too serious, but qi will inevitably be damaged all the same."[10]

2. If the patient has trouble drinking a half cup of a decocted formula, she may also try sipping on the "tea" throughout the day or taking it by the dropper full. She may also hold it under her tongue instead of swallowing it so that the medicinals may be absorbed directly into her blood stream. If the formula has been correctly chosen and it aggravates the woman's nausea right after it is taken, one of these methods usually works. If the woman cannot keep anything down, she should also sip on dilute rice soup or congee (*shi fan*). Eating plain, white flour crackers is the Western equivalent of this.

3. In choosing from the above formulas, one should compare their patient's disease mechanism and signs and symptoms with the ingredients in each formula. The one that is the closest match should be chosen. As one can see from the above formulas, often women suffer from a combination of spleen-stomach vacuity, some phlegm and dampness, some food stagnation, some yin vacuity, some liver qi, and some heat. One may also pick a guiding formula and add and subtract ingredients as necessary to fit the patient's condition as exactly as possible.

4. Often, Chinese internal medicinals ameliorate the nausea but do not completely eliminate it. Commonly, women may stop taking their medicine thinking that it is not working, only to find that, as soon as they stop, their nausea is much worse. This is usually enough incentive to get the woman to continue taking her Chinese medicinals.

5. *Zi Su Ye* (Folium Perillae Frutescentis) is a very useful medicinal in the treatment of nausea and vomiting of pregnancy. It harmonizes the liver and stomach, liver and spleen at the same time as it downbears counterflow and quiets the fetus. Therefore, not only does it alleviate nausea and vomiting, it also protects against miscarriage.

6. Although some Chinese doctors shy away from the use of *Ban Xia* (Rhizoma Pinelliae) during pregnancy for fear that this medicinal's toxins may damage the fetus (see above), it is a common ingredient in formulas routinely

used for this complaint since the late Han dynasty. Personally, I have never seen any problems from the use of this medicinal during pregnancy. However, I routinely use the ginger-processed variety, and ginger-processing this medicinal does lessen its toxicity.

Endnotes:

[1] www.sosmorningsickness.com

[2] www.am-i-pregnant.com/morning.shtml

[3] *Ibid.*

[4] www.alternativeparenting.com/preglaborbirth/morning_sickness.htm

[5] *Ibid.*

[6] Fu Qing-zhu, *Fu Qing-zhu's Gynecology,* trans. by Yang Shou-zhong & Liu Da Wei, Blue Poppy Press, Boulder, CO, 1995, p. 65-66

[7] One can substitute Radix Codonopsitis *(Dang Shen)* for Radix Ginseng *(Ren Shen)* in any of the formulas in this book unless otherwise noted.

[8] Wiseman translates *xian mai* as "stringlike pulse." I prefer "bowstring."

[9] The reader should note that *Zu San Li* is considered one of the prohibited points during pregnancy. Yet it is indicated, warranted, and routinely used for the treatment of NVP. This is yet another example of the fact that the traditional prohibitions during pregnancy are not absolute prohibitions but cautions to the uninitiated.

[10] Fu Qing-zhu, *op. cit.*, p. 66

3
Abdominal Pain During Pregnancy

Abdominal pain during pregnancy is not a disease category in modern Western medicine, although it is a disease category in traditional Chinese gynecology. The first discussion of this disorder in the Chinese medical literature is found in Zhang Zhongjing's late Han dynasty *Jin Gui Yao Lue (Essentials from the Golden Cabinet)*. As used in Chinese medicine, abdominal pain during pregnancy may be located in either the upper or lower abdomen, may be chronic or acute, may be mild or severe, and may or may not have anything to do with gestation *per se*. The Western medical differential diagnosis of abdominal pain during pregnancy includes: gastroenteritis, inflammatory bowel disease, peptic ulcer, appendicitis, herpes zoster and/or genitalia, pneumonia, sickle cell disease, psychogenic somatoform disorders, hernias, adhesions, foreign bodies (including gallstones), fecal impaction, ectopic pregnancy, and threatened abortion. In Chinese gynecology and obstetrics, upper abdominal pain is usually not serious. Lower abdominal pain which extends to the low back, however, may be a premonition of miscarriage and, therefore, requires speedy care. Some premodern Chinese gynecology texts discuss abdominal pain during pregnancy as a separate disease category. Others choose instead to discuss fetus stirring restlessly and fetal leakage. Therefore, the reader is referred to those categories discussed below for further information and formulas for the treatment of threatened abortion.

Chinese medical disease categorization

Bao zu, uterine obstruction, *ren shen fu tong*, abdominal pain during pregnancy

Disease causes & disease mechanisms

The fundamental statement about pain in Chinese medicine is, "[If there is] free flow, [there is] no pain; [if there is] pain, [there is] no free flow." Based on this dictum, abdominal pain indicates by its very nature a lack of free flow in the abdomen.

Zhang Zhong-jing stated essentially this same thing when he wrote that abdominal pain during pregnancy is due to obstruction of the network vessels in the abdomen. However, because there are different areas of the abdomen in which pain may be felt and also different types of pain and discomfort, there are several different disease mechanisms which may cause pain in the abdomen during pregnancy.

Pain in the epigastrium, what in Chinese is referred to as the "large abdomen," is mostly due to food stagnation. This may be due to overeating or may be the result of disharmony of the stomach qi during the first trimester. If kidney yang becomes vacuous, lower abdominal pain may be due to vacuity cold. Because cold's nature is to contract and constrict, such cold obstructs the free flow of the qi in the lower burner giving rise to pain. Since kidney qi secures the fetus and yang is nothing other than a lot of qi, if uncorrected, this disease mechanism may develop into miscarriage. If the central qi becomes too vacuous and weak to lift the abdominal contents, this may cause a heavy, dragging pain in the lower abdomen. This results in a loosening of the fetal ligation and can also prestage miscarriage. On the other hand, emotional frustration and anger may give rise to liver depression and qi stagnation. Since the liver channel traverses the lower abdomen, such stagnation may give rise to lower abdominal pain and distention. And finally, blood stasis may also cause lower abdominal pain during pregnancy. Such blood stasis may be due to traumatic injury during the pregnancy or internal causes preceding the pregnancy.

Because damp heat and other disease mechanisms involving the gastrointestinal tract are associated with non-uterine signs and symptoms, these disease mechanisms and the patterns they manifest are not discussed under the category of abdominal pain during pregnancy even though they may be associated with abdominal pain. Instead, they are discussed under the category of diarrhea and dysentery or constipation during pregnancy.

Patterns common to this condition

Food stagnation
Vacuity cold
Spleen qi vacuity
Liver depression qi stagnation
Blood stasis

Treatment based on pattern discrimination

Food stagnation

Main symptoms: Fullness and pain in the stomach duct, frequent belching, diminished appetite, bad breath, possible loose stools or constipation, slimy, white tongue fur, and a slippery, bowstring pulse

Treatment principles: Disperse food, downbear counterflow, and harmonize the stomach

Guiding formula:

Ping Wei San Jia Wei (Level the Stomach Powder with Added Flavors)
Cang Zhu (Rhizoma Atractylodis), 9g
Hou Po (Cortex Magnoliae Officinalis), 9g
Chen Pi (Pericarpium Citri Reticulatae), 6-9g
Gan Cao (Radix Glycyrrhizae), 3-6g
Sheng Jiang (uncooked Rhizoma Zingiberis), 6g
Da Zao (Fructus Jujubae), 2-3 pieces
Cao Guo (Fructus Amomi Tsao-ko), 6g
Zhi Ke (Fructus Aurantii), 6g
Shen Qu (Massa Medica Fermentata), 6-9g

If there is constipation, add *Da Huang* (Radix Et Rhizoma Rhei) and *Mang Xiao* (Mirabilitum). In this case, add more Radix Glycyrrhizae to prevent injury to the fetus.

Acupuncture & moxibustion: Zhong Wan (CV 12), Liang Men (St 21), Zu San Li (St 36), Nei Ting (St 44)

Vacuity Cold

Main symptoms: Chilly, cold pain in the lower abdomen desiring warmth and pressure, a cold appearance, chilled extremities, facial edema, possible loose stools, white, slimy or thin fur, and a deep, weak pulse, remembering that the definition of a weak pulse includes the fact that it is slow and not just forceless

Treatment principles: Warm the channels, nourish the blood, and quiet the fetus

Guiding formulas:

Jiao Ai Tang (Gelatin & Mugwort Decoction)
Dang Gui (Radix Angelicae Sinensis), 9g
Bai Shao (Radix Albus Paeoniae Lactiflorae), 9g
Shu Di (cooked Radix Rehmanniae), 12g
Chuan Xiong (Radix Ligustici Wallichii), 9g
Ai Ye (Folium Artemesiae Argyii), 9g
E Jiao (Gelatinum Corii Asini), 9g
Gan Cao (Radix Glycyrrhizae), 3-6g
Rice wine, a suitable amount

Although this formula warms the uterus, it does not invigorate yang. In other words, it should not be used unmodified if there is marked kidney yang vacuity. If there is qi vacuity, add *Dang Shen* (Radix Codonopsitis) and *Huang Qi* (Radix Astragali).

***Jiao Ai Tang Jia Wei* (Gelatin & Mugwort Decoction with Added Flavors)**
E Jiao (Gelatinum Corii Asini), 9g
Ai Ye (Folium Artemesiae Argyii), 9g
Dang Gui (Radix Angelicae Sinensis), 9g
Chuan Xiong (Radix Ligustici Wallichii), 9g
Bai Shao (Radix Albus Paeoniae Lactiflorae), 9g
Sheng Di (uncooked Radix Rehmanniae), 12g
Gan Cao (Radix Glycyrrhizae), 3-6g
Ba Ji Tian (Radix Morindae), 9g
Du Zhong (Cortex Eucommiae), 9g
Bu Gu Zhi (Fructus Psoraleae), 9g

This version of this formula does supplement the kidneys and invigorate yang.

***Dang Gui Shao Yao San* (Dang Gui & Peony Powder)**
Dang Gui (Radix Angelicae Sinensis), 9g
Bai Shao (Radix Albus Paeoniae Lactiflorae), 9g
Chuan Xiong (Radix Ligustici Wallichii), 9g
Fu Ling (Poria), 12g
Bai Zhu (Rhizoma Atractylodis Macrocephalae), 9g
Ze Xie (Rhizoma Alismatis), 6-9g

This formula is for vacuity cold abdominal pain accompanied by facial edema due to the spleen's nonmovement and nontransformation of water fluids.

Acupuncture & moxibustion: *San Yin Jiao* (Sp 6), *Tai Xi* (Ki 3), *Shen Shu* (Bl 23), *Ming Men* (GV 4), *Guan Yuan* (CV 4)

Spleen qi vacuity

Main symptoms: A heavy, dragging pain in the lower abdomen which is worse on standing and due to taxation, fatigue, a pale face, shortness of breath, diminished appetite, a pale, fat tongue with thin, white fur, and a fine, forceless, possibly short pulse

Treatment principles: Fortify the spleen and boost the qi

Guiding formulas:

***Bu Zhong Yi Qi Tang* (Supplement the Center & Boost the Qi Decoction)**
Huang Qi (Radix Astragali), 9-18g
Ren Shen (Radix Ginseng), 3-9g
Bai Zhu (Rhizoma Atractylodis Macrocephalae), 9g
mix-fried *Gan Cao* (Radix Glycyrrhizae), 6-9g
Dang Gui (Radix Angelicae Sinensis), 9g
Sheng Ma (Rhizoma Cimicifugae), 3-6g
Chai Hu (Radix Bupleuri), 3-9g
Chen Pi (Pericarpium Citri Reticulatae), 3-9g

To more forcefully upbear the qi and lift the fallen, add *Zhi Shi* (Fructus Immaturus Aurantii).

Dang Gui Shao Yao San Jia Jian
(Dang Gui & Peony Powder with Additions & Subtractions)
Dang Gui (Radix Angelicae Sinensis), 9g
Bai Shao (Radix Albus Paeoniae Lactiflorae), 9g
Chuan Xiong (Radix Ligustici Wallichii), 9g
Fu Ling (Poria), 12g
Bai Zhu (Rhizoma Atractylodis Macrocephalae), 9g
He Shou Wu (Radix Polygoni Multiflori), 9-15g
Sang Ji Sheng (Herba Taxilli), 12-15g

This formula is for dual qi and blood vacuity lower abdominal pain where the blood vacuity is more pronounced than the qi vacuity. In this case, there are the qi vacuity signs and symptoms above plus a sallow, yellow complexion, heart palpitations, a pale tongue with thin, white fur, and a fine, slippery, forceless pulse.

Acupuncture & moxibustion: *Zu San Li* (St 36), *Zhong Wan* (CV 12), *San Yin Jiao* (Sp 6), *Pi Shu* (Bl 20), *Wei Shu* (Bl 21)

For a heavy, dragging pain in the lower abdomen due to middle qi insufficiency, moxa indirectly *Bai Hui* (GV 20) every day.

Liver depression qi stagnation

Main symptoms: Lower abdominal pain and distention, emotional depression, irritability, easy anger, chest oppression, frequent sighing, burping or belching, a dark tongue with thin, slimy or thin, yellow fur, and a bowstring, slippery, possibly rapid pulse

Treatment principles: Course the liver and rectify the qi, resolve depression and stop pain

Guiding formulas:

Xiao Yao San (Rambling Powder)
Chai Hu (Radix Bupleuri), 9g
Bai Zhu (Rhizoma Atractylodis Macrocephalae), 9g
Fu Ling (Poria), 12g
mix-fried *Gan Cao* (Radix Glycyrrhizae), 6-9g
Dang Gui (Radix Angelicae Sinensis), 9g
Bai Shao (Radix Albus Paeoniae Lactiflorae), 9g
Sheng Jiang (uncooked Rhizoma Zingiberis), 6g
Bo He (Herba Menthae Haplocalycis), 3-6g

This formula is for liver depression and spleen vacuity with elements of blood vacuity and dampness, but without any depressive heat.

Dan Zhi Xiao Yao San (Moutan & Gardenia Rambling Powder)
Dan Pi (Cortex Moutan), 9g
Zhi Zi (Fructus Gardeniae), 9g
Chai Hu (Radix Bupleuri), 9g

Bai Zhu (Rhizoma Atractylodis Macrocephalae), 9g
Fu Ling (Poria), 12g
mix-fried *Gan Cao* (Radix Glycyrrhizae), 6-9g
Dang Gui (Radix Angelicae Sinensis), 9g
Bai Shao (Radix Albus Paeoniae Lactiflorae), 9g

This formula is for when there is a liver-spleen disharmony with depressive heat, especially depressive heat in the blood aspect or division.

Acupuncture & moxibustion: *Tai Chong* (Liv 3), *He Gu* (LI 4), *Tian Shu* (St 25), *Qi Hai* (CV 6)

Blood stasis

Main symptoms: Fixed, lancinating, and/or severe abdominal pain, possible fetus stirring restlessly or fetal death, a dark, purplish tongue or possible static macules or spots, and a bowstring, choppy pulse

Treatment principles: Quicken the blood & transform stasis, stop pain & quiet the fetus

Guiding formula:

***Ba Zhen Tang* (Eight Pearls Decoction with Added Flavors)**
Dang Shen (Radix Codonopsitis), 9g
Bai Zhu (Rhizoma Atractylodis Macrocephalae), 9g
Fu Ling (Poria), 12g
mix-fried *Gan Cao* (Radix Glycyrrhizae), 6-9g
Dang Gui (Radix Angelicae Sinensis), 9g
Shu Di (cooked Radix Rehmanniae), 12-15g
Bai Shao (Radix Albus Paeoniae Lactiflorae), 9g
Chuan Xiong (Radix Ligustici Wallichii), 9g
Sheng Jiang (uncooked Rhizoma Zingiberis), 6g
Da Zao (Fructus Jujubae), 2-3 pieces
Du Zhong (Cortex Eucommiae), 9g
Sang Ji Sheng (Herba Taxilli), 12-15g
Ru Xiang (Resina Olibani), 3-6g
Mo Yao (Resina Myrrhae), 3-6g
Su Mu (Lignum Sappan), 9g

Because of the interrelationship of the qi to the blood as well as the fact that blood stasis causes blood vacuity and blood vacuity causes blood stasis, the above formula does more, in fact, than the treatment principles stated above strictly speaking warrant.

Acupuncture & moxibustion: *Xue Hai* (Sp 10), *San Yin Jiao* (Sp 6), *He Gu* (LI 4), *Qi Hai* (CV 6), *Tian Shu* (St 25), *Da Chang Shu* (Bl 25)

Abstract of representative Chinese research

From "The Treatment of 34 Cases of Abdominal Pain during Pregnancy with *Dang Gui Shao Yao San Jia Jian* (Dang Gui & Peony Powder with Additions & Subtractions), *Zhe Jiang Zhong Yi Za Zhi* (Zhejiang Journal of Chinese Medicine), #11, 2001, p. 476

Cohort description:

All 34 patients in this study were diagnosed as suffering from abdominal pain during pregnancy. The oldest was 30 and the youngest was 21 years old. Twenty-eight cases were 21-25 years old and six cases were 26-30, with an average age of 24. The longest pregnancy was 79 days, the shortest was 38 days, and the average was 48 days. There were 16 cases who had been pregnant 38-45 days, 10 cases who had been pregnant 46-55 days, six cases who had been pregnant 56-65 days, and two cases who had been pregnant 66 days or more. The shortest course of disease was one day, the longest was 42 days, and the average was seven days. Twenty-eight cases had been experiencing abdominal pain for 1-10 days, five cases had had pain for 11-20 days, and one case had had pain for more than 21 days. The onset of this abdominal pain was insidious in all cases.

Treatment method:

The basic formula consisted of: *Dang Gui* (Radix Angelicae Sinensis), *Fu Ling* (Poria), and mix-fried *Gan Cao* (Radix Glycyrrhizae), 10g each, *Bai Shao* (Radix Albus Paeoniae Lactiflorae), 20-30g, *Chuan Xiong* (Radix Ligustici Wallichii), 5g, and *Gou Qi Zi* (Fructus Lycii) and *Tu Si Zi* (Semen Cuscutae), 15g each. If there was qi vacuity, *Dang Shen* (Radix Codonopsitis) and *Huang Qi* (Radix Astragali) were added. If there was a dry mouth, *Yu Zhu* (Rhizoma Polygoni Odorati) and *Mai Men Dong* (Tuber Ophiopogonis) were added. If there was nausea and vomiting, either *Zhu Ru* (Caulis Bambusae In Taeniis) or *Sheng Jiang* (uncooked Rhizoma Zingiberis) was added. If there was abdominal distention, *Mu Xiang* (Radix Auklandiae) and *Zi Su Gen* (Caulis Perillae Frutescentis) were added. If the stools were loose or there was diarrhea, *Sha Ren* (Fructus Amomi) and *Shan Yao* (Radix Dioscoreae) were added. If the stools were dry and bound, *Bai Zi Ren* (Semen Platycladi) or uncooked *He Shou Wu* (Radix Polygoni Multiflori) were added. If there was a chilly sensation in the lower abdomen, *Ai Ye* (Folium Artemesiae Argyii) and *Bu Gu Zhi* (Fructus Psoraleae) were added. One packet of these medicinals was administered internally per day.

Treatment outcomes:

Twenty-five cases were judged cured. This meant that, after taking the medicinals for five days, their abdominal pain disappeared, did not recur within two weeks, and their pregnancies continued on normally. Six cases got a marked effect. This meant that, after taking the medicinals for seven days, their abdominal pain disappeared, there was no recurrence within two weeks, and their pregnancies continued on normally. One case got some effect. This meant that, after taking the medicinals for 10 days, their abdominal pain improved and that their pregnancies continued on normally, and one case got no effect. After 10 days of taking the above medicinals, this woman's abdominal pain had not diminished. Therefore, the total amelioration rate was 97.06%.

Representative case histories

Case 1: The patient was a female of undisclosed age who had developed abdominal pain after becoming pregnant. This pain extended to her low back and ribside and hurt so much that sometimes she was not able to eat or sleep. The prescribing physician decided that this pain was due to fetal qi irregularity and qi and blood insufficiency. In order to prevent a miscarriage, he prescribed the following Chinese medicinals: *Dang Gui* (Radix Angelicae Sinensis), 18g, *Bai Shao* (Radix Albus Paeoniae Lactiflorae), 9g, *Bai Zhu* (Rhizoma Atractylodis Macrocephalae), 9g, *Fu Ling* (Poria), 15g, *Shi Chang Pu* (Rhizoma Acori Tatarinowii), 2.4g, *Xiang Fu* (Rhizoma Cyperi), 9g, *Mu Xiang* (Radix Auklandiae), 4.5g, added later, *Chen Pi* (Pericarpium Citri Reticulatae), 9g, *Su Xin Hua* (Flos Jasmini Officinalis), 6g, *Zi Su Gen* (Caulis Perillae Frutescentis), 4.5g, *Zhu Ma Gen* (Radix Boehmeriae Niveae), 9g, and *Sang Ji Sheng* (Herba Taxilli), 15g. After taking these medicinals, the pain decreased and the pregnancy continued on in a healthy manner. Based on an analysis of the medicinals in this formula, another way of stating the pattern discrimination would be a liver-spleen disharmony.

Case 2: The patient was a 27 year-old female who had been pregnant for six months. Due to excessive taxation and stirring, the woman had developed low back and abdominal aching and pain. When examined, there was lower abdominal cramping and her lower back felt as if cut by a knife. Her spirit qi was not good, and there was a profuse, white-colored, mucus discharge from her vagina. Based on these signs and symptoms, the patient was prescribed the following Chinese medicinals in order to guard the fetus and prevent a miscarriage: *E Jiao* (Gelatinum Corii Asini), 6g, *Ai Ye* (Folium Artemisiae Argyii), 2.4g, *Bai Shao* (Radix Albus Paeoniae Lactiflorae), 9g, *Du Zhong* (Cortex Eucommiae), 9g, *Sheng Di* (uncooked Radix Rehmanniae), 9g, *Tu Si Zi* (Semen Cuscutae), 4.5g, *Dang Gui* (Radix Angelicae Sinensis), 4.5g, and *Ren Shen* (Radix Ginseng), 4.5g. After taking these medicinals, the patient was able to sleep and her symptoms greatly decreased. After taking two more packets of these medicinals, her condition was considered cured.

Remarks

One must treat abdominal pain during pregnancy without hesitation. If timely treatment is not provided, abdominal pain may result in restless stirring of the fetus, miscarriage, or possible fetal death. Although blood-quickening, stasis-trsansforming medicinals are nominally prohibited during pregnancy, if there is blood stasis, they must be used.

4

Ectopic Pregnancy

Ectopic pregnancy is a modern Western medical disease category. It refers to the implantation of the fertilized zygote outside of the uterus, most often in the fallopian tubes. However, it may occur in the ovary, abdominal, or pelvic cavities. In 50% of cases tubal implantation is the result of previous tubal infection. The incidence of ectopic pregnancy is one in 100-200 pregnancies. However, this incidence is rising and is higher among non-whites.[1]

The symptoms of ectopic pregnancy are spotting and cramping pain in the lower abdomen not long after the first missed menstrual period. Spotting or leakage may transform into flooding or hemorrhagic bleeding. If that occurs, the woman may lose so much blood as to experience shock. Uterine examination will find the uterus enlarged but not as large as it should be for the date of the pregnancy. Serum and urine tests may be performed and, if positively suggesting ectopic pregnancy, an ultrasound is usually done. In the West, ectopic pregnancy is considered a surgical disease requiring, in most cases, emergency treatment. If not corrected, at about 6-8 weeks of pregnancy, abdominal pain may markedly decrease followed by the patient's fainting. This suggests rupture of the tubes with intra-abdominal hemorrhage. Although the mortality rate for ectopic pregnancy is dropping, it currently stands at one in 826[2] and, left untreated, it is usually fatal.

Chinese medical disease categorization

In Chinese medicine, ectopic pregnancy is most often diagnosed as *shao fu xue yu shi zheng*, lower abdominal repletion blood stasis condition, *jing bi*, menstrual blockage, meaning amenorrhea, *jing lou* or menstrual leakage, or *zheng jia*, abdominal mass.

Disease causes & disease mechanisms

In Chinese medicine, this condition is thought to be due to abnormal growth and, therefore, the shape of the *bao mai* or uterine vessel. Either it is excessively long or excessively fine. This then results in blood stasis, obstruction, and stagnation. When the patient conceives, transportation and movement of the zygote is obstructed. Therefore, the fertilized zygote does not get to the uterus.

Patterns common to this condition

Blood stasis in the lower abdomen
Evils replete, righteous deserted
Unstable type
Blood stasis abdominal lump

Treatment based on pattern discrimination

Blood stasis in the lower abdomen

Main symptoms: Delayed menstruation, dribbling and dripping of blood which does not come easily, violent pain in the lower abdomen that resists pressure, thin tongue fur, and a bowstring, fine, rapid pulse

Note: This pattern typically corresponds to the unruptured stage of ectopic pregnancy.

Treatment principles: Quicken the blood, dispel stasis, and stop pain

Guiding formulas:

Gong Wai Yun Fang Yi Hao **(Ectopic Pregnancy Formula #1)**
Dan Shen (Radix Salviae Miltiorrhizae), 9-15g
Chi Shao (Radix Rubrus Paeoniae Lactiflorae), 9g
Tao Ren (Semen Persicae), 9g
E Jiao (Gelatinum Corii Asini), 9g
San Qi (Radix Notoginseng), 1-3g (taken powdered with the medicinal decoction)

Gong Wai Yun Fang Er Hao **(Ectopic Pregnancy Formula #2)**
Chi Shao (Radix Rubrus Paeoniae Lactiflorae), 9g
Dan Shen (Radix Salviae Miltiorrhizae), 9-15g
Tao Ren (Semen Pruni Persicae), 9g
San Leng (Rhizoma Sparganii), 9g
E Zhu (Rhizoma Curcumae), 9g

Huo Luo Xiao Ling Tang
(Quicken the Network Vessels Magically Effective Decoction)
Dan Shen (Radix Salviae Miltiorrhizae), 9-15g
Chi Shao (Radix Rubrus Paeoniae Lactiflorae), 9g
Ru Xiang (Resina Olibani), 3-6g
Mo Yao (Resina Myrrhae), 3-6g
Tao Ren (Semen Persicae), 9g

If there is simultaneous cold, add *Rou Gui* (Cortex Cinnamomi). If there is simultaneous heat, add *Jin Yin Hua* (Flos Lonicerae), *Lian Qiao* (Fructus Forsythiae), *Pu Gong Ying* (Herba Taraxaci), and *Ban Lan Gen* (Radix Isatidis/Baphicacanthi). If qi and blood have both deserted, add *Ren Shen* (Radix Ginseng). If the four limbs are cold due to counterflow reversal, add *Zhi Fu Zi* (Radix Lateralis Praeparatus Aconiti Carmichaeli). If there is a dripping, dribbling cold sweat, add *Shan Zhu Yu* (Fructus Corni). If the body is habitually vacuous with reduced intake of food and drink, bodily heaviness and fatigue, and a fine, weak pulse, add *Dang Shen* (Radix Codonopsitis). If there is constipation due to replete heat, add *Da Huang* (Radix Et Rhizoma Rhei) and *Mang Xiao* (Mirabilitum).

Evils replete, righteous deserted

Main symptoms: Dribbling and dripping of blood from the vagina which does not stop, violent pain in the lower abdomen which resists pressure, an ashen white facial complexion, chilled limbs, profuse cold sweating, spirit mind vexation and agitation and other such signs and symptoms of desertion, plus a fine, faint, about to be cut off, or exhausted pulse

Note: This pattern corresponds to ruptured ectopic pregnancy with shock.

Treatment principles: Quicken the blood and transform stasis, rescue the yang and stem desertion

Guiding formulas:

Shen Fu Tang (Ginseng & Aconite Decoction) plus
Gong Wai Yun Fang (Ectopic Pregnancy Formula) with added flavors
Ren Shen (Radix Ginseng), 3-9g
Zhi Fu Zi (Radix Lateralis Praeparatus Aconiti Carmichaeli), 3-9g
Dan Shen (Radix Salviae Miltiorrhizae), 9-15g
Chi Shao (Radix Rubrus Paeoniae Lactiflorae), 9g
Tao Ren (Semen Persicae), 9g
uncooked *Long Gu* (Os Draconis), 12-15g
uncooked *Mu Li* (Concha Ostreae), 12-15g
San Qi (Radix Notoginseng), 1-3g (taken powdered with the
    medicinal decoction)

Gong Wai Yun Fang Yi Hao Jia Wei
(Ectopic Pregnancy Formula #1 with Added Flavors)
Chi Shao (Radix Rubrus Paeoniae Lactiflorae), 9g
Dan Shen (Radix Salviae Miltiorrhizae), 9-15g
Tao Ren (Semen Persicae), 9g
Zhi Fu Zi (Radix Lateralis Praeparatus Aconiti Carmichaeli), 3-9g
Ren Shen (Radix Ginseng), 3-9g
Mai Men Dong (Tuber Ophiopogonis), 9-12g
Wu Wei Zi (Fructus Schisandrae), 9g

Unstable type

Main symptoms: Abdominal pain with tenderness which gradually is relieved, a palpable mass with indistinct borders, a small amount of vaginal bleeding, stable blood pressure, and a fine, moderate (*i.e.*, slightly slow) pulse

Note: This pattern corresponds to ruptured ectopic pregnancy but without shock.

Treatment principles: Quicken the blood and disperse conglomeration

Guiding formula:

Gong Wai Yun Fang Yi Hao (Ectopic Pregnancy Formula #1)
Chi Shao (Radix Rubrus Paeoniae Lactiflorae), 9g
Dan Shen (Radix Salviae Miltiorrhizae), 9-15g
Tao Ren (Semen Persicae), 9g

Blood stasis abdominal lump

Main symptoms: Abdominal pain that resists pressure, a palpable mass within the abdomen, scant vaginal bleeding, stable blood pressure, and a fine, slow or fine, choppy pulse

Treatment principles: Quicken the blood and dispel stasis, disperse concretions and scatter nodulation

Guiding formulas:

Gong Wai Yun Fang Jia Wei
(Ectopic Pregnancy Formula with Added Flavors)
Dan Shen (Radix Salviae Miltiorrhizae), 9-15g
Chi Shao (Radix Rubrus Paeoniae Lactiflorae), 9g
Tao Ren (Semen Persicae), 9g
E Jiao (Gelatinum Corii Asini), 9g
San Qi (Radix Notoginseng), 1-3g (taken powdered with the
    medicinal decoction)
San Leng (Rhizoma Sparganii), 9g
E Zhu (Rhizoma Curcumae), 9g
Shan Zha (Fructus Crataegi), 3-4.5g

If there is fear of chill and a desire for warmth with a deep, slow pulse suggesting yang vacuity, add *Rou Gui* (Cortex Cinnamomi) and *Zhi Fu Zi* (Radix Lateralis Praeparatus Aconiti Carmichaeli). If there is generalized lack of strength and shortness of breath, add *Dang Gui* (Radix Angelicae Sinensis) and *Huang Qi* (Radix Astragali). If the chest and rib-sides are distended and full and one has qi stagnation, add *Chuan Lian Zi* (Fructus Toosendan), *Yu Jin* (Tuber Curcumae), *Qing Pi* (Pericarpium Citri Reticulatae Viride), *Xiang Fu* (Rhizoma Cyperi), and *Zhi Ke* (Fructus Aurantii). If there is constipation with a full, distended abdomen, use the basic formula, *Gong Wai Yun Fang* above and add *Da Cheng Qi Tang* (Major Order the Qi Decoction), *i.e., Da Huang* (Radix Et Rhizoma Rhei), *Mang*

Xiao (Mirabilitum), *Hou Po* (Cortex Magnoliae Officinalis), and *Zhi Shi* (Fructus Immaturus Aurantii).

Gong Wai Yun Fang Er Hao Jia Wei
(Ectopic Pregnancy Formula #2 with Added Flavors)
Chi Shao (Radix Rubrus Paeoniae Lactiflorae), 9g
Dan Shen (Radix Salviae Miltiorrhizae), 9-15g
Tao Ren (Semen Persicae), 9g
San Leng (Rhizoma Sparganii), 9g
E Zhu (Rhizoma Curcumae), 9g
Dang Shen (Radix Codonopsitis), 9-15g
Huang Qi (Radix Astragali), 9-18g

Abstracts of representative Chinese research

From "The Chinese Herbal Treatment of Ectopic Pregnancy" by Cui Hua-ming *et al., Si Chuan Zhong Yi (Sichuan Chinese Medicine)*, #7, 1993, p. 43

Cohort description:

In this clinical audit, the authors report on the treatment of 10 cases of ectopic pregnancy seen from June 1990-March 1991. The women ranged in age from 23-35 years old. Their menses had ceased but there was irregular bleeding from the vagina and abdominal pain. Urine pregnancy tests were positive for eight cases and negative for two. The diagnosis of ectopic pregnancy was derived by physical examination.

Treatment method:

The treatment method consisted of two formulas. Formula I: *Tian Hua Fen* (Radix Trichosanthis), 30g, *Wu Gong* (Scolopendra), 2 pieces, *Dan Shen* (Radix Salviae Miltiorrhizae), 15g, *San Leng* (Rhizoma Sparganii), *E Zhu* (Rhizoma Curcumae), *Tao Ren* (Semen Persicae), *Mu Xiang* (Radix Auklandiae), *Xiang Fu* (Rhizoma Cyperi), *Hong Hua* (Flos Carthami), 10g each, processed *Ru Xiang* (Resina Olibani) and *Mo Yao* (Resina Myrrhae), 8g each, *Yi Mu Cao* (Herba Leonuri), 20g, and uncooked *Gan Cao* (Radix Glycyrrhizae), 6g.

Formula II: *Dan Shen* (Radix Salviae Miltiorrhizae), 15g, *Chi Shao* (Radix Rubrus Paeoniae Lactiflorae), *Chuan Xiong* (Radix Ligustici Wallichii), *Yuan Hu* (Rhizoma Corydalis), *Rou Gui* (Cortex Cinnamomi), 9g each, and *San Leng* (Rhizoma Sparganii), *E Zhu* (Rhizoma Curcumae), *Tao Ren* (Semen Persicae), and *Fu Ling* (Poria), 6g each.

If there was qi vacuity, *Huang Qi* (Radix Astragali), 9g, and *Shu Di* (cooked Radix Rehmanniae), 15g, were added. If there was flooding and leaking (*i.e.*, uterine bleeding), *Shi Xiao San* (Loose a Smile Powder) was added. During administration of Formula I, when urine pregnancy tests turned negative or serological markers had lowered on two occasions, Formula I was stopped and Formula II was administered instead. Formula I kills the embryo, quickens the blood, and stops pain, while Formula II is for the purpose of quickening static blood, stopping pain, and freeing the flow of the network vessels.

Treatment outcomes:

In this study, cure was defined as disappearance of the clinical manifestations as well as the physical manifestations revealed on examination. After administering Formula I for three days, three cases' urine pregnancy test turned negative, with another five cases turning negative after five days administration. Nine cases were hospitalized for an average of 21 days for complete cure to be affected. One case was hospitalized for two months because of encysted blood accumulations on both sides of her abdomen which reabsorbed slowly.

From "The Treatment of 15 Cases of Ectopic Pregnancy with *Yi Qi Huo Xue Tang* (Boost the Qi & Quicken the Blood Decoction)" by Ha Xiao-lian & Peng Hui-min, *Tian Jin Zhong Yi (Tianjin Chinese Medicine)*, #3, 1993, p. 12-13

Cohort description:

In this clinical audit, 15 cases of ectopic pregnancy were treated with *Yi Qi Huo Xue Tang*. Four of the women were between 24-26 years of age, eight were between 27-30, and three were between 31-35 years old. In addition, eight were primiparas, six had been pregnant twice, and one had been pregnant three times. Thirteen of the women had tubal pregnancies, one woman had a uterine angle pregnancy, and one woman had an abdominal cavity pregnancy.

Treatment method:

The formula used consisted of: *Dang Gui* (Radix Angelicae Sinensis), 9g, *Chi Shao* (Radix Rubrus Paeoniae Lactiflorae), 9g, uncooked *Pu Huang* (Pollen Typhae), 9g, *Ru Xiang* (Resina Olibani), 6g, mix-fried *Mo Yao* (Resina Myrrhae), 6g, *Wu Yao* (Radix Linderae), 9g, *Xiang Fu* (Rhizoma Cyperi), 10g, *San Leng* (Rhizoma Sparganii), and *E Zhu* (Rhizoma Curcumae), 9g each, *Dang Shen* (Radix Codonopsitis), 15g, *Dan Shen* (Radix Salviae Miltiorrhizae), 15g, and *Tian Hua Fen* (Radix Trichosanthis), 12g. These were decocted down to 300ml and one packet was administered internally per day. The purpose of this formula was to boost the qi and nourish the blood, quicken the blood and transform stasis, and to rectify the qi and stop pain.

If abdominal pain was severe, *Wu Ling Zhi* (Feces Trogopterori Seu Pteromi), 10g, was added and *Wu Yao* was increased to 15g. If hemorrhaging was excessive, *San Leng* and *E Zhu* were removed and *Yi Mu Cao* (Herba Leonuri), 15g, was added. If the appetite was poor, stir-fried *Mai Ya* (Fructus Germinatus Hordei), 10g, and *Nei Jin* (Endothelium Corneum Gigeriae Galli), 6g, were added. And if there was constipation, *Da Huang* (Radix Et Rhizoma Rhei), 10g, or *Fan Xie Ye* (Folium Sennae), 3g, were added.

Treatment outcomes:

Of the 15 cases so treated, all were completely cured except for one who was hemorrhaging greatly and received surgery.

From "The Treatment of 21 Cases of Ectopic Pregnancy with Quickening the Blood & Transforming Stasis Method" by Jia Ying, *Jiang Su Zhong Yi (Jiangsu Chinese Medicine)*, #9, 1993, p.15-16

Cohort description:

The author begins this report by stating that traditionally this condition was discussed under lower abdominal depression of blood, concretions and conglomerations, falling fetus, etc. If, for some reason, surgery cannot be used to treat this condition, one may resort to the methods of quickening the blood and transforming stasis. Of the 21 cases treated by these means by the author, six were between 23-30 years of age and 15 between 31-42. There were 16 cases of fallopian tube pregnancy, three cases of ovarian pregnancy, one case of abdominal cavity pregnancy, and one case of uterine cervix pregnancy.

Treatment method:

The formula employed was *Huo Luo Xiao Ling Dan Jia Wei* (Quickening the Network Vessels Magically Effective Elixir with Added Flavors). It was comprised of: *Chi Shao* (Radix Rubrus Paeoniae Lactiflorae), *Tao Ren* (Semen Pruni Persicae), *Ru Xiang* (Resina Olibani), *Mo Yao* (Resina Myrrhae), *San Leng* (Rhizoma Sparganii), and *E Zhu* (Rhizoma Curcumae).

If there was heat, *Jin Yin Hua* (Flos Lonicerae), *Lian Qiao* (Fructus Forsythiae), *Pu Gong Ying* (Herba Taraxaci), and *Hong Teng* (Caulis Sargentodoxae) were added. If there was cold, *Wu Zhu* (Fructus Evodiae) and *Gui Zhi* (Ramulus Cinnamomi) were added. If there was constipation, *Da Huang* (Radix Et Rhizoma Rhei) and *Mang Xiao* (Mirabilitum) were added. If there was abdominal pain, *Pu Huang* (Pollen Typhae), *Wu Ling Zhi* (Feces Trogopterori Seu Pteromi), and *Yan Hu Suo* (Rhizoma Corydalis) were added. If there was discharge of profuse blood, *Qian Cao* (Radix Rubiae), *Xue Yu Tan* (Crinis Carbonisatus), and carbonized *Shan Zha* (Fructus Crataegi) were added. If there was qi vacuity, *Huang Qi* (Radix Astragali) and *Dang Shen* (Radix Codonopsitis) were added. If the embryo was not dead, *Tian Hua Fen* (Radix Trichosanthis) or *Wu Gong* (Scolopendra) was added. If the absorption and assimilation of the bloody swelling was delayed, *Hong Hua* (Flos Carthami), *Chuan Shan Jia* (Squama Manitis), and *Wang Bu Liu Xing* (Semen Vaccariae) were added. If there was nausea and vomiting, *Chen Pi* (Pericarpium Citri Reticulatae) and *Ban Xia* (Rhizoma Pinelliae) were added. And if appetite was below normal, *Shen Qu* (Massa Medica Fermentata) and *Ji Nei Jin* (Endothelium Corneum Gigeriae Galli) were added.

Treatment outcomes:

In this study, complete cure was defined as disappearance of the signs and symptoms of this condition, disappearance of lower abdominal pain, cessation of blood flowing from the vaginal tract, the menses returning to normal, and serum pregnancy indicators either disappearing or being reduced by 2/3. Based on these criteria, the author reports that all 21 cases were completely cured. The author also says that, in the treatment of this disease, it is typically not appropriate to use heavy doses of blood-stopping medicinals since these might impede the assimilation and reabsorption of static blood.

From "The Treatment of 40 Cases of Unruptured Fallopian Tube Pregnancy by Quickening the Blood & Transforming Stasis" by Wu Lian-zhen, *Zhe Jiang Zhong Yi Za Zhi (Zhejiang Journal of Chinese Medicine)*, #7, 1993, p. 304-305

Cohort description:

Dr. Wu begins this report on the treatment of ectopic pregnancy by saying that the methods of quickening the blood and transforming stasis were used in order to promote miscarriage. Thirty women in this study were between 23-28 years of age and 10 were over 30, with the oldest being 50 years old. In three cases, their menstruation had ceased less than 35 days previously. In 28 cases, their menses had ceased between 35-40 days before, in seven cases, menstruation had ceased 41-45 days before, and in two cases, menstruation had ceased more than 46 days before. Pregnancy was confirmed by cessation of menstruation, urine analysis, serum tests, lower abdominal distention and pain, and pelvic examinations. Based on these criteria, all the women in this group were diagnosed as suffering from tubal pregnancy.

Treatment method:

The medicinals used were: *Dan Shen* (Radix Salviae Miltiorrhizae), *Chi Shao* (Radix Rubrus Paeoniae Lactiflorae), *San Leng* (Rhizoma Sparganii), and *E Zhu* (Rhizoma Curcumae), 15g each, and *Tao Ren* (Semen Persicae), *Ru Xiang* (Resina Olibani), and *Mo Yao* (Resina Myrrhae), 10g each.

If the tongue was pale with a white coating and the pulse was deep and slow, *Rou Gui* (Cortex Cinnamomi), 5g, and *Zhi Fu Zi* (Radix Lateralis Praeparatus Aconiti Carmichaeli), 10g, were added. If the tongue was red with yellow fur and the pulse was bowstring and rapid, *Jin Yin Hua* (Flos Lonicerae) and *Lian Qiao* (Fructus Forsythiae), 15g each, were added. If the abdomen was distended, *Zhi Ke* (Fructus Aurantii) and *Hou Po* (Cortex Magnoliae Officinalis), 5g each, were added, and if there was constipation, uncooked *Da Huang* (Radix Et Rhizoma Rhei), 10g, was added.

Treatment outcomes:

After administration of from 10-30 packets of the above medicinals, 36 cases were cured, meaning their urine pregnancy tests turned negative, their serum pregnancy markers disappeared, and their menses returned to normal. Four cases experienced no result. In other words, their urine pregnancy tests remained positive, their serum pregnancy markers remained, the lumps in their abdomen increased in size, or their tubes ruptured. Among the cases which experienced no result, three were treated surgically when their urine and serum tests did not change and the lumps in their abdomen grew larger. The other case experienced rupture of her tube and fever, at which time she was also treated surgically.

Remarks

It is unlikely that a woman in the West diagnosed with ectopic pregnancy would be treated solely with Chinese medicine. In fact, this would be highly dangerous legally as well as possibly medically. Therefore, the above discussion of the Chinese medical treatment of ectopic pregnancy is offered for informational purposes and perhaps as a stimulant for the development of integrated Chinese-Western medicine in the West.

Endnotes:

[1] Beers, Mark H. & Robert Berkow, *The Merck Manual of Diagnosis and Therapy*, 17th edition, Merck Research Laboratories, Whitehouse Station, NJ, 1999, p. 2055

[2] *Ibid.*, p. 2056

5

Spontaneous Abortion

In Western medicine, abortion (or miscarriage) is defined as loss of pregnancy before the 20th week of gestation. Delivery between 20-37 weeks is considered preterm birth. Twenty to thirty percent of women bleed or experience abdominal cramping some time during the first 20 weeks of pregnancy, with half of these spontaneously aborting. According to Western medicine, in up to 60% of spontaneous abortions, there is either no fetus or the fetus is grossly malformed. In 25-60% of cases, the fetus has chromosomal abnormalities which are incompatible with life. Therefore, spontaneous abortion is often the natural rejection of a maldeveloping fetus. Eight-

ABORTION TERMINOLOGY

4 weeks	Amenorrhea, morning sickness
Type	Definition
Early	Loss of pregnancy before week 12 of pregnancy
Late	Loss of pregnancy between 12-20 weeks of pregnancy
Spontaneous	Spontaneous, noninduced loss of pregnancy
Induced	Deliberate termination of pregnancy for medical reasons or by choice
Therapeutic	Termination of pregnancy for medical reasons
Threatened	Any bleeding or cramping in the first 20 weeks of pregnancy
Inevitable	Bleeding or rupture of the membranes accompanied by pain & dilation of the cervix
Incomplete	Expulsion of only part of the products of conception
Complete	Expulsion of all the products of conception
Habitual	Three or more consecutive spontaneous abortions
Missed	Prolonged delay in expulsion of a dead fetus
Septic	Infection of the uterus before, during, or after an abortion

five percent of spontaneous abortions occur in the first trimester and tend to have fetal causes, whereas those that occur in the second trimester tend to have maternal causes.[1] In the 4.8 million pregnancies that occur in the United States each year which are not artificially terminated, approximately 800,000 end in spontaneous abortion.[2]

In Western medicine, threatened abortions are treated by bed rest. However, this rarely changes the outcome. Inevitable or incomplete abortions are completed by suction curettage or sometimes by D & C. Missed abortion is completed as soon as the diagnosis is certain. Typically, ultrasonography can detect fetal death within 1-2 weeks. In cases of septic abortion, antibiotics and immediate emptying of the uterus are considered essential to prevent life-threatening sepsis.

Chinese medical disease categorization

In Chinese medicine, there are likewise a number of different traditional terms covering different types of abortion and preterm delivery. If, after conception and at a time other than normally scheduled menstruation, a woman has a small amount of bloody fluid discharge from her vagina, this is called *tai lou* or *lou tai*, fetal leakage or leaky fetus. If this is accompanied by low back soreness and abdominal pain and the amount of the discharge is more, this is called *tai dong bu an*, fetus stirring restlessly. If there is low back pain and a heavy, falling feeling in the abdomen, the bloody discharge is even more in quantity, and if the blood has clumps or clots in it, this is called *liu chan*, flowing birth, or *duo tai*, falling or dropping fetus, if it occurs within the first trimester. If it occurs after the first three months of pregnancy, it is called *xiao chan*, small birth, or *ban chan*, half birth. If a woman spontaneously aborts three or more times either before or after three months, this is called *hua tai* or slippery fetus and is discussed separately below. Contemporary Chinese gynecology has also adopted some of the same terms used in modern Western gynecology, such as inevitable abortion, incomplete abortion, and complete abortion.

In clinical practice, one must also distinguish between *tai lou* and miscarriage and *ji jing* and *nao xue*. *Ji jing* means stimulated menses. This refers to menstruation occurring on its regular cycle for several months after conception has taken place. It is distinguished from miscarriage by its occurrence at its normally appointed times and its regular cyclicity. In this case, the woman's affect, appetite, and six pulses are normal and she does not experience any pain in her body. This bleeding is due to exuberance of the woman's blood. *Nao xue* refers to blood in the urine. It is typically due to binding or knotting of heat in the bladder. This causes the blood to move frenetically. The blood enters the water passageways and exits with the urine. If the mother's uterus is normal and the blood flows right before or right after urination, this is usually not a manifestation of threatened abortion.

Disease causes & disease mechanisms

There are five basic mechanisms associated with miscarriage according to Chinese medicine. The first is kidney vacuity. It is kidney qi that secures the fetus and astringes the lower yin, *i.e.*, the anal and vaginal orifices. If, due to congenital weakness and insufficiency, age, chronic disease, extreme and/or prolonged taxation, or lack of restraint in bedroom affairs after conception, the lifegate is insufficient, yin essence is damaged and consumed, or yin and yang are both damaged, the chong and ren may become vacuous and empty. In that case, the fetus may not be secured in place.

Secondly, if food and drink are not well regulated or if one suffers from overtaxation or excessive worry and anxiety, the spleen and stomach may become vacuous and weak. Because spleen qi contains and lifts the abdominal contents and because the spleen is the latter heaven root of blood engenderment and transformation, spleen vacuity may lead to downward falling of central qi and insufficient blood to nourish the fetus. This, likewise, leads to the *chong* and *ren* not securing the fetus and holding it in place. In that case, the fetal ligation may become weak and the fetus may fall downward.

Third, mental agitation and emotional frustration, envy, anger, or excessive jealousy may all give rise internally to depressive heat. This heat may then harass the sea of blood, scorching and damaging the *bao mai*. Yin blood may thus flow frenetically downward, and the fetus may have no place on which to rest and rely.

Fourth, it is possible also for blood stasis to force the blood to move outside its pathways, thus causing fetal leakage. In this case, blood stasis due to past injury, iatrogenesis, or long-term qi stagnation may become aggravated due to the accumulation of qi and blood focused on the lower abdomen. This mechanism of fetal leakage is often overlooked. It often complicates other mechanisms and patterns and is frequently present when treatment methods aimed at other mechanisms fail to stop the bleeding.

And fifth, external injury, such as falling from a height, being hit or struck, or sustaining a sprain or strain, may damage and injure the *chong* and *ren*. In this case, once again the fetus may have no place to tie or fasten.

Ye Heng-yin summarizes these disease mechanisms of spontaneous abortion when he says:

If a pregnant woman's qi and blood are full and sufficient, strong and replete, then the fetus will automatically be quiet and secure. [However,] if the two channels of the *chong* and *ren* are vacuous and weak, there will be detriment to the fetal source. If violent anger damages the liver, bedroom taxation damages the kidneys, or other diseases are engendered by various factors which then attack [the fetus], the fetal qi will not be quiet. It is also possible for knocks, falls, and jolts to damage the fetus.

1. Threatened Abortion

Patterns common to this condition

Kidney yang vacuity
Kidney yin vacuity
Qi and blood dual vacuity
Blood heat
Blood stasis
External injury

Treatment based on pattern discrimination

Kidney yang vacuity

Main symptoms: Constant attacks of dizziness after conception, tinnitus, impaired memory, an increasingly profuse, white vaginal discharge, low back and knee soreness and limpness, frequent urination, lack of warmth in the four limbs, pronounced lower abdominal heaviness and distention, blood flowing from the vagina, a feeling as if the fetus were falling, a dirty-colored facial complexion, a pale, moist tongue, and a deep, weak pulse with the cubit position being especially so

Treatment principles: Supplement the kidneys, invigorate yang, and quiet the fetus

Guiding formulas:

Bu Shen An Tai Yin **(Supplement the Kidneys & Quiet the Fetus Drink)**
Sang Ji Sheng (Herba Taxilli), 12-15g
Tu Si Zi (Semen Cuscutae), 9g
Xu Duan (Radix Dipsaci), 9g
Du Zhong (Cortex Eucommiae), 9-15g
Chong Wei Zi (Semen Leonuri), 9-15g
He Shou Wu (Radix Polygoni Multiflori), 9-15g
E Jiao (Gelatinum Corii Asini), 9-12g
Han Lian Cao (Herba Ecliptae), 12-15g
Bai Zhu (Rhizoma Atractylodis Macrocephalae), 9g
Dang Shen (Radix Codonopsitis), 9-15g
Sheng Ma (Rhizoma Cimicifugae), 3-6g

This formula treats yin and yang dual vacuity.

Jia Wei Bu Shen An Tai Yin
(Added Flavors Supplement the Kidneys & Quiet the Fetus Drink)
Ren Shen (Radix Ginseng), 3-9g
Bai Zhu (Rhizoma Atractylodis Macrocephalae), 9g
Du Zhong (Cortex Eucommiae), 9-15g

Xu Duan (Radix Dipsaci), 9-12g
Sang Ji Sheng (Herba Taxilli), 12-15g
Yi Yi Ren (Semen Coicis), 15-25g
E Jiao (Gelatinum Corii Asini), 9g
Ai Ye (Folium Artemesiae Argyii), 9g
Tu Si Zi (Semen Cuscutae), 9g
Bu Gu Zhi (Fructus Psoraleae), 9g
Ba Ji Tian (Radix Morindae), 9g
Shan Yao (Radix Dioscoreae), 9-15g

This formula treats spleen-kidney yang vacuity.

Kidney yin vacuity

Main symptoms: Constant vaginal bleeding, dizziness, tinnitus, low back pain, knee pain, tidal fever, night sweats, heat in the hearts of the hands and feet, pronounced abdominal heaviness, a flushed red facial complexion, a dry mouth but no desire to drink, a dry, red tongue with no fur, and a bowstring, fine, rapid pulse

Treatment principles: Supplement the kidneys, secure the thoroughfare (vessel), and quiet the fetus

Guiding formulas:

Yu Yin Tang Jia Jian (Heal Yin Decoction with Additions & Subtractions)
Shu Di (cooked Radix Rehmanniae), 12-15g
Shan Zhu Yu (Fructus Corni), 9-18g
Xu Duan (Radix Dipsaci), 9g
Sang Ji Sheng (Herba Taxilli), 12-15g
Du Zhong (Cortex Eucommiae), 9-15g
Mu Li (Concha Ostreae), 12-15g
Long Gu (Os Draconis), 12-15g
Bai Shao (Radix Albus Paeoniae Lactiflorae), 9g
E Jiao (Gelatinum Corii Asini), 9g
Zhi Mu (Rhizoma Anemarrhenae), 9g
Di Gu Pi (Cortex Lycii), 9g
Gui Ban (Plastrum Testudinis), 9g

This formula treats yin vacuity with vacuity heat. If there is bleeding, add *Di Yu* (Radix Sanguisorbae), *Zong Tan* (Folium Et Petriolus Carbonisatus Trachycarpi), and *Shan Yao* (Radix Dioscoreae).

Liu Wei Di Huang Tang (Six Flavors Rehmannia Decoction)
Shu Di (cooked Radix Rehmanniae), 12-15g
Shan Zhu Yu (Fructus Corni), 9-18g
Shan Yao (Radix Dioscoreae), 9-15g
Dan Pi (Cortex Moutan), 9g
Fu Ling (Poria), 12g
Ze Xie (Rhizoma Alismatis), 6-9g

An Dian Er Tian Tang **(Quiet Madness Two Tians Decoction)**
Ren Shen (Radix Ginseng), 3-9g
Shu Di (cooked Radix Rehmanniae), 12-15g
Bai Zhu (Rhizoma Atractylodis Macrocephalae), 9g
Shan Yao (Radix Dioscoreae), 9-15g
Shan Zhu Yu (Fructus Corni), 9-18g
Du Zhong (Cortex Eucommiae), 9-15g
Gou Qi Zi (Fructus Lycii), 9g
Bai Bian Dou (Semen Dolichoris), 9-15g
mix-fried *Gan Cao* (Radix Glycyrrhizae)

This formula treats spleen qi-kidney yin and yang dual vacuity.

An Tai San Jia Wei **(Quiet the Fetus Powder with Added Flavors)**
Shu Di (cooked Radix Rehmanniae), 12-15g
Ai Ye (Folium Artemesiae Argyii), 9g
Bai Shao (Radix Albus Paeoniae Lactiflorae), 9g
Chuan Xiong (Radix Ligustici Wallichii), 9g
Huang Qi (Radix Astragali), 9g
E Jiao (Gelatinum Corii Asini), 9g
Dang Gui (Radix Angelicae Sinensis), 9g
Gan Cao (Radix Glycyrrhizae), 3-6g
Di Yu (Radix Sanguisorbae), 9g
Fu Ling (Poria), 12g
Du Zhong (Cortex Eucommiae), 9-15g
Xu Duan (Radix Dipsaci), 9g

This formula treats spleen qi-kidney yin and yang dual vacuity with bleeding.

Qi & blood dual vacuity

Main symptoms: Scanty vaginal bleeding which is pale red in color, lower abdominal distention and heaviness or insidious pain, lassitude of the spirit, a haggard affect, a lusterless facial complexion, a pale white, ashen face, low back soreness, weak limbs, frequent, profuse urination, a pale tongue with thin, white fur, and a fine, slippery, forceless pulse

Note: It is the qi vacuity which results in the fetal leakage.

Treatment principles: Supplement the qi and nourish the blood, secure the kidneys and quiet the fetus

Guiding formulas:

Si Jun Zi Tang **(Four Gentlemen Decoction)**
Ren Shen (Radix Ginseng), 3-9g
Bai Zhu (Rhizoma Atractylodis Macrocephalae), 9g
Fu Ling (Poria), 12g
Gan Cao (Radix Glycyrrhizae), 3-6g

Wan Mi-zhai recommends this as a guiding formula for qi vacuity fetal leakage. One may also use *Xiang Sha Liu Jun Zi Tang* (Auklandia & Amomum Six Gentlemen Decoction) which is the same formula but with the addition of *Ban Xia* (Rhizoma Pinelliae), *Chen Pi* (Pericarpium Citri Reticulatae), *Mu Xiang* (Radix Auklandiae), and *Sha Ren* (Fructus Amomi).

Bu Zhong Yi Qi Tang Jia Wei
(Supplement the Center & Boost the Qi Decoction with Added Flavors)
Ren Shen (Radix Ginseng), 3-9g
Huang Qi (Radix Astragali), 9-18g
Bai Zhu (Rhizoma Atractylodis Macrocephalae), 9g
mix-fried *Gan Cao* (Radix Glycyrrhizae), 6-9g
Dang Gui (Radix Angelicae Sinensis), 9g
Sheng Ma (Rhizoma Cimicifugae), 3-6g
Chai Hu (Radix Bupleuri), 3-9g
Chen Pi (Pericarpium Citri Reticulatae), 6g
Sang Ji Sheng (Herba Taxilli), 12-15g
Chuan Xu Duan (Radix Dipsaci), 9g

This formula is especially effective for late term miscarriage due to incompetent cervix.

Jiao Ai Si Wu Tang (Donkey Skin Glue & Mugwort Decoction)
E Jiao (Gelatinum Corii Asini), 9g
Ai Ye (Folium Artemesiae Argyii), 9g
Dang Gui (Radix Angelicae Sinensis), 9g
Bai Shao (Radix Albus Paeoniae Lactiflorae), 9g
Shu Di (cooked Radix Rehmanniae), 12-15g
Chuan Xiong (Radix Ligustici Wallichii), 6-9g

This formula is for blood vacuity fetal leakage. However, strictly speaking, there is no blood vacuity fetal leakage. Blood vacuity is not one of the causes of pathological bleeding in Chinese medicine. Although this formula is a very old, very famous one in Chinese medicine, this means that it must be modified in real-life practice.

Acupuncture & moxibustion: For late term threatened abortion due to incompetent cervix in turn due to central qi insufficiency, indirectly moxa *Bai Hui* (GV 20) at least once per day in addition to taking medicinal supplements in high doses.

Blood heat

Main symptoms: Bright red or dark red vaginal bleeding that occurs early in pregnancy and which is thick in nature if it is dark, more severe lower abdominal pain, a feeling of drooping or dropping, heart vexation, disquieted spirit, vexatious heat in the hands and feet, a dry mouth and parched throat, a desire for chilled drinks, possible dizziness and vertigo, yellow-red urination, difficult, bound stools, a red tongue with thin, yellow fur, and a slippery, rapid pulse

Treatment principles: Clear heat, cool the blood, and quiet the fetus

Guiding formulas:

Qing Re An Tai Yin Yi Hao (Clear Heat & Quiet the Fetus Drink #1)
Sheng Di (uncooked Radix Rehmanniae), 12-15g
Bai Shao (Radix Albus Paeoniae Lactiflorae), 9g
Huang Qin (Radix Scutellariae), 9-12g
blackened *Zhi Zi* (Fructus Gardeniae), 6-9g
Han Lian Cao (Herba Ecliptae), 12-15g
Nu Zhen Zi (Fructus Ligustri Lucidi), 12-15g
Xu Duan (Radix Dipsaci), 9g
Zhu Ma Geng (Radix Boehmeriae Niveae), 9-18g
Bai Zhu (Rhizoma Atractylodis Macrocephalae), 9g
E Jiao (Gelatinum Corii Asini), 9g
Sha Ren (Fructus Amomi), 3-4.5g

Qing Re An Tai Yin Er Hao (Clear Heat & Quiet the Fetus Drink #2)
stir-fried *Huang Qin* (Radix Scutellariae), 9-12g
Bai Wei (Radix Cynanchi Atrati), 9g
Bai Shao (Radix Albus Paeoniae Lactiflorae), 9g
Ce Bai Ye (Cacumen Platycladi), 9g
Zhu Ma Geng (Radix Boehmeriae Niveae), 9-18g
Sheng Di (uncooked Radix Rehmanniae), 12-15g
Chen Pi (Pericarpium Citri Reticulatae), 6g
ginger-processed *Zhu Ru* (Caulis Bambusae In Taeniis), 6-9g
Han Lian Cao (Herba Ecliptae), 12-15g

If there is simultaneous low back soreness, add *Sang Ji Sheng* (Herba Taxilli) and *Xu Duan* (Radix Dipsaci). If the tongue fur is peeled in the center, add *Mai Men Dong* (Tuber Ophiopogonis).

Qing Re Yang Yin Tang (Clear Heat & Nourish Yin Decoction)
Sheng Di (uncooked Radix Rehmanniae), 12-15g
Huang Qin (Radix Scutellariae), 9-12g
Di Gu Pi (Cortex Lycii), 9g
Zhi Mu (Rhizoma Anemarrhenae), 9g
Mai Men Dong (Tuber Ophiopogonis), 9-12g
Bai Shao (Radix Albus Paeoniae Lactiflorae), 9g
Du Zhong (Cortex Eucommiae), 9-15g
E Jiao (Gelatinum Corii Asini), 9g
Xu Duan (Radix Dipsaci), 9g
Sang Ji Sheng (Herba Taxilli), 12-15g

If bleeding is profuse add *Di Yu* (Radix Sanguisorbae). If bleeding is due to vacuity heat delete *Huang Qin* and add *Gui Ban* (Plastrum Testudinis).

An Tai Jie Du Yin (Quiet the Fetus & Resolve Toxins Drink)
Gan Cao (Radix Glycyrrhizae), 3-9g

Dou Chi (Semen Praeparatus Sojae), 9-15g
Zhu Ye (Herba Lophatheri), 9-15g

This formula is for the treatment of fetus stirring restlessly due to the mistaken administration of toxic medicinals. It clears heat and resolves toxins, harmonizes the stomach and quiets the fetus.

Blood stasis

Main symptoms: Unstoppable vaginal bleeding during the first three months of pregnancy accompanied by rigidity of the muscles of the lower left quadrant, lumbar soreness, a pale, lusterless facial complexion, a dark tongue with static spots or macules with thin, white fur, and a fine, choppy, and/or deep pulse

Treatment principles: Quicken the blood, transform stasis, and stop bleeding

Guiding formula:

Gui Zhi Fu Ling Wan (Cinnamon & Poria Pills)
Gui Zhi (Ramulus Cinnamomi), 6-9g
Fu Ling (Poria), 12g
Dan Pi (Cortex Moutan), 9g
Tao Ren (Semen Persicae), 9g
Chi Shao (Radix Rubrus Paeoniae Lactiflorae), 9g

External injury

Main symptoms: History of recent fall or injury, overwork, or excessive fatigue, low back and abdominal aching and pain, lower abdominal distention and pain with a heavy, dragging feeling, blood flowing from the vagina, an ashen white facial complexion, dizziness, blurred vision, shortness of breath, a pale, moist tongue, and a forceless, slippery pulse

Treatment principles: Boost the qi and nourish the blood, secure, restrain, and quiet the fetus

Note: Although neither the name of the pattern says so or the treatment principles, this pattern is a combination of qi and blood vacuity with blood stasis.

Guiding formulas:

Jiu Sun An Tai Tang (Rescue Detriment & Quiet the Fetus Decoction)
Dang Gui (Radix Angelicae Sinensis), 9g
Bai Shao (Radix Albus Paeoniae Lactiflorae), 9g
Sheng Di (uncooked Radix Rehmanniae), 12-15g
Chuan Xiong (Radix Ligustici Wallichii), 9g
mix-fried *Gan Cao* (Radix Glycyrrhizae), 6-9g
Ren Shen (Radix Ginseng), 3-9g
Su Mu (Lignum Sappan), 6-9g
Ru Xiang (Resina Olibani), 3-6g
Mo Yao (Resina Myrrhae), 3-6g

Tai Shan Pan Shi San (Mt. Tai Bedrock Powder)
Ren Shen (Radix Ginseng), 3-9g
Huang Qi (Radix Astragali), 9-18g
Xu Duan (Radix Dipsaci), 9g
Huang Qin (Radix Scutellariae), 9-12g
Chuan Xiong (Radix Ligustici Wallichii), 9g
Shu Di (cooked Radix Rehmanniae), 12-15g
Bai Shao (Radix Albus Paeoniae Lactiflorae), 9g
Bai Zhu (Rhizoma Atractylodis Macrocephalae), 9g
Sha Ren (Fructus Amomi), 3-4.5g
Nuo Mi (glutinous rice), 15-30g

Tai Shan Pan Shi San Jia Jian
(Mt. Tai Bedrock Powder with Additions & Subtractions)
Dang Shen (Radix Codonopsitis), 9-18g
Bai Zhu (Rhizoma Atractylodis Macrocephalae), 9g
Bai Shao (Radix Albus Paeoniae Lactiflorae), 9g
Huang Qi (Radix Astragali), 9-18g
Dang Gui (Radix Angelicae Sinensis), 9g
Shu Di (cooked Radix Rehmanniae), 12-15g
Sha Ren (Fructus Amomi), 3-4.5g
Xu Duan (Radix Dipsaci), 9g
Du Zhong (Cortex Eucommiae), 9-15g
Sang Ji Sheng (Herba Taxilli), 12-15g

Sheng Yu Tang (Sagelike Healing Decoction)
Huang Qi (Radix Astragali), 9-18g
Ren Shen (Radix Ginseng), 3-9g
Dang Gui (Radix Angelicae Sinensis), 9g
Shu Di (cooked Radix Rehmanniae), 12-15g
Chuan Xiong (Radix Ligustici Wallichii), 6-9g
Bai Shao (Radix Albus Paeoniae Lactiflorae), 9g

One may add *Xu Duan* (Radix Dipsaci), *Sang Ji Sheng* (Herba Taxilli), *Du Zhong* (Cortex Eucommiae), and *E Jiao* (Gelatinum Corii Asini) to secure the *chong* and supplement the kidneys. If bleeding is profuse, add stir-fried *Di Yu* (Radix Sanguisorbae). If there is lancinating pain in the abdomen with scant bleeding, add *Xiang Fu* (Rhizoma Cyperi) to move depression and stagnation.

Sheng Yu Tang Jia Wei (Sagelike Healing Decoction with Added Flavors)
Ren Shen (Radix Ginseng), 3-6g
Huang Qi (Radix Astragali), 9-18g
Dang Gui (Radix Angelicae Sinensis), 9g
Chuan Xiong (Radix Ligustici Wallichii), 6-9g
Shu Di (cooked Radix Rehmanniae), 12-15g
Sheng Di (uncooked Radix Rehmanniae), 12-15g
Tu Si Zi (Semen Cuscutae), 9g
Sang Ji Sheng (Herba Taxilli), 12-15g

Xu Duan (Radix Dipsaci), 9g

An Tai Shen Ying Fang (Quiet the Fetus Divinely Responding Formula)
Dang Gui (Radix Angelicae Sinensis), 9g
earth stir-fried *Bai Zhu* (Rhizoma Atractylodis Macrocephalae), 9g
Huang Qin (Radix Scutellariae), 9-12g
Chuan Xiong (Radix Ligustici Wallichii), 6-9g
wine stir-fried *Bai Shao* (Radix Albus Paeoniae Lactiflorae), 9g
Fu Ling (Poria), 12g
mix-fried *Huang Qi* (Radix Astragali), 9-18g
Du Zhong (Cortex Eucommiae), 9-15g
Shu Di (cooked Radix Rehmanniae), 12-15g
E Jiao (Gelatinum Corii Asini), 9g
Gan Cao (Radix Glycyrrhizae), 3-9g

Remarks

Wan Mi-zhai, in *Wan Shi Fu Ren Ke (Master Wan's Gynecology),* gives a very interesting breakdown on threatened abortion or fetus stirring restlessly which is different from the above contemporary Chinese pattern discrimination. Master Wan begins by giving formulas for spleen vacuity and kidney vacuity types of threatened abortion but then goes on to give a number of variations of *Si Wu Tang* (Four Materials Decoction), each variation associated with internal damage due to one of the seven affects.

For anger damaging the liver and the uterine network vessels, add *Huang Qin* (Radix Scutellariae), *Ren Shen* (Radix Ginseng), *Chai Hu* (Radix Bupleuri), and mix-fried *Gan Cao* (Radix Glycyrrhizae).

For sadness and melancholy damaging the lungs, add *Huang Qin* (Radix Scutellariae), *E Jiao* (Gelatinum Corii Asini), *Zi Su Ye* (Folium Perillae Frutescentis), *Wu Wei Zi* (Fructus Schisandrae), and mix-fried *Gan Cao* (Radix Glycyrrhizae).

For fear damaging the kidneys affecting the fetal ligation, add *Xu Duan* (Radix Dipsaci), stir-fried *Huang Bai* (Cortex Phellodendri), stir-fried *Du Zhong* (Cortex Eucommiae), and *Wu Wei Zi* (Fructus Schisandrae).

For worry and unresolved anxiety damaging the spleen, add *Bai Zhu* (Rhizoma Atractylodis Macrocephalae), *Ren Shen* (Radix Ginseng), *Chen Pi* (Pericarpium Citri Reticulatae), *Xiang Fu* (Rhizoma Cyperi), and mix-fried *Gan Cao* (Radix Glycyrrhizae).

For excessive joy damaging the heart, add *Huang Qin* (Radix Scutellariae), *Huang Lian* (Rhizoma Coptidis), *Bai Zhu* (Rhizoma Atractylodis Macrocephalae), *Mai Men Dong* (Tuber Ophiopogonis), and mix-fried *Gan Cao* (Radix Glycyrrhizae).

Further, if fetus stirring restlesly is caused by fall or strike, use *An Tai He Qi Yin* (**Quiet the Fetus & Harmonize the Qi Drink**): *Dang Gui* (Radix Angelicae Sinensis), *Bai Shao* (Radix Albus Paeoniae Lactiflorae), *Bai Zhu* (Rhizoma Atractylodis Macrocephalae), *Huang Qin* (Radix Scutellariae), *Zi Su Ye* (Folium Perillae Frutescentis), *Sha Ren* (Fructus Amomi), mix-fried *Gan Cao* (Radix Glycyrrhizae), *Sheng Jiang* (uncooked Rhizoma Zingiberis), and *Da Zao* (Fructus Jujubae).

But, if fetus stirring restlessly is caused by lack of restraint in bedroom affairs, use *Jia Jian Si Wu Tang* (**Additions & Subtractions Four Materials Decoction**): *Dang Gui* (Radix Angelicae Sinensis), *Shu Di* (cooked Radix Rehmanniae), stir-fried *E Jiao* (Gelatinum Corii Asini), mix-fried *Gan Cao* (Radix Glycyrrhizae), *Sha Ren* (Fructus Amomi), and *Zhu Ru* (Caulis Bambusae In Taeniis).

2. Inevitable Abortion

Main symptoms: The signs and symptoms of threatened abortion continue. Blood exits from the vagina and its amount increases. In addition, there may be blood clots. The amount continues to increase until it becomes as much or more than normal menstruation. There may either be violent, convulsive pains in the lower abdomen or a heavy, falling, distended feeling. Gynecological examination reveals the cervix is dilated wide open. Although excessive bleeding typically results in blood vacuity, excessive use of blood-stopping medicinals to prevent miscarriage can cause blood stasis.

Note: The above description presupposes that one has already tried to treat a threatened abortion with bleeding-stopping medicinals.

Treatment principles: Quicken the blood and dispel stasis, warm, open, drive out, and descend

Guiding formula:

Shao Fu Zhu Yu Tang Jia Wei
(**Lower Abdomen Dispel Stasis Decoction with Added Flavors**)
Xiao Hui Xiang (Fructus Foeniculi), 9-15g
Dang Gui (Radix Angelicae Sinensis), 9g
Rou Gui (Cortex Cinnamomi), 6-9g
Yan Hu Suo (Rhizoma Corydalis), 9-15g
Mo Yao (Resina Myrrhae), 3-6g
Chuan Xiong (Radix Ligustici Wallichii), 6-18g
Pao Jiang (blast-fried Rhizoma Zingiberis), 6-9g
uncooked *Pu Huang* (Pollen Typhae), 9-15g
Chi Shao (Radix Rubrus Paeoniae Lactiflorae), 9g
Chuan Niu Xi (Radix Cyathulae), 9-15g

Wu Ling Zhi (Feces Trogopterori Seu Pteromi), 9-12g
Da Huang (Radix Et Rhizoma Rhei), 3-9g

3. Incomplete Abortion

Main symptoms: Discharge of some fetal matter, either insidious pain in the lower abdomen or violent pain, both of which resist pressure, profuse vaginal bleeding with blood clots mixed with large amounts of body fluids. In this case, stagnation and stasis in the uterus lead to lower abdominal aching and pain.

Treatment principles: Quicken the blood and dispel stasis

Guiding formula:

Shi Xiao San Jia Wei (Loose a Smile Powder with Added Flavors)
Dang Gui (Radix Angelicae Sinensis), 9g
Chuan Xiong (Radix Ligustici Wallichii), 6-18g
uncooked *Pu Huang* (Pollen Typhae), 9-15g
Wu Ling Zhi (Feces Trogopterori Seu Pteromi), 9g
Yi Mu Cao (Herba Leonuri), 9-15g
Dan Shen (Radix Salviae Miltiorrhizae), 9-15g

4. Complete Abortion

After abortion, either bleeding may continue on abnormally or pain may be felt in the lower abdomen. These are two common sequelae of miscarriage. They are treated in Chinese medicine essentially the same as excessive or prolonged lochiorrhea and abdominal pain after delivery. If bleeding continues on abnormally after spontaneous or induced abortion, this is mostly due to damage of the *chong* and *ren* which fail to secure the lower yin and essence. If there is an abnormally scanty discharge and more intense abdominal pain after miscarriage, this is due to blood stasis and stagnation. It is also possible for blood stasis following abortion or miscarriage to prevent the engenderment of fresh blood. Thus blood stasis may be simply replete or may be mixed with and the cause of vacuity.

Chong & ren damage & detriment

Main symptoms: Heavy blood loss following abortion or miscarriage, fainting,

Patterns common to this condition

Chong & ren damage & detriment
Blood stasis obstructing internally

unchecked leakage of blood, low back soreness and limpness, weakness of the four limbs, abdominal pain which desires pressure, a pale tongue with thin fur, and a weak pulse

Treatment principles: Greatly supplement the qi and blood

Guiding formulas:

Shi Sheng Tang (10 Sagelike [Medicinals] Decoction)
Ren Shen (Radix Ginseng), 3-9g
Huang Qi (Radix Astragali), 9-18g
Bai Zhu (Rhizoma Atractylodis Macrocephalae), 9g
Shu Di (cooked Radix Rehmanniae), 12-15g
Sha Ren (Fructus Amomi), 3-4.5g
carbonized *Dang Gu* (Radix Angelicae Sinensis), 9g
Chuan Xiong (Radix Ligustici Wallichii), 6-9g
wine stir-fried *Bai Shao* (Radix Albus Paeoniae Lactiflorae), 9-18g
Xu Duan (Radix Dipsaci), 9g
Gan Cao (Radix Glycyrrhizae), 3-9g

Gui Pi Tang (Restore the Spleen Decoction)
Ren Shen (Radix Ginseng), 3-9g
Huang Qi (Radix Astragali), 9-18g
Dang Gui (Radix Angelicae Sinensis), 9g
Long Yan Rou (Arillus Euphoriae Longanae), 9-12g
Bai Zhu (Rhizoma Atractylodis Macrocephalae), 9g
Mu Xiang (Radix Auklandiae), 6-9g
Fu Ling (Poria), 12g
Yuan Zhi (Radix Polygalae), 6-9g
Suan Zao Ren (Semen Zizyphi Spinosae), 12-15g
mix-fried *Gan Cao* (Radix Glycyrrhizae), 6-9g
Sheng Jiang (uncooked Rhizoma Zingiberis), 6g
Da Zao (Fructus Jujubae), 2-3 pieces

Blood stasis obstructing internally

Main symptoms: Prolonged bleeding, violently intense abdominal pain with excessive blood flow or continuous dribbling. The entire embryo is discharged. Bleeding from the vagina gradually stops but the abdominal pain persists.

Treatment principles: Quicken the blood and transform stasis assisted by boosting the qi

Guiding formulas:

Sheng Hua Tang Jia Yi Mu Cao
(Engendering & Transforming Decoction plus Lenourus)
Dang Gui (Radix Angelicae Sinensis), 9g
Chuan Xiong (Radix Ligustici Wallichii), 6-9g
Yi Mu Cao (Herba Leonuri), 9-15g
Tao Ren (Semen Persicae), 9g
Pao Jiang (blast-fried Rhizoma Zingiberis), 6-9g
mix-fried *Gan Cao* (Radix Glycyrrhizae), 6-9g

Sheng Hua Tang Jia Wei Er Hao
(Engendering & Transforming Decoction with Added Flavors #2)
Dang Gui (Radix Angelicae Sinensis), 9g
Chuan Xiong (Radix Ligustici Wallichii), 6-9g
Tao Ren (Semen Persicae), 9g
Pao Jiang (blast-fried Rhizoma Zingiberis), 6-9g
mix-fried *Gan Cao* (Radix Glycyrrhizae), 6-9g
Niu Xi (Radix Achyranthis Bidentatae), 9-15g
Bai Shao (Radix Albus Paeoniae Lactiflorae), 9g
Yi Mu Cao (Herba Leonuri), 9-15g
San Qi (Radix Notoginseng), 1-3g
    (taken powdered with the medicinal decoction)

Abstracts of representative Chinese research

From "The Treatment of 51 Cases of Fetal Leakage with *Shou Tai Wan* (Long-life Fetus Pills)" by Ying Ying, *Zhe Jiang Zhong Yi Za Zhi (Zhejiang Journal of Chinese Medicine)*, #6, 1994, p. 261

Cohort description:

The author treated 51 women with fetal leakage or breakthrough bleeding during pregnancy with *Shou Tai Wan* with additions and subtractions with good results. All 51 women were seen as outpatients. They ranged in age from 23-32 years old. Forty-five were primiparas; six had been pregnant twice. The course of disease ranged from 2-5 days.

Treatment method:

Shou Tai Wan Jia Jian was comprised of: *Tu Si Zi* (Semen Cuscutae), *Xu Duan* (Radix Dipsaci), *Sang Ji Sheng* (Herba Taxilli), *Dang Shen* (Radix Codonopsitis), scroched *Bai Zhu* (Rhizoma Atractylodis Macrocephalae), 10g each, *E Jiao* (Gelatinum Corii Asini), 12g, stir-fried *Du Zhong* (Cortex Eucommiae), 15g, *Ba Yue Zha* (Fructus Akebiae Trifoliatae), 8g, mix-fried *Gan Cao* (Radix Glycyrrhizae), 3g, *He Ye* (Folium Nelumbinis), 1 length. One packet of these medicinals was decocted in water and administered in two divided doses per day. If qi vacuity was marked, mix-fried *Huang Qi* (Radix Astragali), 15g, and *Sheng Ma* (Rhizoma Cimicifugae), 3g, were added. If there was blood heat, carbonized *Huang Qin* (Radix Scutellariae), 5g, and *Zhu Ma Gen* (Radix Boehmeriae Niveae) were added.

Treatment outcomes:

In 40 cases, the leakage stopped after taking two packets of the medicinals. In 10 other cases, bleeding stopped after taking five packets of these medicinals. In one case there was no result. In that case, ultrasonography showed that abortion had not yet occurred. However, after taking two packets of the above medicinals, the women did abort.

From "A Clinical Report on 61 Cases of Protecting the Fetus with *Jia Wei Shou Tai Wan* (Added Flavors Long-life Fetus Pills)" by Wang Bei-ju, *Gan Su Zhong Yi (Gansu Chinese Medicine)*, #7, 1994, p. 41

Cohort description:

The author of this clinical audit treated 61 cases of protecting the fetus with *Jia Wei Shou Tai Wan*. Of these 61 cases, their ages ranged from 20-38 years old. Thirty-eight were workers, 14 were office workers, nine were cadres, and 10 were farm workers. Fifty-five had previously had abortions, nine had had preterm deliveries, and seven had been diagnosed with habitual abortion.

Treatment method:

Jia Wei Shou Tai Wan was comprised of: *Xu Duan* (Radix Dipsaci), *Sang Ji Sheng* (Herba Taxilli), *Tu Si Zi* (Semen Cuscutae), *E Jiao* (Gelatinum Corii Asini), *Dang Shen* (Radix Codonopsitis), *Huang Qi* (Radix Astragali), *Bai Zhu* (Rhizoma Atractylodis Macrocephalae*)*, *Sha Ren* (Fructus Amomi), *Huang Qin* (Radix Scutellariae), *Du Zhong* (Cortex Eucommiae), *Su Gen* (Caulis Perillae Frutescentis), and *Gan Cao* (Radix Glycyrrhizae). On the basis of whether the disease was light or heavy, relaxed or acute, 1-2 packets were administered per day.

If there was profuse vaginal bleeding, carbonized *Sheng Di* (uncooked Radix Rehmanniae) and carbonized *Di Yu* (Radix Sanguisorbae) were added. If there was a heavy downward feeling in the lower abdomen, *Sheng Ma* (Rhizoma Cimicifugae) and *Chai Hu* (Radix Bupleuri) were added. If there was severe abdominal pain, *Bai Shao* (Radix Albus Paeoniae Lactiflorae) was added. And if there was emotional tension, stir-fried *Zao Ren* (Semen Zizyphi Spinosae) was added.

Treatment outcomes:

If the pregnant woman was able to carry her baby to full term, this was defined as a cure. If not, this was defined as no result. Based on these criteria, 45 patients or 74% were cured and 16 cases or 26% got no result. The longest course of treatment was 128 days and the shortest was seven days, with the average being 67.5 days.

From "The Treatment of 60 Cases of Threatened Abortion" by Lin Zhen-lian, *Shang Hai Zhong Yi Yao Za Zhi (Shanghai Journal of Chinese Medicine & Medicinals)*, #9, 1995, p. 33

Cohort description:

Based on the author's many years of clinical experience, he has treated 60 cases with self-composed *Yi Mu Bao Tai Tang* (Leonurus Protect the Fetus Decoction) with good results. Of these 60 cases, the youngest was 22 and the oldest was 37 years old. All were confirmed to be in the early stage of pregnancy through ultrasound. Thirty of these cases had experienced vaginal tract bleeding 40-50 days after the cessation of menstruation. Eighteen had experienced the bleeding 51-60 days after their last menstruation. And 12 cases had experienced bleeding 61 days to three months after stopping their last menstruation. In 31 cases, the bleeding had lasted

1-5 days, in 21 cases, 6-10 days, and in eight cases, over 10 days. Fifty-one of these cases had either previously undergone an artificial abortion or were having a spontaneous abortion, while seven cases suffered from habitual miscarriage.

Treatment method:

Yi Mu Bao Tai Tang was composed of: *Dang Shen* (Radix Codonopsitis), 15g, *Huang Qi* (Radix Astragali), 15-50g, *Bai Zhu* (Rhizoma Atractylodis Macrocephalae), 10g, *Sang Ji Sheng* (Herba Taxilli), 12g, *Xu Duan* (Radix Dipsaci), 12g, stir-fried *Du Zhong* (Cortex Eucommiae), 12g, *Qian Shi* (Semen Euryalis), 10g, *Tu Si Zi* (Semen Cuscutae), 10g, and stir-fried *Huang Qin* (Radix Scutellariae), 10g.

If there was obvious abdominal pain, *Bai Shao* (Radix Albus Paeoniae Lactiflorae), 10g, and *Dang Gui* (Radix Angelicae Sinensis), 6g, were added. If bleeding was profuse, *Dan Pi* (Cortex Moutan), 10g, *Xian He Cao* (Herba Agrimoniae), 12g, *Zhu Ma Gen* (Radix Boehmeriae Niveae), 20g, and *Sheng Di* (uncooked Radix Rehmanniae), 10g, were added. If there was low back pain and marked lower abdominal downward sagging, *Bu Gu Zhi* (Fructus Psoraleae) and *Jin Ying Zi* (Fructus Rosae Laevigatae), 10g each, were added. If there was vomiting, ginger-processed *Ban Xia* (Rhizoma Pinelliae) and *Zhu Ru* (Caulis Bambusae In Taeniis), 6g each, were added.

Treatment outcomes:

Of the 60 cases in this study, 56 were cured. This meant that any abortion was forestalled. In 10 cases, bleeding stopped in one day of taking these medicinals, in 18 cases, in two days, in 26 cases, in three days, and in three cases, within seven days. In three cases, there was no effect. In two of those three cases, external injury precipitating bleeding had damaged the fetus. In the other cases, ultrasonography showed no fetal heartbeat and a D & C was performed.

From "An Analysis of the Effectiveness of Treating 95 Cases of Threatened Abortion with the Methods of Supplementing the Kidneys & Tranquilizing the Heart" by Gao Yue-ping, *Si Chuan Zhong Yi (Sichuan Chinese Medicine)*, # 5, 1995, p. 38

Cohort description:

The author treated 95 cases of threatened abortion mainly with the methods of supplementing the kidneys and tranquilizing the heart with additions and subtractions. Seventy-three cases were 23-30 years old and 22 cases were 31-40 years old. Twenty-six had never had an abortion, 62 had had 1-2 abortions, and seven had had 3-5 abortions. Seventy-four cases had ceased menstruation anywhere from several to 60 days and 21 had ceased menstruation for 61-100 days. Sixty-nine cases had vaginal tract bleeding, 76 had abdominal pain, and 80 had low back soreness. Urine analysis was positive for pregnancy in all these cases. Of the women who had had three or more abortions, all had some degree of low back pain, while all the women in this study had some degree of mental-emotional disquietude.

Treatment method:

The formula consisted of: *E Jiao* (Gelatinum Corii Asini), *Shu Di* (cooked Radix Rehmanniae), *Bai Shao* (Radix Albus Paeoniae Lactiflorae), *He Huan Pi* (Cortex Albizziae), *Bai He* (Bulbus Lilii), stir-fried *Xu Duan* (Radix Dipsaci), *Tu Si Zi* (Semen Cuscutae), *Du Zhong* (Cortex Eucommiae), stir-fried *Shan Yao* (Radix Dioscoreae), *Bai Zhu* (Rhizoma Atractylodis Macrocephalae), 10g each, and *Huang Qin* (Radix Scutellariae), 6g. If there was simultaneous vaginal bleeding, *Zhu Ma Gen* (Radix Boehmeriae Niveae), 30g, was added. If there was abdominal pain, *Su Gen* (Caulis Perillae Frutescentis), 10g, was added. If there was emotional tension and agitation, *Gou Teng* (Ramulus Uncariae Cum Uncis), 15g, was added. If there was nausea and vomiting, ginger-processed *Zhu Ru* (Caulis Bambusae In Taeniis), 10g, was added. Patients were advised to lie in bed resting their body, and they were prohibited from sexual activity.

Treatment outcomes:

Some effect was defined as cessation of vaginal bleeding, disappearance of the symptoms of low back soreness and abdominal pain, ultrasound showing a normal fetal heart beat, and pregnancy continuing till full term delivery. Based on these criteria, this treatment was effective in 68 cases. No effect meant that this treatment was not able to eliminate either the vaginal tract bleeding or the other symptoms and that a spontaneous abortion did occur. Twenty-seven women got no effect from this treatment. Therefore, the total effectiveness rate was 71.58%. Of the 73 women 30 years old or younger, 19 cases (26.03%) did not get any result. Whereas, of the 22 cases 31-40 years old, eight cases (36.36%) did not get any result. Of the 62 women who had had two abortions or less, 12 cases (19.36%) got no result. Whereas, of the seven cases who had had three or more abortions, five cases (71.43%) got no result. And, of the 74 women who had ceased menstruating within 60 days, 15 cases (20.27) got no result, while, of the 21 cases who had ceased menstruating between 61-100 days, 12 cases (57.13%) got no result.

From "The Treatment of 73 Cases of Threatened Abortion with *Bu Shen An Tai Tang Jia Jian* (Supplement the Kidneys & Quiet the Fetus Decoction with Additions & Subtractions)" by Zhang Xiao-ping, *Zhong Yi Za Zhi (The Journal of Chinese Medicine)*, #8, 1995, p. 486

Cohort description:

The author of this article treated 73 cases of threatened abortion with *Bu Shen An Tai Tang*. All the women in this group were diagnosed as suffering from threatened abortion based on the criteria in *Shi Yong Fu Ke Xue (A Study of Practical Gynecology)*. All were outpatients. The oldest was 36 and the youngest was 20 years old with an average age of 28. Thirty-three had already had spontaneous abortions. Of these, 16 had had one miscarriage, 11 had had two miscarriages, and six suffered from habitual miscarriage, with one woman having miscarried six times. The other 40 women had not previously had any miscarriages. Five women had been treated for infertility and, after conceiving, showed symptoms of threatened miscarriage. In 59 cases, the women were 5-12 weeks pregnant, and in 14 cases, they were 12-20 weeks pregnant. The longest time any of these women had been bleeding was 10 days and the shortest was two hours.

Treatment method:

Self-composed *Bu Shen An Tai Tang* was composed of: *Tu Si Zi* (Semen Cuscutae), 20g, *Sang Ji Sheng* (Herba Taxilli), 15g, *Xu Duan* (Radix Dipsaci), 15g, *E Jiao* (Gelatinum Corii Asini), 10g, *Shan Zhu Yu* (Fructus Corni), 10g, *Du Zhong* (Cortex Eucommiae), 15g, and *Xian He Cao* (Herba Agrimoniae), 30g. If there was qi vacuity, *Dang Shen* (Radix Codonopsitis) or *Hong Shen* (red Radix Ginseng), *Huang Qi* (Radix Astragali), and *Bai Zhu* (Rhizoma Atractylodis Macrocephalae) were added. If there was yang vacuity, *E Jiao* was removed and *Lu Jiao Jiao* (Gelatinum Cornu Cervi) and *Ai Ye* (Folium Artemisiae Argyii) were added. If there was yin vacuity, *Shi Hu* (Herba Dendrobii) was added. If there was blood vacuity, *Bai Shao* (Radix Albus Paeoniae Lactiflorae) was added. If there was blood heat, *Sheng Di* (uncooked Radix Rehmanniae), *Han Lian Cao* (Herba Ecliptae), and *Zhu Ma Gen* (Herba Boehmeriae Niveae) were added. If there was traumatic injury due to fall or strike, *Mu Xiang* (Radix Auklandiae), *Chuan Lian Zi* (Fructus Toosendan), and *Lian Fang* (Receptaculum Nelumbinis) were added. If suffering from fright and fear or if, after bleeding, psychological fear developed, uncooked *Mu Li* (Concha Ostreae) was added. One packet was decocted in water each day and administered in divided doses in the morning and at night. Once the vaginal tract bleeding stopped, these medicinals were continued for 1-2 months in order to secure the treatment effect.

Treatment outcomes:

After taking these medicinals, the vaginal tract bleeding stopped, the symptoms disappeared or diminished, urine pregnancy test was positive or HCG levels were normal, and ultrasound showed an active fetus in 69 patients or 94.5%. Four cases (5.5%) got no result. The smallest number of packets needed for successfully protecting the fetus was 35 and the largest was 69. In 64 cases, parturition was normal and there was no deformity or poor development of the fetus. On follow-up after half a year, the children's intelligence, strength, and development was normal. Five cases did not end in successful childbirth. However, ultrasound tallied with the pregnancy and fetus, and regular prenatal checkups had all been normal.

Representative case histories

Case 1: The patient was a 31 year-old female teacher. This woman had had superficial edema for more than one year. Her facial complexion was sallow yellow and sometimes she had heart palpitations, shortness of breath, and lack of strength in the four extremities. In the preceding year, she had had one artificial abortion, after which she had not had any regulating treatment. Three months prior to her visit, the patient had become pregnant. After becoming pregnant she had developed a continuous, dilute vaginal discharge. In addition, there was lower and upper back pain, and she was commonly dizzy and had tinnitus. In the prior two days, there was a downward sagging sensation in her lower abdomen, abdominal pain, and red leakage. Her tongue was pale and her pulse was soggy, fine, and rapid, with both cubit positions being slightly weak.

Based on these signs and symptoms, the patient's Chinese medical pattern was categorized as spleen disease reaching the kidneys with poor fetal qi and threatened abortion. Therefore, she was prescribed three packets of the following medicinals: *Dang Shen* (Radix Codonopsitis), *Huang Qi* (Radix Astragali), *Shan Yao* (Radix Dioscoreae), *Bai Zhu* (Rhizoma Atratylodis Macrocephalae), *Du Zhong* (Cortex Eucommiae), *Gou Ji* (Rhizoma Cibotii), carbonized *Dang Gui* (Radix Angelicae Sinensis), *Sang Ji Sheng* (Herba Taxilli), *E Jiao* (Gelatinum Corii Asini), *Zhu Ma Gen* (Radix Boehmeriae Niveae), *Shu Di* (cooked Radix Rehmanniae), and *Hong Shen* (red Radix Ginseng). The amounts of these medicinals was undisclosed.

On the second examination, the red leakage and abdominal pain had stopped. However, the low back pain and lower abdominal downward sagging feeling had not yet been eliminated. There was also still dizziness, tinnitus, facial edema, lack of strength, and a soggy, rapid pulse. Therefore, *E Jiao* was removed from the original prescription and *Sheng Ma* (Rhizoma Cimicifugae) and *Nan Gua Di* (Pedunculus Melonis) were added. Three more packets were prescribed.

On the third examination, the low back pain, lower adominal downward sagging, dizziness, and tinnitus were all improved. The pulse was soggy and the cubit positions were soft. Therefore, in order to regulate and rectify the spleen and kidneys in order to secure the fetal qi, four packets of the following medicinals were prescribed: *Ren Shen* (Radix Ginseng), *Bai Zhu* (Rhizoma Atractylodis Macrocephalae), *Du Zhong* (Cortex Eucommiae), *Xu Duan* (Radix Dipsaci), *Sang Ji Sheng* (Herba Taxilli), *Shu Di* (cooked Radix Rehmanniae), *Gou Qi Zi* (Fructus Lycii), *Zhu Ma Gen* (Radix Boehmeriae Niveae), *Shan Yao* (Radix Dioscoreae), *Sha Ren* (Fructus Amomi), and *Da Zao* (Fructus Jujubae). On the fourth and fifth visits, everything was fine.

Case 2: The patient was a 27 year-old married worker. The patient had been married for two years, and her last menses had stopped 72 days before. Urine analysis confirmed that she was pregnant. One week before, she had developed vomiting, a bitter taste in her mouth, constipation, and lower abdominal pain and downward sagging. The previous evening, she had experienced abdominal contractions and there was a scanty red seepage from her vagina. The patient's tongue fur was slightly yellow and her pulse was slippery and rapid.

Based on these signs and symptoms, this patient's Chinese medical pattern was categorized as fetal heat scorching and burning. Therefore, she was prescribed the following medicinals: carbonized *Huang Qin* (Radix Scutellariae), *E Jiao* (Gelatinum Corii Asini), and stir-fried *Bai Shao* (Radix Albus Paeoniae Lactiflorae), 9g each, *Zhu Ma Gen* (Radix Boehmeriae Niveae), *Sang Ji Sheng* (Herba Taxilli), mix-fried *Huang Qi* (Radix Astragali), and *Dang Shen* (Radix Codonopsitis), 12g each, carbonized *Sheng Di* (uncooked Radix Rehmanniae), 15g, *Xian He*

Cao (Herba Agrimoniae), 30g, *Zi Su Gen* (Caulis Perillae Frutescentis), 4.5g, and mix-fried *Gan Cao* (Radix Glycyrrhizae), 2.4g.

On the second examination, the patient reported that, after taking two packets of the above medicinals, her bleeding had stopped, theabdominal pain had remitted, and the vomiting had calmed. Therefore, she was prescribed three more packets of the original medicinals. On the third examination, all the patient's symptoms were improved. *Huang Qi*, *Sheng Di*, and *E Jiao* were, therefore, removed from the prescription and *Shan Yao* (Radix Dioscoreae), *Da Zao* (Fructus Jujubae), and *Long Yan Rou* (Arillus Euphoriae Longanae) were added. The patient took another 10 packets of medicinals and all her symptoms were judged cured, her affect was revitalized, and she stopped taking the herbs.

Case 3: The patient was a 25 year-old female. It had been 46 days since this woman's last menstruation had stopped. Urine analysis confirmed that she was pregnant. Two days previously some blood had begun exiting her vaginal tract. Its amount was scant and its color was pale red. This was accompanied by low backache. Her tongue was pale red and had the indentations of her teeth on its edges and thin, white fur. Her pulse was fine and slippery. She was diagnosed as suffering from fetal leakage and her pattern was categorized as detriment of the qi and blood with *chong* and *ren* not securing. Therefore, she was treated with the following formula: *Tu Si Zi* (Semen Cuscutae), *Xu Duan* (Radix Dipsaci), *Sang Ji Sheng* (Herba Taxilli), *Dang Shen* (Radix Codonopsitis), and scorched *Bai Zhu* (Rhizoma Atractylodis Macrocephalae), 10g each, *E Jiao* (Gelatinum Corii Asini), 12g, stir-fried *Du Zhong* (Cortex Eucommiae), 15g, *Ba Yue Zha* (Fructus Akebiae Trifoliatae), 8g, mix-fried *Gan Cao* (Radix Glycyrrhizae), 3g, and *He Ye* (Folium Nelumbinis), 1 length. After one packet of these medicinals, the bleeding had diminished, and, after two packets, it had stopped. After three packets, the patient's symptoms had improved, and after five packets, these medicinals were stopped. On follow-up some time later, it was found that she had given birth to a baby boy.

Remarks

1. In attempting to treat threatened abortion, besides basing internal medicinals on a correct, comprehensive pattern discrimination, it is also important to use large doses and many packets for emergency quieting of the fetus. If qi vacuity is one of the disease mechanisms, as it usually is, one should also not skimp on cost by using *Dang Shen* instead of *Ren Shen*. In addition, if there is bleeding, bleeding-stopping medicinals should be used charred or carbonized for greater styptic effect also based on the branch principle of stopping leakage. Further, the patient should remain in bed while abortion is threatening, and treatment should be commenced without delay as soon as the patient experiences any lower abdominal pain, vaginal bleeding, or low back pain. Early and aggressive treatment are the keys to forestalling a threatened abortion.

2. Because Western physicians inform their patients that most abortions are due to genetic malformation of the fetus and their subsequent nonviability, many women are confused whether or not to undergo Chinese medical treatment to attempt to forestall a threatened abortion. In my experience, every threatened abortion should be treated according to a Chinese medical pattern discrimination since there are a number of other factors besides malformation of the fetus that can cause a spontaneous abortion. It is my assumption that if the fetus is not genetically viable, no amount of Chinese medicinals are going to save it and continue the pregnancy. I know of no case where treatment by Chinese medicine for threatened abortion has resulted in the birth of a malformed baby, and I have successfully forestalled a number of threatened abortions in my more than 23 years of clinical practice.

3. Late term miscarriages are often due to incompetence of the cervix. In this case, the cervix is not sufficiently toned to remain closed in the presence of the growing weight of the fetus. Both the Chinese medical literature and my own clinical experience suggest that such late term miscarriages are primarily due to insufficiency of central or spleen qi. In such cases, modified *Bu Zhong Yi Qi Tang* (Supplement the Center & Boost the Qi Decoction) plus moxibustion at *Bai Hui* (GV 20), bed rest, and a proper diet can be very effective in forestalling an abortion or preterm delivery. In my experience, women with incompetent cervices do eventually deliver prematurely, but the longer the pregnancy continues, usually the better it is for the child.

4. If a pregnant woman passes a large amount of blood and even blood containing copious clots, she should not immediately assume that she has miscarried. A pregnancy test can be done, followed by a gynecological exam and ultrasonography. It is my experience that a woman may think she has miscarried when, in fact, she has not. In general, the prognosis is best for those women who have not experienced pronounced low back soreness and pain even if they have passed considerable blood. This is even so if the woman experienced considerable lower abdominal pain. Therefore, it is important to inform pregnant women that low back pain is a symptom for which they should seek Chinese medical treatment during the first part of pregnancy.

5. Certain Chinese medicinals are believed to have a special empirical effect of quieting the fetus and thus forestalling a threatened abortion. *Huang Qin* (Radix Scutellariae) and *Zhu Ma Gen* (Radix Boehmeriae Niveae) clear heat and quiet the fetus. *Bai Zhu* (Rhizoma Atractylodis Macrocephalae) fortifies the spleen and quiets the fetus. *Su Gen* (Caulis Perillae Frutescentis) and *Sha Ren* (Fructus Amomi) rectify the qi and

quiet the fetus. *Du Zhong* (Cortex Eucommiae) supplements the kidneys, invigorates yang, and quiets the fetus, while *Sang Ji Sheng* (Herba Taxilli) supplements the kidneys, enriches yin, and quiets the fetus. And *Shi Nan Teng* (Caulis Photiniae Serrulatae) quickens the blood and quiets the fetus. As the reader will see, these medicinals are used over and over again in the above formulas and research protocols for the treatment of threatened abortion.

Endnotes:

1 Beers, Mark H. & Robert Berkow, *The Merck Manual of Diagnosis and Therapy*, 17th edition, Merck Research Laboratories, Whitehouse Station, NJ, 1999, p. 2053

2 Harger, James H., "Recurrent Spontaneous Abortion and Pregnancy Loss," *Gynecology & Obstetrics: A Longitudinal Approach, op. cit.*, p. 247

6
Hydatidiform Mole

Hydatidiform mole is a neoplasm which originates from trophoblast cells. It can follow either intra- or extrauterine pregnancy. A hydatidiform mole is typically the end stage of a degenerating pregnancy in which the villi have become hydropic and the trophoblastic elements have undergone variable amounts of proliferation. They are called moles because *mola* means mass. Essentially, they are a conceptus lacking an intact fetus. Western medicine identifies two basic types: benign hydatidiform mole and malignant hydatidiform mole. Malignant moles can be further divided into chorioadenoma which are only locally invasive of the myometrium and choriocarcinoma which are highly metastatic.

Hydatidiform moles are more common among older women. They occur at a rate of about one in 2,000 pregnancies in the United States and one in 200 pregnancies in Asia. This large difference in incidence may be due to this condition's being associated with repeated artificial abortions, and artificial abortions are used as a method of birth control in the People's Republic of China. Eighty percent of hydatidiform moles are benign, 15% are malignant but localized, and 5% are metastatic. Signs and symptoms of hydatidiform mole can include a uterus which grows too fast for the number of days pregnant, vaginal bleeding, lack of fetal heart tones by Doppler ultrasonography, severe nausea and vomiting, and passage of grape-like molar tissue. Histological examination of this tissue confirms the diagnosis.

The complications of a hydatidiform mole can include intrauterine infection, septicemia, hemorrhage, toxemia of pregnancy, and development of choriocarcinoma or metastatic disease. Modern Western medicine considers evacuation of the mole essential via suction curettage followed by oxytocin stimulation and D&C. After evacuation, chest x-rays are suggested to check the lungs for metastases. Malignant moles are mostly treated by chemotherapy with hysterectomies typically reserved for women over 40. The remission rate after therapy is between 75-85%.

Chinese medical disease categorization

In Chinese medicine, this condition is mostly diagnosed as *tai lou xia xue*, fetal leakage of blood downward, and *ban chan hou xu xia xue bu zhi*, half birth with bleeding downward which does not stop.

Disease causes & disease mechanisms

This disease is mostly due to damp heat filth and turbidity evils assailing and raiding the lower burner. These smolder and bind in the uterus, obstructing and stagnating the movement and transportation of the qi and blood. This leads to stasis and heat mutually binding. This then damages the fetal origin, producing ghost fetus. At the same time, evil toxins also easily assail and raid the lungs. The lungs face the hundreds of vessels. Hence such disease can affect (*i.e.*, metastasize to) the entire body.

Treatment based on pattern discrimination

Damp heat stasis & stagnation

Main symptoms: A rapidly enlarging uterus 10-16 weeks after conception accompanied by vaginal bleeding, severe nausea and vomiting, passage of a grape-like mass from the vagina, a red tongue with slimy, yellow fur, and a slippery, rapid, bowstring pulse

Treatment principles: Resolve evil toxins and clear lung heat, clean the uterus and dispel stasis and stagnation

Guiding formula:

Jie Du Hua Yu Zhuan Fang
(Resolve Toxins & Transform Stasis Special Formula)
Ban Zhi Lian (Radix Scutellariae Barbatae), 9-15g
Hong Teng (Caulis Sargentodoxae), 15-18g
Bai Hua She She Cao (Herba Hedyotis Diffusae), 15-18g
Pu Gong Ying (Herba Taraxaci), 15-18g
Yu Xing Cao (Herba Houttuyniae), 15-18g
Dan Shen (Radix Salviae Miltiorrhizae), 9-15g
Che Qian Zi (Semen Plantaginis), 9g
Long Kui (Herba Solani Nigri), 9g
Dang Gui Wei (Extremitas Radicis Angelicae Sinensis), 9g
Fu Ling (Poria), 12g
Huang Qin (Radix Scutellariae), 9-15g
Huang Bai (Cortex Phellodendri), 9g
Chi Shao (Radix Rubrus Paeoniae Lactiflorae), 9g
Dan Pi (Cortex Moutan), 9g
Zhi Zi (Fructus Gardeniae), 6-9g
uncooked *Da Huang* (Radix Et Rhizoma Rhei), 3-6g
Long Dan Cao (Radix Gentianae), 3-6g

Remarks

Although some Chinese sources talk about curing this condition by using Chinese medicinals and without resorting to hysterectomy, Chinese medicinals are mainly used as adjuncts in the chemotherapy treatment of metastases. If the practitioner suspects this condition, the patient should be referred to a Western MD for further diagnosis and treatment.

7

Habitual Abortion

Recurrent loss of pregnancy is also referred to as habitual abortion. This refers to three or more consecutive spontaneous abortions. According to James H. Harger, the actual incidence of three or four consecutive spontaneous abortions is unknown.[1] The Western medical causes of habitual abortion include genetic abnormalities, Müllerian duct developmental abnormalities, chronic intrauterine infection, endocrine disorders, such as a luteal phase deficiency and hypothyroidism, and autoimmune disorders, such as systemic lupus erythmatosus (SLE), rheumatoid arthritis (RA), scleroderma, and polymyositis/dermatomyositis. Because there is no single cause of habitual abortion, Western medical diagnosis includes physical and especially pelvic examination and a variety of laboratory evaluations in order to make a differential diagnosis between the foregoing causes. While some Western clinicians focus on luteal phase defect (LPD) as the main cause of habitual abortion, this is controversial. Luteal phase defect may be due to simple aging of the ovaries or it may be due to an autoimmune ovaritis with or without concomitant autoimmune thyroiditis. In terms of Western medical therapy, uterine morphological abnormalities can sometimes be corrected by surgery. When endocrine disorders are diagnosed these can be treated medically. For those with autoimmune disorders, prednisone and aspirin therapy have both been tried with inconclusive results.

Chinese medical disease categorization

Three or more spontaneous abortions are traditionally referred to as *hua tai*, slippery fetus. Another Chinese term for this condition is *shu duo tai*, repeated fallen fetus.

Disease causes & disease mechanisms

In Chinese medicine, there is a single main mechanism responsible for habitual abortion. This is insufficiency of the *chong* and *ren* which leads to lack of securing of the fetal source. Such insufficiency of the *chong* and *ren* is tantamount to a spleen-kidney-liver vacuity. In this case, the spleen qi is vacuous and weak, the liver suffers from blood and yin vacuity, and the kidneys suffer from yin and yang dual vacuity. In addition, the liver qi is typically depressed and stagnant. These vacuities may be due to former heaven natural endowment insufficiency, aging, enduring disease, excessive sex, drug abuse, and prolonged and extreme stress and taxation. The liver depression is due to a variable combination of emotional stress and malnourishment and non-warming affecting coursing and discharge. In addition, depression or vacuity may also force the blood to move frenetically outside its pathways. In individual patients, various of these disease mechanisms will be more or less prominent.

Patterns common to this condition

Qi & blood vacuity weakness
Liver-kidney yin vacuity
Spleen-kidney dual vacuity
Liver-kidney vacuity with stasis & stagnation
Liver-kidney depletion vacuity with qi & blood damage & detriment

Treatment based on pattern discrimination

Qi & blood vacuity weakness

Main symptoms: A history of repeated spontaneous abortion, scanty menstruation, if severe, blocked menstruation, a somber white or sallow yellow facial complexion, dizziness, heart palpitations, lassitude of the spirit, weak limbs, a pale tongue with thin fur, and a fine, forceless pulse

Treatment principles: Fortify the spleen and boost the qi, nourish the blood and regulate the *chong*

Guiding formula:

Tai Shan Pan Shi Yin **(Mt. Tai Bedrock Drink)**
Ren Shen (Radix Ginseng), 3-9g
Huang Qi (Radix Astragali), 9-18g
Dang Gui (Radix Angelicae Sinensis), 9g
Xu Duan (Radix Dipsaci), 9g
Huang Qin (Radix Scutellariae), 6-12g
Chuan Xiong (Radix Ligustici Wallichii), 6-12g
Bai Shao (Radix Albus Paeoniae Lactiflorae), 9-18g
Shu Di (cooked Radix Rehmanniae), 12-15g
Bai Zhu (Rhizoma Atractylodis Macrocephalae), 9g
mix-fried *Gan Cao* (Radix Glycyrrhizae), 6-9g
Sha Ren (Fructus Amomi), 3-4.5g
Nuo Mi (glutinous rice), 15g

Acupuncture & moxibustion: Zu San Li (St 36), San Yin Jiao (Sp 6), Ge Shu (Bl 17), Gan Shu (Bl 18), Pi Shu (Bl 20)

Liver-kidney yin vacuity

Main symptoms: A history of habitual abortion, low back and knee soreness and limpness, dry mouth with no thought of drinking, yellow urination, constipation, a fine, possibly rapid pulse, and a red tongue with thin, yellow or scanty fur

Treatment principles: Enrich yin and clear heat

Guiding formula:

Er Zhi Wan Jia Wei (Two Ultimates Pills with Added Flavors)
Nu Zhen Zi (Fructus Ligustri Lucidi), 12-15g
Han Lian Cao (Herba Ecliptae), 12-15g
Sheng Di (uncooked Radix Rehmanniae), 12-15g
Bai Shao (Radix Albus Paeoniae Lactiflorae), 9-18g
Huang Qin (Radix Scutellariae), 6-12g
Shan Yao (Radix Dioscoreae), 9g
Sang Ji Sheng (Herba Taxilli), 12-15g
Tu Si Zi (Semen Cuscutae), 9g
Xu Duan (Radix Dipsaci), 9g
Sheng Ma (Rhizoma Cimicifugae), 3-6g

Acupuncture & moxibustion: *San Yin Jiao* (Sp 6), *Tai Xi* (Ki 3), *Shen Shu* (Bl 23), *Guan Yuan* (CV 4)

If there is dry mouth, add *Zhao Hai* (Ki 6) and *Lie Que* (Lu 7). If there is constipation, add *Zhao Hai, Tian Shu* (St 25), and *Da Chang Shu* (Bl 25).

Spleen-kidney dual vacuity

Main symptoms: A history of habitual abortion, low back and knee soreness and limpness, fatigue, lack of strength, possible edema of the four limbs, abdominal distention, torpid intake, loose stools, a pale red, fat tongue with teeth-marks on its edges and thin, white fur, and a deep, fine, forceless pulse

Treatment principles: Fortify the spleen and boost the qi, supplement the kidneys and invigorate yang

Guiding formula:

**Bu Shen Qiang Yang Fang
(Supplement the Kidneys & Invigorate Yang Formula)**
Sang Ji Sheng (Herba Taxilli), 12-15g
Tu Si Zi (Semen Cuscutae), 9g
Xu Duan (Radix Dipsaci), 9g
Du Zhong (Cortex Eucommiae), 9-15g
Shan Yao (Radix Dioscoreae), 9g
Qian Shi (Semen Euryalis), 9g
Bai Zhu (Rhizoma Atractylodis Macrocephalae), 9g
Sheng Ma (Rhizoma Cimicifugae), 3-6g

Fu Ling (Poria), 12g
Sha Ren (Fructus Amomi), 3-4.5g

Acupuncture & moxibustion: *Pi Shu* (Bl 20), *Shen Shu* (Bl 23), *Zu San Li* (St 36), *Qi Hai* (CV 6), *Guan Yuan* (CV 4)

Liver-kidney vacuity with stasis & stagnation

Main symptoms: A history of habitual abortion, lower abdominal discomfort or aching and pain, chest, breast, and/or rib-side distention and pain, low back and knee soreness and limpness, a dry mouth with no thought to drink, a dark tongue with possible static macules or spots and thin or scanty fur, and a bowstring, fine, possibly choppy pulse

Treatment principles: Supplement the liver and boost the kidneys, rectify the qi and quicken the blood

Guiding formulas:

Si Wu Tang Jia Jian
(Four Materials Decoction with Additions & Subtractions)
Dang Gui (Radix Angelicae Sinensis), 9g
Chuan Xiong (Radix Ligustici Wallichii), 6-12g
Bai Shao (Radix Albus Paeoniae Lactiflorae), 9-18g
Mu Xiang (Radix Auklandiae), 6-9g
Yi Mu Cao (Herba Leonuri), 9-15g
Sang Ji Sheng (Herba Taxilli), 12-15g
Xu Duan (Radix Dipsaci), 9g
Du Zhong (Cortex Eucommiae), 9-15g
Tu Si Zi (Semen Cuscutae), 9g
Sheng Ma (Rhizoma Cimicifugae), 3-6g
Sha Ren (Fructus Amomi), 3-4.5g
Shan Yao (Radix Dioscoreae), 9-12g

Unnamed formula given by Zhang Xue-wen in Yu Xue Zheng Zhi
(Proven Treatments for Blood Stasis)
Shu Di (cooked Radix Rehmanniae), 12-15g
Shan Yao (Radix Dioscoreae), 9-12g
Shan Zhu Yu (Fructus Corni), 9g
Fu Ling (Poria), 12g
Gou Qi Zi (Fructus Lycii), 9g
Ju Hua (Flos Chrysanthemi), 9g
Dan Pi (Cortex Moutan), 6-9g
Dan Shen (Radix Salviae Miltiorrhizae), 9-15g
Yu Jin (Tuber Curcumae), 9g
Xiang Fu (Rhizoma Cyperi), 9g
Yi Mu Cao (Herba Leonuri), 9-15g
Hong Hua (Flos Carthami), 9g

Acupuncture & moxibustion: San Yin Jiao (Sp 6), *Tai Xi* (Ki 3), *Shen Shu* (Bl 23), *Guan Yuan* (CV 4), *Xue Hai* (Sp 10), *He Gu* (LI 4)

Liver-kidney depletion vacuity with qi & blood damage & detriment

Main symptoms: A history of habitual abortion, a habitually vacuous and weak body, a lusterless facial complexion, low back soreness, weakness of the limbs, loss of appetite after conception, lower abdominal heaviness and distention, dizziness, a cold body, fat tongue with teeth-marks on its edges and thin fur, and a fine, bowstring pulse. If there is depressive, damp, or vacuity heat, the tongue may be red with yellow fur.

Treatment principles: Boost the liver and kidneys and supplement the qi and blood assisted by clearing vacuity heat and eliminating dampness if necessary

Guiding formula:

Er Xian Tang Jia Jian
(Two Immortals Decoction with Additions & Subtractions)
Xian Mao (Rhizoma Curculiginis), 9g
Xian Ling Pi (Herba Epimedii), 9g
Dang Gui (Radix Angelicae Sinensis), 9g
Dang Shen (Radix Codonopsitis), 9-12g
Bai Zhu (Rhizoma Atractylodis Macrocephalae), 9g
Wu Yao (Radix Linderae), 9g
Mu Xiang (Radix Auklandiae), 6-9g
Xiang Fu (Rhizoma Cyperi), 9g
Ze Xie (Rhizoma Alismatis), 6-9g

If there is vacuity heat and stirring of ministerial fire, add *Zhi Mu* (Rhizoma Anemarrhenae) and *Huang Bai* (Cortex Phellodendri). If there is more pronounced spleen vacuity, add *Huang Qi* (Radix Astragali). If there is more pronounced kidney yang vacuity with low back pain, add *Du Zhong* (Cortex Eucommiae) and *Xu Duan* (Radix Dipsaci). If there is more pronounced liver depression qi stagnation, add *Chai Hu* (Radix Bupleuri) and *Chuan Lian Zi* (Fructus Toosendan). If there is early menstruation due to qi vacuity, add *Sheng Ma* (Rhizoma Cimicifugae), *Chai Hu* (Radix Bupleuri), *Huang Qi* (Radix Astragali), and *E Jiao* (Gelatinum Corii Asini). If there is dysmenorrhea accompanied by diarrhea that is watery, acidic, and/or explosive due to damp heat evils, add *Bai Tou Weng* (Radix Pulsatillae). If there is nausea and vomiting accompanying menstruation, add *Wu Mei* (Fructus Mume) and *Gan Jiang* (dry Rhizoma Zingiberis). If there is intense dysmenorrhea with pain on the sides of the abdomen, add *Ma Xian Cao* (Herba Verbena Officinalis), *Hong Teng* (Caulis Sargentodoxae), *Ju He* (Semen Citri Reticulatae), and *Xiao Hui Xiang* (Fructus Foeniculi). If there are clots in the menstrual discharge which then dribbles on past its time, add *Dan Shen* (Radix Salviae Miltiorrhizae), *Yi Mu Cao* (Herba Leonuri), and *Ce Bai Ye* (Cacumen Platycladi).

Acupuncture & moxibustion: *Zu San Li* (St 36), *San Yin Jiao* (Sp 6), *Ge Shu* (Bl 17), *Gan Shu* (Bl 18), *Pi Shu* (Bl 20), *Shen Shu* (Bl 23), *Guan Yuan* (CV 4)

Abstracts of representative Chinese research

From "A Clinical Survey of the Effectiveness of *Shou Tai Wan* (Long-life Fetus Pills) in the Treatment of Habitual Miscarriage" by Li Xin-hua & Song Mei-hua, *Shan Xi Zhong Yi (Shanxi Chinese Medicine)*, #4, 1995, p. 13-14

Cohort description:

The patients in this study were divided into two groups. One group was the treatment group and consisted of 140 women who received *Shou Tai Wan* with additions and subtractions depending on their symptoms. This group ranged in age from 24-42 years old. Eighty of these women had had three spontaneous abortions, 50 had had four spontaneous abortions, and 10 had had five or more spontaneous abortions. The other group was the comparison group. Patients in this group received Western medication (vitamin C, vitamin E, and intramuscular progesterone shots). The ages of the women in this group ranged from 24-39 years old. Forty women in this group had had three spontaneous abortions, three had had four spontaneous abortions, and two had had five or more spontaneous abortions. The diagnosis of pregnancy in both groups was confirmed by both positive urine HCG and ultrasonography of their uteri. Chromosomal analysis and gynecological examination were not abnormal. In terms of clinical symptoms, in the treatment group, 70 women had some degree of lumbosacral soreness and encumbrance, lower abdominal sagging pain, and psychoemotional withering and devitalization. In the comparison group, 38 women had these same symptoms. In the treatment group another 50 women had a somber white facial complexion, lassitude of the spirit, fatigued limbs, scanty intake, and loose stools. There were four cases in the comparison group with these same symptoms. In the treatment group, there were another 20 women with vexatious heat in the five hearts, a dry mouth and parched throat, dizziness, and tinnitus. In the comparison group, there were three women with these same symptoms. Further, there were 80 women who had some degree of vaginal tract bleeding.

Treatment method:

Shou Tai Wan was composed of: *Tu Si Zi* (Semen Cuscutae), *Sang Ji Sheng* (Herba Taxilli), *Xu Duan* (Radix Dipsaci), and *E Jiao* (Gelatinum Corii Asini). If there was qi vacuity, *Dang Shen* (Radix Codonopsitis) and *Huang Qi* (Radix Astragali) were added. If there was blood vacuity, *Dang Gui* (Radix Angelicae Sinensis) and *Bai Shao* (Radix Albus Paeoniae Lactiflorae) were added. If there was blood heat, *Huang Qin* (Radix Scutellariae) was added. If there was yin vacuity with internal heat, *Sheng Di* (uncooked Radix Rehmanniae), *Nu Zhen Zi* (Fructus Ligustri Lucidi), and *Han Lian Cao* (Herba Ecliptae) were added. If nausea and vomiting of pregnancy were severe, *Chen Pi* (Pericarpium Citri Reticulatae), *Sha Ren* (Fructus Amomi), and *Zi Su Gen* (Caulis Perillae Frutescentis) were added. If there was spleen vacuity, *Bai Zhu* (Rhizoma Atractylodis Macrocephalae) was added. And if there was excessive bleeding from the vaginal tract, *Xian He Cao* (Herba Agrimoniae), carbonized *Zong Lu* (Petiolus Trachycarpi), and calcined *Long Gu* (Os Draconis) and *Mu Li* (Concha Ostreae) were added. One packets was decocted in water and administered each day. Ten packets were administered in this manner each month during the latter half of the cycle from the end of the previous miscarriage to the beginning of becoming pregnant. After becoming pregnant, three packets were administered each week for 12 weeks. A few women continued these medicinals till they were 16 weeks pregnant.

Treatment outcomes:

Cure was defined as the disappearance of clinical symptoms and the continuation of pregnancy to full term. Marked effect meant that the clinical symptoms either disappeared or were well reduced but, although the pregnancy exceeded 12 weeks, birth was still early. No effect meant that the symptoms did not change for the better and that there was another spontaneous abortion. In the treatment group, 120 women (85.71%) were cured, 15 women (10.71%) got a marked effect, and five cases (3.57%) got no result. Thus the total amelioration rate in the treatment group was 96.42%. In the comparison group, 32 women (71.11%) were cured, 6 cases (13.33%) got a marked result, and seven cases (15.56%) got no result. Therefore, the total amelioration rate in the comparison group was 84.44%.

From "The Treatment of 8 Cases of Habitual Miscarriage with *Dang Gui Tang* (Dang Gui Decoction)" by Zhang Yun-sheng, *Hu Bei Zhong Yi Za Zhi (Hubei Journal of Chinese Medicine)*, #4, 1995, p. 18

Cohort description:

Of the eight women in this clinical survey, three were between 24-30 years old, four were between 31-35, and one was 37 years old. Four had had spontaneous abortions three times occurring before the 8th week of pregnancy. Two had had spontaneous abortions four times occurring before the 10th week of pregnancy. And another two had had spontaneous abortions more than four times occurring before the 12th week of pregnancy.

Treatment method:

All eight women received *Dang Gui Tang* (Dang Gui Decoction) which was composed of: *Dang Gui* (Radix Angelicae Sinensis), 4.5g, *Chuan Xiong* (Radix Ligustici Wallichii), 4.5g, uncooked *Huang Qi* (Radix Astragali), 2.4g, *Bai Shao* (Radix Albus Paeoniae Lactiflorae), 4.5g, *Jing Jie* (Herba Schizonepetae), 2.4g, *Tu Si Zi* (Semen Cuscutae), 3g, *Gan Cao* (Radix Glycyrrhizae), 1.5g, and *Sheng Jiang* (uncooked Rhizoma Zingiberis), 3 slices. These were decocted in water and administered warm on an empty stomach, one packet per day.

Treatment outcomes:

In five cases, after administering these medicinals for one day, the vaginal tract bleeding had diminished and had stopped after three days. In two cases, the vaginal tract bleeding had diminished after two days of administering these medicinals and had stopped after five days, and, in one case, the vaginal tract bleeding had become scanty after five days of treatment. After their bleeding had stopped, they were administered these medicinals for three more days to secure the treatment and then were discharged from the hospital. Subsequently, six women carried their babies to full term. In two cases, after the bleeding stopped, later it returned again.

From "The Treatment of 40 Cases of Habitual Miscarriage with *Zhi Ke An Tai Yin* (Aurantium Quiet the Fetus Drink)" by Chen Yun-wang & Wu Chun-tao, *Si Chuan Zhong Yi (Sichuan Chinese Medicine)*, #12, 1995, p. 35

Cohort description:

Of the 40 women in this clinical audit, 22 were 23-30 and 18 were 31-42 years old. Seventeen cases had had three spontaneous abortions, 21 had had four spontaneous abortions, and two had had five or more spontaneous abortions. All these women were three months pregnant or more. Their clinical symptoms included lumbosacral and lower abdominal sagging and distention or soreness and pain, scanty or no vaginal tract bleeding, chest and rib-side distention and fullness, a susceptibility to sighing, a pale red or tender, red tongue with thin, white or thin, yellow fur, and a bowstring, slippery, forceless pulse.

Treatment method:

Zhi Ke An Tai Yin was composed of: *Zhi Ke* (Fructus Aurantii), *Jie Geng* (Radix Platycodi), *E Jiao* (Gelatinum Corii Asini), 12g each, *Qiang Huo* (Radix Et Rhizoma Notopterygii), 3g, *Huang Qi* (Radix Astragali), *Xu Duan* (Radix Dipsaci), *Tu Si Zi* (Semen Cuscutae), 15g each, *Sang Ji Sheng* (Herba Taxilli), 20g, and *Dang Gui* (Radix Angelicae Sinensis), 10g. One packet of these medicinals was decocted in water and administered per day. First 20 packets were administered, and, if there were no apparent symptoms, the formula was then given every other day for another 20 packets. After that, two packets were given each week up until parturition.

Treatment outcomes:

Cure meant that the symptoms disappeared, there were no abnormal reactions during pregnancy, pregnancy continued up till the due date, the baby was healthy at birth, and the birth went normally. Based on these criteria, 36 women or 95% were cured.

Representative case histories

Case 1: The patient was a 35 year-old female who was initially examined on May 30, 1958. The woman had been married for 12 years but had had either miscarriage or premature delivery five times. The first time that she had miscarried, it had been during the fourth month of pregnancy. All the rest of the times it was in the fifth and sixth months. Each time, after the woman had been pregnant for one month, she had developed leakage for 10 days. In addition, she had low blood pressure, dizziness, and low back pain for 3-4 months. During her fourth pregnancy, she had been treated with *Tai Chan Jin Dan* (Fetus Birth Golden Elixir) but without effect. Currently, the woman had been pregnant for two months and, for the last 20 days, had had nausea, vomiting, poor appetite, dry stools, and a slightly poor affect. Her left bar position pulse was deep, bowstring, and short, while the right was deep and slippery. Her tongue was normal and without fur.

Based on the above, the patient's Western medical diagnosis was habitual abortion, her Chinese medical diagnosis was slippery fetus, and her pattern was discriminated as spleen, liver, and kidney vacuity. The formula she was prescribed for this consisted of: *Dang Shen* (Radix Codonopsitis), 6g, *Bai Zhu* (Rhizoma Atractylodis Macrocephalae), 6g, *Fu Ling* (Poria), 6g, mix-fried *Gan Cao* (Radix Glycyrrhizae), 3g, *Chen Pi* (Pericarpium Citri Reticulatae), 4.5g, *Sha Ren* (Fructus Amomi), 3g, *Huo Xiang* (Herba Pogostemonis), 6g, *Shan Yao* (Radix Dioscoreae), 9g, *Sheng Jiang* (uncooked Rhizoma Zingiberis), 3 slices, and *Da Zao* (Fructus Jujubae), 3 pieces.

After taking three packets of this formula, the patient's nausea had stopped. Therefore, she was switched to the following formula: *Shu Di* (cooked Radix Rehmanniae), 12g, *Bai Zhu* (Rhizoma Atractylodis Macrocephalae), 6g, *Zhi Fu Zi* (Radix Lateralis Praeparatus Aconiti Carmichaeli), 3g, *Ren Shen* (Radix Ginseng), 3g, *Du Zhong* (Cortex Eucommiae), 9g, *Dang Gui* (Radix Angelicae Sinensis), 3g, *Sang Ji Sheng* (Herba Taxilli), 9g, *Ba Ji Tian* (Radix Morindae), 9g, *Rou Cong Rong* (Herba Cistanchis), 9g, *Xu Duan* (Radix Dipsaci), 6g, and *Zhu Ma Gen* (Radix Boehmeriae Niveae), 9g. The patient boiled each packet of this formula two times, each time for one hour. This resulted in 400ml of medicinal liquid. The patient divided this amount into two doses which she took warm. Each week she took one packet of these medicinals. She eventually got to full term and gave birth normally to a healthy child.

Case 2: The patient was a 35 year-old female who was in the first two months of pregnancy. This was accompanied by slight low back soreness, dizziness, restless sleep at night, a dry mouth, constipation, a crimson red tongue, and fine, slippery, bowstring pulse. The woman had had three previous miscarriages. Her Chinese medical pattern was categorized as yin vacuity with internal heat and she was prescribed the following medicinals in order to prevent slippery fetus: *Sheng Di* (uncooked Radix Rehmanniae), 20g, *Bai Shao* (Radix Albus Paeoniae Lactiflorae), 9g, *Shan Yao* (Radix Dioscoreae), 12g, carbonized *Huang Qin* (Radix Scutellariae), 6g, *Huang Bai* (Cortex Phellodendri), 2.4g, *Gan Cao* (Radix Glycyrrhizae), 2.4g, *Sang Ji Sheng* (Herba Taxilli), 9g, mix-fried *Mai Men Dong* (Tuber Ophiopogonis), 9g, *Shi Hu* (Herba Dendrobii), 9g, *Zi Zhu Cao* (Herba Callicarpae Pedunculatae), 15g, and *Sang Ye* (Folium Mori), 30g. After taking these medicinals for three whole months, the patient stopped, she achieved full term, and she gave birth to a healthy child.

Remarks

1. In treating slippery fetus, one should distinguish between prophylactic treatment given before pregnancy to forestall a possible miscarriage in a woman with a previous history of habitual miscarriage and remedial treatment given to an already pregnant woman who is presenting signs and symptoms of threatened abortion. In clinical practice, it is far easier to prevent miscarriage by supplementing the woman before conception than trying to frantically forestall a miscarriage once a woman displays signs of fetal leakage or fetus stirring restlessly.

2. In my experience, many women with histories of habitual miscarriage also have histories of infertility. In addition, most of these same women also suffer from early periods coming from 22-25 days apart. This suggests that the cause of their habitual abortions is a luteal phase defect. Typically, such women suffer from both yin and yang vacuities, including spleen qi vacuity, and liver depression qi stagnation as well. In such cases, it is necessary not only to supplement the yin and yang of the kidneys but also to fortify the spleen and lead ministerial fire back down to its lower source.

3. In women with a history of habitual abortion and early menstruation, once the menses come at 28 days without premenstrual breast distention or other signs of PMS, they may safely become pregnant without unduly worrying about the likelihood of miscarriage. Typically, this requires 3-6 months or cycles of therapy with the above medicinals which are mostly given from day 18 on. At other phases in the cycle, one should use other treatment methods as necessary, such as nourishing yin post-menstrually, quickening the blood at ovulation and again during menstruation, etc.

4. It is of utmost importance that the woman suffering from habitual miscarriage be made to understand that her condition requires several months of herbal supplementation therapy and that she should by all means not allow herself to get pregnant before the signs and symptoms associated with her cycle have all become normal according to the parameters of Chinese medicine. Should she become pregnant too soon before all her menstrual signs and symptoms have returned to normal, there is every likelihood of her miscarrying again. Since such repeated abortions engender blood stasis, damage the kidneys, and disquiet the spirit, and the more the woman suffers from repeated abortions, the more difficult it will be to eventually get the right result. Therefore, such women must be counselled on forbearance and patience.

Endnote:

[1] Harger, James H., "Recurrent Spontaneous Abortion and Pregnancy Loss," *Gynecology & Obstetrics: A Longitudinal Approach, op. cit.*, p. 247

8

Fetal Growth Disorders

In Western medicine, the terms "small for gestational age" (SGA) and "small for dates" describe a fetus whose size is considered smaller than normal for the number of days or weeks of gestation. Such smaller than normal size may be due to differences in genetic and biological potential of the individual or any of a number of regulating and modulating influences on fetal growth. The term "intrauterine growth retardation" (IUGR) specifically refers to retarded growth due to failure of oxygen and nutrient supply.[1] According to Gruenwald et al., IUGR develops because of a fixed and limited placental capacity to transfer nutrients to the fetus.[2] During the initial stage of gestation, the placenta supplies sufficient nutrients to the fetus to allow it to grow normally. However, as the fetus grows in size, its demand for nutrients may exceed the ability of the placenta to supply these. In this case, growth initially slows and eventually stops. A mild restriction in fetal nourishment may compromise growth but not affect other aspects of the fetus's well-being, such as oxygenation, vascular volume, and hydration. However, such restriction may be so severe as to lead to abrupt fetal death. Other negative consequences of arrested growth in utero include fetal distress in labor, asphyxia and low Apgar score, polycythemia, thrombocytopenia, hypoglycemia, hypocalcemia, respiratory distress, and kidney failure. Long-term problems with neurological development appear to be directly related to early onset of growth retardation and immaturity at birth. However, small infants born at term appear to have little such risk as long as there is no concomitant hypoxemia.

Risk factors of IUGR include extremes of maternal age, low socioeconomic status, addictions, poor past obstetric history, and multiple pregnancy. Some of the specific causes of IUGR in Western medicine include maternal disease, such as hypertension, kidney disease, collagen disorders, chronic respiratory disorders, and chronic bowel disorders, placental disease, such as chorioangioma, single umbilical artery, and velamentous insertion of the umbilical cord, and maternal nutritional deficiency. Western medical diagnosis of IUGR consists of clinical examination of the fetus at antenatal visits. Measuring symphysis-fundal height with a tape measure allows the obstetrician to compare fetal growth with standard charts. Once IUGR is confirmed, a number of subsequent tests may be performed to monitor fetal health and help determine the course of therapy. These tests include umbilical Doppler studies, fetal heart rate monitoring, fetal movement monitoring, serial ultrasound measurements, amniotic fluid volume assessment, establishing fetal karyotype, and percutaneous umbilical blood sampling to determine blood gas tension and pH.

In terms of Western medical treatment, early delivery is effected whenever the risk of fetal death *in utero* or asphyxial injury is greater than that of premature delivery. Commonly, such preterm delivery is accomplished by Cesarean section. If there is a specific underlying maternal disease, such as hypertension or diabetes, treatment is directed at remedying or reducing the negative effects of that disease. Aspirin has been shown to increase birth weight in fetuses identified by abnormal umbilical artery Doppler studies after 28 weeks.[3] While there is much anecdotal evidence that bed rest may be of benefit, this is currently unsupported by clinical trial.

Chinese medical disease categorization

If, after 4-5 months of pregnancy, the mother's uterus is not the size it should be for the stage in pregnancy but the fetus continues to move, this is called *tai wei bu chang*, fetal decline and failure to grow, or *ren shen tai wei zao*, withering and parching of the fetus.

Disease causes & disease mechanisms

In Chinese medicine, this condition is due to the fetus not getting enough nourishment. Either the woman's viscera and bowel function or her dietary nourishment is insufficient. This leads to insufficiency of the qi and blood and thus insufficient fetal nourishment. In terms of insufficient viscera and bowel function, this may be due to former heaven natural endowment insufficiency, age, enduring disease, or overtaxation. In terms of inadequate dietary nourishment, either the mother is not eating sufficiently nourishing foods or is overeating uncooked, chilled foods. Therefore, the spleen becomes weak and fails to engender sufficient qi and blood. Lack of fetal nourishment may also occur after fetal leakage, in which case, the blood, having been lost, is not adequate to nourish both the mother and child.

Patterns common to this condition

Qi & blood dual vacuity
Spleen-kidney dual vacuity

Treatment based on pattern discrimination

Qi & blood dual vacuity

Main symptoms: Smaller than normal uterine size after 4-5 months of pregnancy but fetal movements continue, mother's body emaciated and weak, a sallow yellow or pale facial complexion, dizziness, shortness of breath, a pale tongue with thin fur, and a fine, forceless pulse

Treatment principles: Supplement the qi, boost the blood, and nourish the fetus

Guiding formula:

Ba Zhen Tang (Eight Pearls Decoction)
Dang Shen (Radix Codonopsitis), 9-18g
Shu Di (cooked Radix Rehmanniae), 12-15g
Bai Zhu (Rhizoma Atractylodis Macrocephalae), 9g
Dang Gui (Radix Angelicae Sinensis), 9g
Bai Shao (Radix Albus Paeoniae Lactiflorae), 9-18g
Chuan Xiong (Radix Ligustici Wallichii), 6-15g
Fu Ling (Poria), 12g
mix-fried *Gan Cao* (Radix Glycyrrhizae), 3-9g

Spleen-kidney dual vacuity

Main symptoms: Lower abdominal size smaller than it should be for the number of months pregnant, low back soreness and chill, diminished appetite, loose stools, a cold body and chilled limbs, cold hands and feet, a pale tongue with white fur, and a deep, slow pulse

Treatment principles: Fortify the spleen and boost the qi, supplement the kidneys and warm yang

Guiding formulas:

Wen Tu Shui Tang Fa Shen Qu
(Warm Earth & Water Decoction Minus Massa Medica Fermentata)
Ba Ji Tian (Radix Morindae), 9g
Bai Zhu (Rhizoma Atractylodis Macrocephalae), 9g
Ren Shen (Radix Ginseng), 3-9g
Shan Yao (Radix Dioscoreae), 9-12g
Fu Pen Zi (Fructus Rubi), 9g

Bu Tai Tang (Supplement the Fetus Decoction)
Dang Gui (Radix Angelicae Sinensis), 9g
Shu Di (cooked Radix Rehmanniae), 12-15g
stir-fried *Bai Shao* (Radix Albus Paeoniae Lactiflorae), 9-18g
earth stir-fried *Bai Zhu* (Rhizoma Atractylodis Macrocephalae), 9g
Tu Si Zi (Semen Cuscutae), 9g
Xu Duan (Radix Dipsaci), 9g
stir-fried *Du Zhong* (Cortex Eucommiae), 9-15g
Gou Ji (Rhizoma Cibotii), 9g
Chen Pi (Pericarpium Citri Reticulatae), 6g
Shi Hu (Herba Dendrobii), 9g

Dang Shen (Radix Codonopsitis), 9-15g

mix-fried *Huang Qi* (Radix Astragali), 9-18g

mix-fried *Gan Cao* (Radix Glycyrrhizae), 6-9g

Representative case history

The patient was 25 years old. Her initial examination occurred on March 2, 1970. Her menses had stopped for 5 whole months. Pregnancy tests were positive. However, her abdominal region did not feel normal. Her lower abdomen also was without normal signs of swelling. Gynecological examination showed no clear sign of the fetus and there were no fetal movements. The pulse was slippery and rapid. The patient was diagnosed as fetus withering and not growing and was treated with more than 10 packets of: *Dang Gui* (Radix Angelicae Sinensis), 15g, *Shu Di* (cooked Radix Rehmanniae), 15g, stir-fried *Bai Shao* (Radix Albus Paeoniae Lactiflorae), 10g, earth stir-fried *Bai Zhu* (Rhizoma Atractylodis Macrocephalae), 9g, *Tu Si Zi* (Semen Cuscutae), 10g, *Xu Duan* (Radix Dipsaci), 12g, stir-fried *Du Zhong* (Cortex Eucommiae), 15g, *Gou Ji* (Rhizoma Cibotii), 12g, *Chen Pi* (Pericarpium Citri Reticulatae), 9g, *Shi Hu* (Herba Dendrobii), 9g, *Dang Shen* (Radix Codonopsitis), 12g, mix-fried *Huang Qi* (Radix Astragali), 15g, and mix-fried *Gan Cao* (Radix Glycyrrhizae), 6g. The fetus then gradually began to develop and finally she gave birth to a boy at sufficient months. His body was healthy and without disease.

Endnotes:

[1] Trudinger, Brian, "Fetal Growth Disorders," *Gynecology & Obstetrics: A Longitudinal Approach, op. cit.*, p. 488

[2] *Ibid.*, p. 488

[3] *Ibid.*, p. 496

9

Missed Abortion

Fetal death may occur at any time during gestation. Missed abortion refers to a prolonged delay in the expulsion of a dead fetus. In modern Western medicine, missed abortion is suspected when the uterus fails to enlarge, when fetal heart sounds cannot be heard, or when previously present fetal heart sounds are absent. Missed abortion is confirmed by serum and/or urine tests for HCG or ultrasonography which fails to show cardiac activity. If fetal death occurs in the second trimester or later, missed abortion may lead to dead fetus syndrome. This refers to disseminated intravascular coagulation, progressive hypofibrinogenemia, and possible massive bleeding when delivery eventually occurs. In terms of stimulating delivery of the dead fetus, the current standard of care in Western medicine is the vaginal, intra-cervical, extra-amniotic, or intra-amniotic administration of prostaglandins. Delivery by Cesarean section in this case is rarely indicated.

Chinese medical disease categorization

If the fetus dies inside the uterus and, after more than one month, is not naturally expelled, this is traditionally called *tai si bu xia*, dead fetus does not descend.

Disease causes & disease mechanisms

In Chinese medicine, if something that should be discharged is not, there can only two main mechanisms responsible. Either there is insufficient qi to move that something out of the body or something is blocking and obstructing that outward movement. Therefore, if the fetus dies *in utero*, this is mostly because of the mother's contraction of a warm heat disease that damages the fetus, trauma that injures the fetus, or vacuity of the mother's body that fails to nourish the fetus. If the fetus fails to descend, this is because either there is insufficient qi to move the dead fetus down and out or blood stasis is blocking the precipitation of the dead fetus.

Patterns common to this condition

Qi & blood vacuity weakness
Blood stasis

Treatment based on pattern discrimination:

Qi & blood vacuity weakness

Main symptoms: Dead fetus within the abdomen, lower abdominal aching and pain or a chilled feeling, lassitude of the spirit, a somber white facial complexion, shortness of breath, a faint voice and disinclination to speak, diminished food intake, bad breath, a pale tongue with white, glossy fur, and a large, vacuous, choppy pulse

Treatment principles: Nourish and quicken the blood, boost the qi and descend the fetus

Guiding formula:

Jiu Mu Dan **(Rescue the Mother Elixir)**
Ren Shen (Radix Ginseng), 3-9g
Dang Gui (Radix Angelicae Sinensis), 9g
Chuan Xiong (Radix Ligustici Wallichii), 6-15g
Yi Mu Cao (Herba Leonuri), 9-15g
Chi Shi Zhi (Hallyositum Rubrum), 9g
carbonized *Jing Jie* (Herba Schizonepetae), 9g

Blood stasis

Main symptoms: Cessation of fetal movements, discharge of purple or black bloody fluids from the vagina, bad breath, lower abdominal aching and pain, a dark, greenish facial complexion, greenish lips, a dark purple tongue, and a deep, choppy pulse

Treatment principles: Quicken the blood and move the qi, dispel stasis and descend the fetus

Guiding formulas:

Tuo Hua Jian Jia Mang Xiao
(Out-Thrust & Gloss Decoction Plus Mirabilitum)
Dang Gui (Radix Angelicae Sinensis), 9g
Chuan Xiong (Radix Ligustici Wallichii), 6-15g
Rou Gui (Cortex Cinnamomi), 6-9g
Che Qian Zi (Semen Plantaginis), 6-9g
Niu Xi (Radix Achyranthis Bidentatae), 9-12g
Hong Hua (Flos Carthami), 9g
Mang Xiao (Mirabilitum), 3-6g

Tao Ren Cheng Qi Tang Jia Wei
(Persica Order the Qi Decoction with Added Flavors)

Tao Ren (Semen Persicae), 9g
Da Huang (Radix Et Rhizoma Rhei), 3-9g
Gui Zhi (Ramulus Cinnamomi), 9g
Mang Xiao (Mirabilitum), 3-6g
Gan Cao (Radix Glycyrrhizae), 3-9g
Chi Shao (Radix Rubrus Paeoniae Lactiflorae), 9-18g
Yi Mu Cao (Herba Leonuri), 9-15g

Xue Fu Zhu Yu Tang Jia Jian
(Blood Mansion Dispel Stasis Decoction with Additions & Subtractions)

Dang Gui (Radix Angelicae Sinensis), 9g
Sheng Di (uncooked Radix Rehmanniae), 12-15g
Chi Shao (Radix Rubrus Paeoniae Lactiflorae), 9g
Chuan Xiong (Radix Ligustici Wallichii), 6-15g
Tao Ren (Semen Persicae), 9g
Niu Xi (Radix Achyranthis Bidentatae), 9-12g
Hong Hua (Flos Carthami), 9g
Chai Hu (Radix Bupleuri), 9g
Zhi Ke (Fructus Aurantii), 6g

Acupuncture & moxibustion:

Rx 1. *He Gu* (LI 4), *San Yin Jiao* (Sp 6), *Xue Hai* (Sp 10), *Guan Yuan* (CV 4), *Shi Men* (CV 5)

Formula rationale: *He Gu* is the source point of the hand *yang ming* large intestine channel. It is able to free the flow of the channels, dispel stasis, and precipitate the dead fetus. *San Yin Jiao* homes to the foot *tai yin*. It is an intersection point of all three foot yin. Of these two points, if one is supplemented and one is drained, then together they have the power to free the channels and dispel stasis. These are combined with *Xue Hai* in order to quicken the blood and with *Guan Yuan* in order to free the flow of the channels. *Shi Men* homes to the conception vessel and is the alarm point of the three burners. According to the *Zhen Jiu Da Cheng (Great Compendium of Acupuncture & Moxibustion)*, it can treat women's birth lochia which does not stop, clots, and flooding and leaking diseases. Therefore, it is combined with these other points in order to dispel and precipitate the dead fetus.

Rx 2. *Tai Chong* (Liv 3), *He Gu* (LI 4), *San Yin Jiao* (Sp 6), *Jian Jing* (GB 21), *Zhong Wan* (CV 12), *Qi Hai* (CV 6)

Formula rationale: *Tai Chong* and *He Gu* are used in order to move and regulate the qi. *San Yin Jiao* is able to quicken and move the blood. *Jian Jing*, *Zhong Wan*, and *Qi Hai* are able to free the flow and downbear the triple burner qi mechanism. When all these points are combined together, they are able to move the qi, quicken the blood, and precipitate the fetus.

Representative case histories:

Case 1: The patient was a 25 year-old female who was initially examined during August 1952. The woman had come to full term and her amniotic sac had broken 6-7 days before. However, the fetus had not been delivered. It was determined that the child had died *in utero*. The woman's facial complexion was purplish, dark, and had scanty spirit. Her pulse was deep and tight, while her tongue was purple with thin, white fur. Therefore, the patient was prescribed *Liao Er San* (Treat the Child Powder): *Dang Shen* (Radix Codonopsitis), 30g, *Dang Gui* (Radix Angelicae Sinensis), 60g, *Chuan Niu Xi* (Radix Cyathulae), 15g, *Gui Mu* (Fructus Rumicis Japonici), 9g, and *Ru Xiang* (Resina Olibani), 6g. After administering these medicinals, the woman felt stirring in the fingertips of both hands as well as abdominal pain. The dead fetus was precipitated and the mother lived. Afterwards, she was treated with *Sheng Hua Tang* (Engendering & Transforming Decoction) in order to dispel stasis and engender the new.

Case 2: The patient was a 35 year-old female who had given birth normally six times before. This time the woman had felt the fetal movements become decreased and weaker after five months of pregnancy. Examination for fetal heart tones were negative and the fetus was deemed dead. Chinese medicinals were prescribed. These were not effective, but the woman had not been re-examined. After eight months of pregnancy, the patient developed a fever of 38°C and came again for examination. There were still no fetal heart tones and the cervix had not dilated. Now the diagnosis was fetal death compounded by infection. Because the woman refused to be treated with surgery, Chinese medicinals were again prescribed. At the time of prescription, the woman's mind was clear, her body was emaciated, and there was fever and aversion to cold. Her two excretions were freely flowing and uninhibited. Her pulse was deep, fine, and choppy, and her tongue was pale with static spots and moist, white fur.

Based on the above, this woman's pattern was categorized as blood vacuity and qi stagnation mixed with blood stasis, for which she was prescribed: *Dang Gui Wei* (Extremitas Radicis Angelicae Sinensis), 15g, *Chuan Xiong* (Radix Ligustici Wallichii), *Chuan Niu Xi* (Radix Cyathulae), *Che Qian Zi* (Semen Plantaginis), *Hong Hua* (Flos Carthami), *Tai Zi Shen* (Radix Pseudostellariae), and *Hou Po* (Cortex Magnoliae Officinalis), 10g each, and *Rou Gui* (Cortex Cinnamomi), 5g. At 9 PM that evening, the patient took the first decoction. At 10:30, she took the second decoction. At 11 PM, she felt uterine contractions, aching, and pain and a small amount of dark red bloody fluids was discharged from her vagina. At 5:30 AM, her water broke and an oily, soysauce colored fluid was discharged with a foul odor. This was followed by delivery of the dead fetus whose flesh was putrefied and purplish black in color. This was followed by explusion of the placenta. The woman lost approximately 300mL of blood.

Because there was still a feeling of pain in her abdomen and her temperature was 37.7°C, she was administered *Tao Hong Si Wu Tang Jia Jian* (Persica & Carthamus Four Materials Decoction with Additions & Subtractions): *Dang Gui* (Radix

Angelicae Sinensis) and *Dan Shen* (Radix Salviae Miltiorrhizae), 10g each, *Chuan Xiong* (Radix Ligustici Wallichii), *Chi Shao* (Radix Rubrus Paeoniae Lactiflorae), *Tao Ren* (Semen Persicae), *Hong Hua* (Flos Carthami), and *Gan Cao* (Radix Glycyrrhizae), 5g each. After one packet of these medicinals, the lochia became scanty, the abdominal pain was eliminated, the body temperature returned to normal (36.9°C), the deep pulse rose back upward, but the tongue was still pale white. Therefore, the woman was prescribed three packets of: *Dang Gui* (Radix Angelicae Sinensis), *Dan Shen* (Radix Salviae Miltiorrhizae), carbonized *Shan Zha* (Fructus Crataegi), and *Bai Shao* (Radix Albus Paeoniae Lactiflorae), 10g each, *Chuan Xiong* (Radix Ligustici Wallichii), 5g, and *Hong Hua* (Flos Carthami), 3g. At this point, the woman was judged cured and discharged from the hospital.

Remarks:

1. Acupuncture might be a reasonable first choice for treatment of missed abortion since its unwanted side effects are so minimal.

2. In the West, most cases of missed abortion are going to be treated by Western medical means. However, even after delivery has been induced, it makes sense to treat the mother postpartum for residual blood stasis if signs and symptoms indicate, as in case #2 above.

3. There are several traditional teachings concerning the prognostication of maternal and/or fetal death. For instance, if the mother's face is red and she has heart vexation with a dark greenish tongue, this signifies the fetus has died. If the mother's face is green with a red tongue and if there is vomiting of frothy saliva, heaviness and distention within the abdomen, and a dirty turbid liquid flows from the vagina, this signifies the death of the mother. If there is no turbid, dirty flow from the vagina, but heart vexation like insanity, with the lips and tongue both green, and vomiting frothy saliva, this signifies that the lochia is attacking above and that both mother and child will die.

10

Edema During Pregnancy

Edema is the collection of fluid in the tissue, and a certain amount of swelling during pregnancy is normal. This occurs as a result of the hormonal changes of pregnancy which lead to sodium and, therefore, fluid retention. Thus the pregnant woman is by nature hypervolemic. In addition, as the uterus enlarges, it puts pressure on the pelvic veins and vena cava. This slows down the circulation in the pelvis and causes the blood to pool in the lower half of the body. The pressure from this trapped blood forces water into the tissues of the lower extremities. This is why edema typically occurs in the legs of pregnant women, worsens as the day progresses, and usually disappears in the morning after bed rest. By itself, edema during pregnancy is not considered a disease category in its own right in modern Western medicine. Rather it is a symptom of a number of other conditions. In Chinese medicine, edema during pregnancy is considered a disease category. While edema during pregnancy may arise from the natural physiologic and mechanical consequences of pregnancy, it may, in a small percentage of cases, be due to pathological causes. For instance, when edema during pregnancy is accompanied by proteinuria and hypertension, this triad of symptoms is referred to by the acronym EPH. This triad is characteristic of pre-eclampsia. Therefore, edema during pregnancy may be nothing more than a temporary inconvenience or symptoms of a life-threatening condition. The Western medical treatment of this complaint depends on its severity and its underlying cause and runs the gamut from medical treatment to induction of delivery.

Chinese medical disease categorization

Edema during pregnancy is discussed under a number of different headings in modern Chinese gynecology texts. *Ren shen fu zhong* means edema during pregnancy. *Ren shen shui zhong* means water swelling during pregnancy. *Ren shen zhong zhang* means swelling and distention during pregnancy. And *tai shui zhong man* means fetal water swelling and fullness. In the premodern Chinese gyneoclogical literature, edema during pregnancy is referred to as *zi zhong* or child swelling, *zi qi* or child qi, and *zi man* or child fullness. Since this edema tends to especially affect the lower limbs, two other traditional pathoconditions are also spoken of in the premodern literature. These are *zhou jiao*, wrinkled feet, *i.e.*, swelling of the feet in which the skin of the feet and ankles is thickened and looks like leather, and *cui jiao*, fragile feet, *i.e.*, swelling of the feet in which the skin looks especially smooth, shiny, and thin. In addition, some contemporary Chinese medical authors append a section called *yang shui guo duo* or excessive sheep water. This covers excessive amniotic fluid.

Although modern Chinese medical authors lump *zi zhong*, *zi qi*, and *zi man* together, in fact, these are slightly different conditions. If the head and face and the entire body are edematous and swollen and urination is short and scant, this is categorized as *zi zhong*. If one's knees and legs are swollen and distended and one's urination is long, this is categorized as the damp qi disease called *zi qi*. If, at around 6-7 months, a pregnant woman's entire body is swollen and her abdomen is larger than normal accompanied by wheezing, this is called *zi man, qi man*, or *tai shui,* fetal water. However, although these are all traditionally distinct conditions, their disease mechanisms are essentially the same.

Disease causes & disease mechanisms

These related conditions all arise due to loss of normalcy of qi transformation. Water dampness is not able to be diffused and discharged. Therefore, it seeps into the flesh and skin. The qi transformation function is based on the lungs' diffusion and downbearing above, on kidney yang's warm transformation below, and on the spleen qi's movement and transformation as the pivot in the middle. During gestation, essence and blood gather to nourish the fetus below. Since essence and blood are part of systemic yin fluids, such growth and accumulation of yin may hinder or harm yang qi. If the kidneys are weak, this may obstruct kidney yang's warm transformation. Or it may obstruct spleen yang's promotion of water transportation. If either spleen or kidney yang is hindered and obstructed, dampness is not moved and transformed properly and will accumulate as evil yin. In addition, the growth of fetal qi in the lower burner may also hinder and obstruct the liver qi. Since the liver governs the coursing and discharge of the qi and since the qi moves water fluids, this may also cause accumulation of water dampness.

Patterns common to this condition

Spleen qi vacuity

Kidney yang vacuity

Qi stagnation & phlegm obstruction

Treatment based on pattern discrimination:

Spleen qi vacuity

Main symptoms: Due to a habitually weak spleen or to excessive intake of chilled, uncooked foods, as the months of pregnancy mount, the face, eyes, body, and limbs become edematous and swollen. There is also abdominal distention, loose stools, bodily fatigue, lack of warmth in the four limbs, diminished intake of food and drink, a weak voice and disinclination to speak, lack of strength, a sallow, yellow facial complexion, a pale, moist tongue with white, glossy fur, and a slippery, moderate (*i.e.*, relaxed or slightly slow), forceless pulse

Treatment principles: Fortify the spleen and disinhibit water

Guiding formulas:

Bai Zhu San Jia Jian (Atractylodes Powder with Additions & Subtractions)
Bai Zhu (Rhizoma Atractylodis Macrocephalae), 9g
Fu Ling (Poria), 12g
Da Fu Pi (Pericarpium Arecae), 6-9g
Sheng Jiang Pi (uncooked Cortex Rhizomatis Zingiberis), 6g
Chen Pi (Pericarpium Citri Reticulatae), 6g
Sha Ren (Fructus Amomi), 3-4.5g
Shan Yao (Radix Dioscoreae), 9-12g

Jia Jian Bu Zhong Yi Qi Tang
(Modified Supplement the Center & Boost the Qi Decoction)
Dang Shen (Radix Codonopsitis), 9-15g
Huang Qi (Radix Astragali), 9-18g
Dang Gui (Radix Angelicae Sinensis), 9g
scorched *Bai Zhu* (Rhizoma Atractylodis Macrocephalae), 9g
Fu Ling (Poria), 12g
Sheng Ma (Rhizoma Cimicifugae), 3-6g
Chai Hu (Radix Bupleuri), 3-9g
Chen Pi (Pericarpium Citri Reticulatae), 6g
mix-fried *Gan Cao* (Radix Glycyrrhizae), 6-9g

Liu Jun Zi Tang (Six Gentlemen Decoction)
Ren Shen (Radix Ginseng), 3-9g
Bai Zhu (Rhizoma Atractylodis Macrocephalae), 9g
Fu Ling (Poria), 12g
Chen Pi (Pericarpium Citri Reticulatae), 6g
Ban Xia (Rhizoma Pinelliae), 9g
mix-fried *Gan Cao* (Radix Glycyrrhizae), 6-9g

If there is pronounced abdominal distention, add *Da Fu Pi* (Pericarpium Arecae) and uncooked *Sheng Jiang Pi* (Cortex Rhizomatis Zingiberis) to warm the center and move the qi. If there is chest oppression and wheezing with difficulty breathing when lying down, add *Ting Li Zi* (Semen Descurianiae) and *Xing Ren* (Semen Armeniacae) to precipitate lung water.

Acupuncture & moxibustion: *Pi Shu* (Bl 20), *San Jiao Shu* (Bl 22), *Shui Fen* (CV 9), *Zu San Li* (St 36), *Yin Ling Quan* (Sp 9)

Kidney yang vacuity

Main symptoms: As the months of pregnancy increase, there is facial edema, swelling of the limbs, heart palpitations, shortness of breath, low back and knee soreness and limpness, frequent but scant urination, lack of warmth in the four limbs, a dark, dusky facial complexion, a pale, moist tongue with white, glossy fur, and a deep, weak, slippery pulse

Treatment principles: Warm the kidneys, invigorate yang, and move water

Guiding formulas:

Zhen Wu Tang (True Warrior Decoction)
Zhi Fu Zi (Radix Lateralis Praeparatus Aconiti Carmichaeli), 3-9g
Fu Ling (Poria), 12g
stir-fried *Bai Zhu* (Rhizoma Atractylodis Macrocephalae), 9g
Bai Shao (Radix Albus Paeoniae Lactiflorae), 9-18g
Sheng Jiang (uncooked Rhizoma Zingiberis), 6g

Ling Gui Zhu Gan Tang Jia Wei
(Poria, Cinnamon, Atractylodes & Licorice Decoction with Added Flavors)
Gui Zhi (Ramulus Cinnamomi), 6-9g
stir-fried *Bai Zhu* (Rhizoma Atractylodis Macrocephalae), 9g
Fu Ling (Poria), 12g
mix-fried *Gan Cao* (Radix Glycyrrhizae), 6-9g
Bu Gu Zhi (Fructus Psoraleae), 9-12g
Du Zhong (Cortex Eucommiae), 9-15g
stir-fried *Ze Xie* (Rhizoma Alismatis), 6-9g
Chen Pi (Pericarpium Citri Reticulatae), 6g

Shen Qi Wan (Kidney Qi Pills)
Shu Di (cooked Radix Rehmanniae), 12-15g
Shan Yao (Radix Dioscoreae), 9-12g
Ze Xie (Rhizoma Alismatis), 6-9g
Fu Ling (Poria), 9-12g
Shan Zhu Yu (Fructus Corni), 9-15g
Dan Pi (Cortex Moutan), 6-9g
Zhi Fu Zi (Radix Lateralis Praeparatus Aconiti Carmichaeli), 3-9g
Rou Gui (Cortex Cinnamomi), 3-9g

Acupuncture & moxibustion: *Shen Shu* (Bl 23), *San Jiao Shu* (Bl 22), *Qi Hai* (CV 6), *San Yin Jiao* (Sp 6)

Qi stagnation & phlegm obstruction

Main symptoms: After 3-4 months of pregnancy and especially in the last trimester, there is swelling and distention of the whole body with both feet edematous and swollen. There are also dizziness, distention and pain of the head, chest oppression, rib-side distention, heart palpitations, heart vexation, easy anger, shortness of breath, inhibited urination, a somber, pale facial complexion, thick, slimy tongue fur, and a bowstring, slippery pulse.

Treatment principles: Regulate the qi and move stagnation

Guiding formula:

Fu Ling Dao Shui Tang Jia Jian
(Poria Abduct Water Decoction with Additions & Subtractions)
Fu Ling (Poria), 9-12g
Bai Zhu (Rhizoma Atractylodis Macrocephalae), 9g
Zhu Ling (Polyporus), 9-12g
Sha Ren (Fructus Amomi), 3-4.5g
Mu Xiang (Radix Auklandiae), 6-9g
Chen Pi (Pericarpium Citri Reticulatae), 6g
Su Gen (Caulis Perillae Frutescentis), 9-15g
Da Fu Pi (Pericarpium Arecae), 6-9g
Sang Bai Pi (Cortex Mori), 9g
Mu Gua (Fructus Chaenomelis), 9g

Acupuncture & moxibustion: Tai Chong (Liv 3), *He Gu* (LI 4), *San Yin Jiao* (Sp 6), *Feng Long* (St 40), *Zhong Wan* (CV 12), *Nei Guan* (Per 6), *Yang Ling Quan* (GB 34)

Remarks:

Edema of the lower extremities during the last trimester is considered normal as long as it is unaccompanied by other discomfort and as long as gynecological examination reveals no other abnormalities. Generally, one should begin treatment using a formula that disinhibits water, such as *Fu Ling Dao Shui Tang* (Poria Abduct Water Decoction). After water dampness has been eliminated, then one can switch to a spleen-fortifying, qi-boosting formula, such as *Liu Jun Zi Tang* (Six Gentlemen Decoction) or *Bu Zhong Yi Qi Tang* (Supplement the Center & Boost the Qi Decoction) to secure and consolidate the therapeutic results. Women suffering from or prone to edema during pregnancy should reduce their intake of salty, fatty foods, should not drink chilled water with meals, and should not eat chilled, uncooked foods. Frequent urine tests and blood pressure readings are also suggested to detect and prevent eclampsia.

11

Polyhydramnios

At full term, usually the amount of amniotic fluid is around 1000ml. However, in some women, the amount becomes excessive. This is referred to as polyhydramnios or excessive amniotic fluid in Western medicine. In some cases it may reach 2000 ml. Generally, this becomes a problem in the 7-10th months. Increased amniotic fluid may be due to either increased production or decreased removal. Although this condition may be associated with fetal gastrointestinal anomalies or maternal diabetes mellitus, many cases are idiopathic. For instance, gestational diabetes is complicated by polyhydramnios in 29% of cases.[1] Polyhydramnios may cause premature labor, placenta abruptio praecox, or excessive postpartum bleeding. Recently, repeated amniocentesis reduction has been used to treat this condition.

Chinese medical disease categorization

Excessive amniotic fluid is referred to as *yang shui guo duo*, excessive sheep water. Traditionally, this condition corresponds to *zi man*, fullness while with child or child fullness.

Disease causes & disease mechanisms

This condition is mostly due to insufficiency of spleen and/or kidney yang. During pregnancy, if the fetal body becomes excessively large, this obstructs and hinders the spleen's function of promoting the movement of water fluids and/or the kidney qi's transformation. This results in water dampness collecting and accumulating. If these damp evils stagnate and accumulate inside the uterus, it results in excessive amniotic fluid.

Patterns common to this condition

Spleen-kidney yang vacuity
Lifegate fire debility

Treatment based on pattern discrimination:

Spleen-kidney yang vacuity

Main symptoms: During the last trimester, the abdominal area may become excessively large. There is stuffiness and oppression inside the chest causing difficulty breathing, panting and wheezing, cyanotic lips and cheeks, swollen and edematous external genitalia, generalized edema, short, scanty urination, constipation, a pale tongue with thin, white, moist fur, and a slippery pulse.

Treatment principles: Fortify the spleen and boost the kidneys, disinhibit water and disperse swelling

Guiding formulas:

Wu Pi Yin Jia Jian **(Five Skins Drink with Additions & Subtractions)**
Bai Zhu (Rhizoma Atractylodis Macrocephalae), 9g
Fu Ling (Poria), 9-12g
Da Fu Pi (Pericarpium Arecae), 6-9g
Jiang Pi (Cortex Rhizomatis Zingiberis), 6-9g
Chen Pi (Pericarpium Citri Reticulatae), 6g
Gui Zhi (Ramulus Cinnamomi), 6-9g
Tu Si Zi (Semen Cuscutae), 9g
Zhu Ling (Polyporus), 9-12g

Wu Ling San Jia Wei
(Five [Ingredients] Poria Powder with Added Flavors)
Huang Qi (Radix Astragali), 9-18g
scorched *Bai Zhu* (Rhizoma Atractylodis Macrocephalae), 9g
Fu Ling (Poria), 12g
Jiang Pi (Cortex Rhizomatis Zingiberis), 6-9g
Da Fu Pi (Pericarpium Arecae), 6-9g
Zhu Ling (Polyporus), 9-12g
Ze Xie (Rhizoma Alismatis), 9g
Gui Zhi (Ramulus Cinnamomi), 6-9g
Tu Si Zi (Semen Cuscutae), 9g
Mu Xiang (Radix Auklandiae), 6-9g
Sha Ren (Fructus Amomi), 3-4.5g

Fu Ling Dao Shui Tang **(Poria Abduct Water Decoction)**
Fu Ling (Poria), 12g

Zhu Ling (Polyporus), 9-12g
Ze Xie (Rhizoma Alismatis), 9g
Bing Lang (Semen Arecae), 6-9g
Mu Xiang (Radix Auklandiae), 6-9g
Da Fu Pi (Pericarpium Arecae), 6-9g
Sha Ren (Fructus Amomi), 3-4.5g
Sang Bai Pi (Cortex Mori), 9g
Bai Zhu (Rhizoma Atractylodis Macrocephalae), 9g
Mu Gua (Fructus Chaenomelis), 9g
Zi Su Zi (Fructus Perillae Frutescentis), 9-12g

In terms of all the above formulas, spleen vacuity is primary and kidney yang vacuity is secondary and not very prominent.

Life gate fire debility

Main symptoms: An abnormally enlarged abdomen, superficial edema of the whole body, chest oppression, rapid breathing, if severe, inability to lie down flat, fear of cold, chilled limbs, a somber white facial complexion, lower and upper back aching and weakness, scanty, white-colored urination, a pale, fat tongue with thin fur, and a deep, fine, forceless pulse

Note: In the case of this pattern, kidney yang vacuity is marked and primary and spleen vacuity is negligible if present at all.

Treatment principles: Supplement the kidneys and warm yang, transform the qi and move water

Guiding formula:

**Jin Gui Shen Qi Wan Jia Wei
(Golden Cabinet Kidney Qi Pills with Added Flavors)**
Zhi Fu Zi (Radix Lateralis Praeparatus Aconiti Carmichaeli), 3-9g
Rou Gui (Cortex Cinnamomi), 6-9g
Shan Yao (Radix Dioscoreae), 9-12g
Fu Ling (Poria), 9-12g
Shan Zhu Yu (Fructus Corni), 9g
Shu Di (cooked Radix Rehmanniae), 12-15g
Dan Pi (Cortex Moutan), 6-9g
Che Qian Zi (Semen Plantaginis), 9g
Da Fu Pi (Pericarpium Arecae), 6-9g
Jiang Pi (Cortex Rhizomatis Zingiberis), 6-9g

If qi and yin are both vacuous, add *Nu Zhen Zi* (Fructus Ligustri Lucidi) and *Tian Dong* (Tuber Asparagi).

Acupuncture & moxibustion: See preceding chapter on edema during pregnancy.

Abstract of representative Chinese research:

From "The Treatment of Acute Excessive Amniotic Fluid Using *Ling Gui Zhu Gan Tang Jia Wei* (Poria, Cinnamon, Atractylodes & Licorice Decoction with Added Flavors)" by Chu Guan-jin & Yue Jia-yi, *Shang Hai Zhong Yi Yao Za Zhi (Shanghai Journal of Chinese Medicine & Medicinals)*, #11, 1993, p. 22-23

Cohort description:

The authors report that they had treated 32 cases of acute excessive amniotic fluid with *Ling Gui Zhu Gan Tang Jia Wei* between 1980-1989. The ages of these 32 cases ranged from 24-35 years. Twenty-four were between 24-30 and eight were between 31-35, with most of these being between 28-30. Twenty-eight were primiparas and the rest were multiparas. The onset of this condition typically manifested between the 4-6th months of pregnancy, with 24 of these women developing this condition in the 5th month. Symptoms of this condition included abnormal enlargement of the abdomen, fullness and oppression of the chest and diaphragm, forced, urgent breathing, and dyspnea counterflow which, in severe cases, prohibited lying flat. Twenty-five of the women in this study also had edematous swelling of their lower extremities and external genitalia, while seven cases had generalized edema. These women's tongues were pale and fat with white, slimy fur, and their pulses were deep, slippery, and forceful.

Treatment method:

The formula consisted of: *Gui Zhi* (Ramulus Cinnamomi), 5g, *Fu Ling* (Poria), 12g, *Bai Zhu* (Rhizoma Atractylodis Macrocephalae), 12g, *Dang Gui* (Radix Angelicae Sinensis), 10g, *Bai Shao* (Radix Albus Paeoniae Lactiflorae), 10g, *Sheng Jiang Pi* (uncooked Cortex Rhizomatis Zingiberis), 5g, *Da Fu Pi* (Pericarpium Arecae), 10g, *Sang Bai Pi* (Cortex Mori), 10g, *Gan Cao* (Radix Glycyrrhizae), 5g, and carp, 1 tailpart (*i.e.*, approximately 1/2 kilo with viscera removed). These were added to a suitable amount of water and decocted into soup. The medicinals were removed and the remaining liquid was divided into two drinks per day. If there was severe abdominal distention, *Ze Xie* (Rhizoma Alismatis), 10g, and *Che Qian Zi* (Semen Plantaginis, wrapped during decoction), 10g, were added. If there was lassitude of the spirit and lack of strength with qi vacuity, *Huang Qi* (Radix Astragali), 15g, was added. If there was kidney vacuity with low backache, *Tu Si Zi* (Semen Cuscutae) and *Sang Ji Sheng* (Herba Taxilli), 12g each, were added. If the face was whitish and there was blood vacuity, Gelatinum Corii Asini (*E Jiao*), 10g, and *He Shou Wu* (Radix Polygoni Multiflori), 10g, were added. And if there was severe, urgent dyspneic breathing, *Xing Ren* (Semen Armeniacae), 10g, was added.

Treatment outcomes:

After seven days of treatment, 22 cases were cured, meaning that their symptoms disappeared. After 15 days, another seven cases were cured. However, three cases experienced no result after 15 days of treatment.

Representative case history:

The patient was a 28 year-old married worker who had been married since she was 22. Two years previous, she had been pregnant. However, during her fifth month, she had developed polyhydramnios, the fetus died *in utero*, and labor was induced. Now she was six months pregnant and had developed a sensation of distention in her abdomen which was difficult to bear. This had gone on for one week without healing and was accompanied by slight edema of the lower extremities. Her intake was torpid and her two excretions were scanty. Gynecological examination diagnosed polyhydramnios again, and the fetal heart tones were faint and weak. The woman was advised to terminate her pregnancy. However, she refused to do so. Over the next week, her symptoms increased; they did not decrease. When the woman was seen on Aug. 26, 1980, the woman was not able to sleep lying down, there was generalized bodily heaviness, torpid intake, and a bland, tastelessness in her mouth. Her facial complexion was somber white and there was abdominal drum distention as if nine months pregnant. Fetal heart tones were faint and weak, her tongue was pale white and moist, and her pulse was slippery and rapid but forceless with heavy pressure.

Based on the above signs and symptoms, it was decided that it was necessary to fortify the spleen and move water, nourish the blood and quiet the fetus, for which the following formula was prescribed: *Dang Shen* (Radix Codonopsitis) and *Fu Ling* (Poria), 30g each, *Bai Zhu* (Rhizoma Atractylodis Macrocephalae) and *Sheng Jiang* (uncooked Rhizoma Zingiberis), 15g each, *Da Fu Pi* (Pericarpium Arecae), *Dang Gui* (Radix Angelicae Sinensis), and *Bai Shao* (Radix Albus Paeoniae Lactiflorae), 10g each, and carp (*Li Yu*), 500g. These medicinals were decocted together, the fish was removed, and the liquid was reserved. Then the liquid was administered while warm.

The patient was seen again on Aug. 29 after having taken three packets of the above formula. Her abdominal distention was greatly reduced and her appetite was good. Her two excretions were freely and easily flowing. Fetal heart tones were now normal. After this, the woman was advised to drink a soup made from 30 grams each of *Dang Shen* and *Fu Ling* with one carp, afterwards also eating the carp. A half month later, the woman had returned to normal. In November, the patient gave birth normally to a healthy baby boy.

Remarks:

As the above Chinese research and case history suggest, Chinese medicine can, at least in some cases, treat polyhydramnios.

Endnote:

[1] Gilbert, William M., "Anatomy and Physiology of the Placenta, Fetal Membranes, and Amniotic Fluid," *Gynecology & Obstetrics: A Longitudinal Approach, op. cit.*, p. 221

12

Lower Limb Cramping & Pain During Pregnancy

Lower limb cramping and pain during pregnancy is not a disease category in Western medicine. However, it can be in Chinese medical gynecology. Usually, this condition is experienced as involuntary cramping of the calf muscles at night and not infrequently during sleep.

Chinese medical disease categorization

Lower leg cramping and pain during pregnancy are referred to in Chinese as *ren shen xia zhi ji tong*.

Disease causes & disease mechanisms

There is only one main disease mechanism in Chinese medicine for this condition and it is malnourishment of the sinew vessels. The liver stores the blood and the liver rules the sinews. During the later stage of pregnancy, blood gathers and nourishes the fetus. If blood is vacuous, this may lead to the sinews not being nourished and this may result in spasms and pain of the lower limbs. At the same time, during the later stage of pregnancy, the uterus enlarges. Thus the blood vessels in the lower limbs are affected and cannot transport and move smoothly.

Treatment based on pattern discrimination:

Blood vacuity malnourishing the sinews

Main symptoms: In the later stage of pregnancy, the foot or lower leg may have cramps and pain. If severe, this may reach the upper leg and buttocks and there may be difficulty walking. Commonly, this worsens at night or during sleep. The tongue is somewhat pale with thin fur, and the pulse is fine.

Treatment principles: Nourish the blood, emolliate the sinews, and relax cramping

Guiding formula:

Shao Yao Gan Cao Tang (Peony & Licorice Decoction)
Bai Shao (Radix Albus Paeoniae Lactiflorae), 18g
mix-fried *Gan Cao (*Radix Glycyrrhizae), 9g

These ingredients can generally be added to other formulas if leg cramps complicate other conditions during pregnancy.

13

Lower Limb Varicose Veins During Pregnancy

Similar to lower limb cramping and pain during pregnancy, lower limb varicose veins during pregnancy are also not considered a separate disease in Western medicine. Nevertheless, they are a common complaint. They are due to the systemic hypervolemia of pregnancy complicated by mechanical pressure from the growing fetus on the veins in the lower abdomen thus affecting the venous return in the lower legs. Other than staying off one's feet and shunning of restrictive clothing on the lower half of the body, Western medicine has no particular treatment for varicose veins during pregnancy.

Chinese medical disease categorization

Varicose veins of the lower limbs during pregnancy are referred to in Chinese as *ren shen xia zhi jing mai qu zhang*.

Disease causes & disease mechanisms

Varicose veins in the lower limbs during pregnancy which typically appear and become more numerous as one gets closer to delivery are due to the fetal child's gradual enlargement. This puts pressure on the blood vessels. This then leads to the blood aspect in the lower limbs becoming depressed and stagnant. Therefore, the pressure in the network vessels become elevated and there is the onset of distention and pain. Thus the main disease mechanism of varicose veins during pregnancy is blood stasis. However, because the kidney qi governs the low back and lower limbs and because the spleen qi upbears and lifts, women with severe varicosities typically also suffer from spleen and kidney vacuities which allow the blood stasis to occur.

Treatment based on pattern discrimination:

Blood stasis complicated by spleen-kidney dual vacuity

Main symptoms: Distended, painful, tortuous, dark-colored veins in the lower legs accompanied by fatigue, lack of strength, and low back pain

Guiding formula:

Unnamed experiential formula
Du Zhong (Cortex Eucommiae), 9-15g
Xu Duan (Radix Dipsaci), 9g
Gou Ji (Rhizoma Cibotii), 9g
Wu Wei Zi (Fructus Schisandrae), 9g
Huang Qi (Radix Astragali), 9-18g
Bai Zhu (Rhizoma Atractylodis Macrocephalae), 9g
Bai Shao (Radix Albus Paeoniae Lactiflorae), 9-18g
Dang Gui (Radix Angelicae Sinensis), 9g
processed *He Shou Wu* (Radix Polygoni Multiflori), 9-15g
Si Gua Luo (Retinervus Luffae Cylindricae), 9-15g
Chen Pi (Pericarpium Citri Reticulatae), 6g

Representative case history:

The patient was a 31 year-old, married female whose initial examination occurred in July 1959. This woman had been pregnant for three months. Her facial complexion was a somber white and her affect was haggard and dull. When pressed, her pulse was slippery and forceless, while her tongue was pale with thin, moist fur. The veins on her lower legs were elevated and engorged like earthworms. These were purplish black in color. When these were pressed by hand or during bending and contraction, they were severely painful. In addition, the lower limbs also felt heavy. At the same time, eating and drinking were devitalized, the patient felt psychologically tired and weak, and her lower back sometimes felt sore and distressed. Urination was frequent and numerous. When the area of the fetus was pressed, it felt comparatively weak, and the lower abdomen had a sensation of downward sagging. This pattern was connected to kidney qi vacuity weakness, with lower limb qi and blood stasis and stagnation. Treatment, therefore, was in order to secure the kidneys and boost the qi, nourish the blood and quicken the network vessels. The formula prescribed consisted of:

Du Zhong (Cortex Eucommiae), 9g, *Xu Duan* (Radix Dipsaci), 9g, *Gou Ji* (Rhizoma Cibotii), 9g, *Wu Wei Zi* (Fructus Schisandrae), 4.5g, *Huang Qi* (Radix Astragali), 9g, *Bai Zhu* (Rhizoma Atractylodis Macrocephalae), 6g, *Bai Shao* (Radix Albus Paeoniae Lactiflorae), 9g, *Dang Gui* (Radix Angelicae Sinensis), 6g, processed *He Shou Wu* (Radix Polygoni Multiflori), 9g, *Si Gua Luo* (Retinervus Luffae Cylindricae), 9g, and *Chen Pi* (Pericarpium Citri Reticulatae), 6g

After administering six packets of the above formula with additions and subtractions, the low back soreness and generalized symptoms were diminished. The varicose veins in the lower leg area were also good. The heavy feeling in the lower abdomen and the lower legs had disappeared. Because the pattern had turned for the better, the treatment methods which were then used were to supplement the qi and boost the blood, fortify the spleen and quicken the network vessels: *Dang Shen* (Radix Codonopsitis), 6g, *Shan Yao* (Radix Dioscoreae), 9g, *Bai Zhu* (Rhizoma Atractylodis Macrocephalae), 6g, *Fu Ling* (Poria), 9g, *Chen Pi* (Pericarpium Citri Reticulatae), 6g, *Wu Wei Zi* (Fructus Schisandrae), 2.4g, stir-fried *Zhi Ke* (Fructus Aurantii), 3g, and *Du Zhong* (Cortex Eucommiae), 9g.

Remarks:

1. Varicose veins during pregnancy only typically require remedial treatment if severe. Otherwise, they spontaneously remit after delivery.

2. *Si Gua Luo* is empirically specific for varicose veins in the lower limbs.

14

Pruritic Urticarial Papules & Plaques of Pregnancy

Pruritic urticarial papules and plaques of pregnancy (PUPP) are a common pruritic eruption of unknown etiology which occur during pregnancy. These consist of intensely itchy, erythematous, hive-like papules and plaques which typically begin on the abdomen and spread to the thighs, buttocks, and, occassionally, to the arms. Some of these lesions may have minute vesicles in their center and there are often white halos surrounding the papules. These lesions most often occur in the last 2-3 weeks of pregnancy, and sometimes in the last several days. However, they may begin any time during the third trimester. Because of the intense itching, the patient's sleep may be disturbed. Nevertheless, the eruption usually resolves spontaneously after delivery and does not usually recur in subsequent pregnancies. Western medical treatment consists of topical corticosteroids and, when necessary, orally administered steroids as well.

Another type of pruritic dermatological condition which occurs during pregnancy is herpes gestationis. These lesions tend to be polymorphic and also intensely itchy. Typically, there are vesicles and bullae, and, like PUPP, these lesions often start on the abdomen and spread from there. These lesions may be annular similar to herpes zoster or simplex, thus the name. However, the term herpes is a misnomer since this eruption is not associated with the herpes virus or any other virus for that matter. This condition usually begins in the second or third trimesters, probably due to autoimmune factors. The eruption commonly worsens immediately postpartum but remits within a few weeks to a few months of delivery. Unlike PUPP, herpes gestationis often does recur in subsequent pregnancies or with oral contraceptive use. Western medical treatment of this condition is similar to PUPP in that it relies on topical and possibly oral use of corticosteroids. Fortunately, this condition is extremely uncommon, occurring in one in 50,000 pregnancies.

Chinese medical disease categorization

These conditions are referred to as *ren shen pi fu yang* in Chinese.

Disease causes & disease mechanisms

There are two main disease mechanisms of itching during pregnancy according to Chinese medicine. These are damp heat and blood vacuity. After conception, the blood gathers to nourish the fetus. Since the blood and fluids share a common source, water fluids in the body also increase. These may collect and transform into damp evils. If these damp evils cause depression to transform heat, damp heat may be engendered internally. This damp heat steams the skin and may cause itching, especially if there is concomitant blood vacuity. On the other hand, if there is habitual bodily blood vacuity or essence blood insufficiency, blood vacuity may engender wind transforming dryness, thus also giving rise to itching.

Patterns common to this condition

Damp heat
Blood vacuity

Treatment based on pattern discrimination:

Damp heat

Main symptoms: Itching of the skin around the body which is worse when hot or at night, if severe, difficulty sleeping at night, dizziness, torpid intake, lack of strength of the four limbs, a dry mouth but no desire to drink, yellow urination, constipation, a pale red tongue with slimy, yellow fur, and a bowstring, rapid pulse

Treatment principles: Nourish the blood and clear heat, eliminate dampness and stop itching

Guiding formula:

Unnamed experiential formula
Yin Chen Hao (Herba Capillaris), 9-15g
Fu Ling (Poria), 12g
Zhu Ling (Polyporus), 9-12g
Ze Xie (Rhizoma Alismatis), 9g
Bai Zhu (Rhizoma Atractylodis Macrocephalae), 9g
Ku Shen (Radix Sophorae Flavescentis), 9g
Bai Xian Pi (Cortex Dictamni), 9g
Dang Gui (Radix Angelicae Sinensis), 9g
Chuan Xiong (Radix Ligustici Wallichii), 6-9g
Bai Shao (Radix Albus Paeoniae Lactiflorae), 9-18g
Sheng Di (uncooked Radix Rehmanniae), 12-15g

Di Gu Pi (Cortex Lycii), 9g
Jing Jie (Herba Schizonepetae), 6-9g
Huang Qin (Radix Scutellariae), 9-12g

Blood vacuity

Main symptoms: Dryness and itching of the skin around the body, many scratch marks, restless sleep at night, dizziness, tinnitus, lassitude of the spirit, lack of strength, low back and knee soreness and limpness, a lusterless facial complexion, no flavor when eating grains, a somewhat pale, fat tongue with thin, white fur, and a fine, slippery pulse

Treatment principles: Nourish the blood and extinguish wind, dispel wind and stop itching

Guiding formula:

Unnamed experiential formula
Sheng Di (uncooked Radix Rehmanniae), 12-15g
Bai Shao (Radix Albus Paeoniae Lactiflorae), 9-18g
Lu Dou Yi (Testa Munginis), 9-15g
Bai Ji Li (Fructus Tribuli), 9-15g
Fang Feng (Radix Sapshnikoviae), 9g
Tai Zi Shen (Radix Pseudostellariae), 9g
Shan Yao (Radix Dioscoreae), 9-12g
Ye Jiao Teng (Caulis Polygoni Multiflori), 9-15g
Gan Cao (uncooked Radix Glycyrrhizae), 3-6g
Gou Teng (Ramulus Uncariae Cum Uncis), 9-15g
Wu Mei (Fructus Mume), 6-9g

Remarks:

If there is urticaria-like angioedema or fluid-filled vesicles and the lesions are also red, there is damp heat. In fact, damp heat is the main disease mechanism of both PUPP and herpes gestationis. Itching during pregnancy associated with blood vacuity tends not to be given a Western medical name.

15
Colds & Flus
During Pregnancy

Any woman might catch a cold or flu during pregnancy. In Chinese medicine, it is believed that, if one catches a cold while pregnant, one must use medicinals that clear heat and harmonize the fetus at the same time as eliminating the evil qi. Thus this condition is considered an obstetrical one in Chinese gynecology and this category of disease is often dealt with as a separate chapter in Chinese gynecology texts.

Chinese medical disease categorization

Cold and flus during pregnancy are referred to as *ren shen shan han*, damage [due to] cold during pregnancy.

Disease causes & disease mechanisms

External contraction of wind evils. In Chinese medicine, maturation and development is due to warm transformation, *i.e.*, the transformation of yin substance by yang qi. Therefore, in general, maturation and development are thought of as a kind of cooking (*cheng re*). As an extension of this conceit, women's ministerial fire tends to be exuberant during pregnancy in order to cook or mature and develop the fetus. Hence, women are especially likely to transform heat if any evil qi become depressed in the body, and, although more than usual heat is required to mature and develop the fetus, too much heat is a main cause of damage to the fetus. Thus the importance of clearing heat and harmonizing the fetus in the treatment of cold damage conditions during pregnancy.

Patterns common to this condition

Tai yang aspect disease
Shao yang aspect disease
Tai yin aspect disease

Treatment based on pattern discrimination:

Tai yang aspect disease

Main symptoms: Acute onset and recent contraction of disease, fear of cold, headache, fever, and a floating, slippery pulse

Treatment principles: Course wind and resolve the exterior, clear heat and harmonize the fetus

Guiding formula:

Si Wei Zi Su He Tai Yin (Four Flavors Perilla Harmonize the Fetus Drink)
Zi Su Ye (Folium Perillae Frutescentis), 9-12g
Huang Qin (Radix Scutellariae), 9-12g
Bai Zhu (Rhizoma Atractylodis Macrocephalae), 9g
Gan Cao (Radix Glycyrrhizae), 3-9g

If there is marked stiff neck with upper back pain, add *Qiang Huo* (Radix Et Rhizoma Notopterygii), *Gao Ben* (Rhizoma Ligustici), *Chuan Xiong* (Radix Ligustici Wallichii), *Fang Feng* (Radix Sapshnikoviae), *Cong Bai* (Bulbus Allii Fistulosi), and *Sheng Jiang* (uncooked Rhizoma Zingiberis). If there is no fever, slight headache, a dry nose, and possible stiff neck, add *Ge Gen* (Radix Puerariae), *Bai Zhi* (Radix Angelicae Dahuricae), *Fang Feng* (Radix Sapshnikoviae), *Cong Bai* (Bulbus Allii Fistulosi), and *Dan Dou Chi* (Semen Praeparatus Sojae). If there is fever and fear of cold with pronounced coughing, add *Ma Huang* (Herba Ephedrae), *Xing Ren* (Semen Armeniacae), *Cong Bai* (Bulbus Allii Fistulosi), and *Sheng Jiang* (uncooked Rhizoma Zingiberis).

Shao yang aspect disease

Main symptoms: Alternating hot and cold, *i.e.*, fever and chills, dizziness, vomiting, vexation below the heart, chest and rib-side fullness and distention, white fur on one half of the tongue and yellow fur on the other half, and a bowstring, slippery pulse

Treatment principles: Harmonize the constructive and defensive, clear heat and harmonize the fetus

Guiding formula:

Si Wei Zi Su He Tai Yin Jia Wei
(Four Flavors Perilla Harmonize the Fetus Drink with Added Flavors)
Zi Su Ye (Folium Perillae Frutescentis), 9-12g
Huang Qin (Radix Scutellariae), 9-12g
Bai Zhu (Rhizoma Atractylodis Macrocephalae), 9g
Gan Cao (Radix Glycyrrhizae), 3-9g
Chai Hu (Radix Bupleuri), 9g
Ren Shen (Radix Ginseng), 3-9g

If there is chest and flank fullness, add *Zhi Ke* (Fructus Aurantii) and *Jie Geng* (Radix Platycodi). If there is dizziness, add *Chuan Xiong* (Radix Ligustici Wallichii), *Sheng Jiang* (uncooked Rhizoma Zingiberis), and *Da Zao* (Fructus Jujubae).

Tai yin aspect disease

Main symptoms: Fear of cold, no fever, abdominal pain, vomiting, diarrhea, no thirst, and the hands and feet have counterflow chill

Treatment principles: Course wind and warm the spleen, clear heat and harmonize the fetus

Guiding formula:

Si Wei Zi Su He Tai Yin Jia Wei
(Four Flavors Perilla Harmonize the Fetus Drink with Added Flavors)
Su Ye (Folium Perillae Frutescentis), 9-12g
Huang Qin (Radix Scutellariae), 9-12g
Bai Zhu (Rhizoma Atractylodis Macrocephalae), 9g
Gan Cao (Radix Glycyrrhizae), 3-9g
Ren Shen (Radix Ginseng), 3-9g
Gan Jiang (dry Rhizoma Zingiberis), 3-6g
wine stir-fried *Bai Shao* (Radix Albus Paeoniae Lactiflorae), 9-18g
Sheng Jiang (uncooked Rhizoma Zingiberis), 6g
Da Zao (Fructus Jujubae), 6-9g

Remarks:

The main reasons for including this condition in this book is to emphasize the tendency to transform heat during pregnancy and the importance of harmonizing or quieting the fetus. The above formulas are all premodern ones recommended by Wan Mi-zhai in his *Wan Shi Fu Ren Ke (Master Wan's Gynecology)*. Contemporary practitioners may choose different formulas with different ingredients. However, practitioners should note that *Zi Su Ye*, *Bai Zhu*, and *Huang Qin* are all famous spirit-quieting medicinals no matter whatever else they do. Therefore, they are especially appropriate during pregnancy.

16

Cough During Pregnancy

A woman may develop a cough for a variety of reasons during pregnancy. As with some of the other preceding conditions, many Chinese gynecological texts consider cough an obstetrical condition when it occurs during pregnancy.

Chinese medical disease categorization

Coughing during pregnancy which will not stop and may occur in any of the four seasons is called *zi sou*, child cough, or *ren shen ke sou*, coughing during pregnancy.

Disease causes & disease mechanisms

Coughing during pregnancy may be due to external contraction of wind cold evils which disturb the lungs' depurative downbearing. Although these external evils may begin as wind cold, they typically transform into heat evils within the body based on Liu Wan-su's law of similar transformation and the fact that women's yang qi tends to be exuberant during gestation. Cough may also be due to habitual bodily yin vacuity that becomes exacerbated during pregnancy. In this case, vacuity heat flames upwards, harassing the lungs' network vessels. Thus lungs lose their normal control of descending and downbearing. On the other hand, if the spleen and stomach become vacuous and weak, movement and transformation may lose their normalcy. In that case, phlegm fluids may stagnate and accumulate and again upbearing and downbearing may lose their normalcy, giving rise to upward counterflow of qi and coughing. Thus Ye Heng-yin states, "[Cough due to] yin vacuity fire stirring, phlegm rheum counterflowing upward, and external contraction of wind cold are not the same."

Patterns common to this condition

External contraction of wind evils
Yin vacuity-lung dryness
Spleen vacuity with phlegm fluids
Kidneys not grasping the qi
Phlegm fire assailing the lungs

Treatment based on pattern discrimination:

External contraction of wind evils

Main symptoms: Cough during pregnancy, aversion to wind, fever, inhibited breathing, nasal congestion and/or runny nose, chest oppression, hoarseness, a somber white facial complexion with bilateral flushing of the cheeks, a moist tongue with thin, white fur, and a slippery, rapid pulse

Treatment principles: Clear heat and resolve the exterior, quiet the fetus and stop coughing

Guiding formulas:

Xing Su Jie Biao Tang (Armeniaca & Perilla Resolve the Exterior Decoction)
Xing Ren (Semen Armeniacae), 6-9g
Zi Su Ye (Folium Perillae Frutescentis), 9-12g
Qian Hu (Radix Peucedani), 6-9g
Jie Geng (Radix Platycodi), 6-9g
Zhi Ke (Fructus Aurantii), 6g
Mai Men Dong (Tuber Ophiopogonis), 9-12g
Chen Pi (Pericarpium Citri Reticulatae), 6g
Qing Pi (Pericarpium Citri Reticulatae Viride), 6g
Fu Ling (Poria), 9-12g
Gan Cao (Radix Glycyrrhizae), 3-9g
Sheng Jiang (uncooked Rhizoma Zingiberis), 6g
Da Zao (Fructus Jujubae), 6-9g

Jia Jian Shen Su Yin (Modified Ginseng & Perilla Drink)
Ren Shen (Radix Ginseng), 3-9g
Zi Su Ye (Folium Perillae Frutescentis), 9-12g
Chen Pi (Pericarpium Citri Reticulatae), 6g
Bai Fu Ling (Poria), 9-12g
Gan Cao (Radix Glycyrrhizae), 3-9g
Zhi Ke (Fructus Aurantii), 6g
Jie Geng (Radix Platycodi), 6-9g
Qian Hu (Radix Peucedani), 6-9g

Huang Qin (Radix Scutellariae), 9-12g
Bo He (Herba Menthae Haplocalycis), 3-9g

Acupuncture & moxibustion: *Lie Que* (Lu 7), *He Gu* (LI 4), *Wai Guan* (TB 5), *Feng Men* (Bl 12), *Fei Shu* (Bl 13)

Yin vacuity-lung dryness

Main symptoms: Repeated attacks of dry cough after conception, no expectoration or vomiting of phlegm, a dry, scratchy throat, hoarseness, chest oppression, tidal fever, night sweats, heat in the hands, feet, and heart, scanty, red urination, a red face and cheeks, a dry, red tongue with no fur, and a fine, rapid pulse

Treatment principles: Nourish yin and moisten the lungs, quiet the fetus and stop coughing

Guiding formulas:

***Bai He Gu Jin Tang* (Lily Secure Metal Decoction)**
Bai He (Bulbus Lilii), 9-12g
Sheng Di (uncooked Radix Rehmanniae), 12-15g
Shu Di (cooked Radix Rehmanniae), 12-15g
Xuan Shen (Radix Scrophulariae), 9-15g
Zhe Bei Mu (Bulbus Fritillariae Thunbergii), 6-9g
Jie Geng (Radix Platycodi), 6-9g
Mai Men Dong (Tuber Ophiopogonis), 9-12g
Bai Shao (Radix Albus Paeoniae Lactiflorae), 9g
Dang Gui (Radix Angelicae Sinensis), 9g
Gan Cao (Radix Glycyrrhizae), 3-9

Ren Shen Qing Fei Tang Jia Jian
(Ginseng Clear the Lungs Decoction with Additions & Subtractions)
Dang Shen (Radix Codonopsitis), 9-15g
E Jiao (Gelatinum Corii Asini), 6-9g
Sang Bai Pi (Cortex Mori), 9g
Di Gu Pi (Cortex Lycii), 9g
Zhi Mu (Rhizoma Anemarrhenae), 9g
Wu Mei (Fructus Mume), 6-9g
Xing Ren (Semen Armeniacae), 6-9g
Bai Bu (Radix Stemonae), 9g
uncooked *Gan Cao* (Radix Glycyrrhizae), 3-6g

This formula treats a qi and yin vacuity with more marked lung heat.

Acupuncture & moxibustion: *Lie Que* (Lu 7), *Zhao Hai* (Ki 6), *Fei Shu* (Bl 13), *Zhong Fu* (Lu 1)

If there are night sweats, add *Yin Xi* (Ht 6). If there is tidal flushing, add *Da Zhui* (GV 14). If there is concomitant kidney yin vacuity, add *San Yin Jiao* (Sp 6) and *Shen Shu* (Bl 23).

Spleen vacuity with phlegm fluids

Main symptoms: Coughing which will not stop after conception, occasional vomiting of phlegmy saliva, chest oppression, hasty breathing, more coughing when lying down and an inability to breathe when lying down, a somber white facial complexion, facial edema, a pale, moist tongue with white, slimy fur, and a slippery, moderate (*i.e.*, relaxed, slightly slow) pulse

Treatment principles: Fortify the spleen and wash away phlegm, quiet the fetus and stop coughing

Guiding formulas:

Liu Jun Zi Tang Jia Wei (Six Gentlemen Decoction with Added Flavors)
Ren Shen (Radix Ginseng), 3-9g
Bai Zhu (Rhizoma Atractylodis Macrocephalae), 9g
Fu Ling (Poria), 9-12g
Chen Pi (Pericarpium Citri Reticulatae), 6g
Ban Xia (Rhizoma Pinelliae), 9g
Gan Cao (Radix Glycyrrhizae), 3-9g
Jie Geng (Radix Platycodi), 6-9g
Zhi Ke (Fructus Aurantii), 6g

Acupuncture & moxibustion: *Feng Long* (St 40), *Zhong Wan* (CV 12), *Dan Zhong* (CV 17), *Fei Shu* (Bl 13), *Pi Shu* (Bl 20), *Wei Shu* (Bl 21)

Kidneys not grasping the qi

Main symptoms: Cough during pregnancy which had endured for days, no force in expectorating phlegm, chest oppression, shortness of breath, frequent urination, low back pain, abdominal sagging, a pale tongue with thin fur, and a bowstring, slippery pulse

Treatment principles: Warm the kidneys and grasp the qi, stop coughing and quiet the fetus

Guiding formula:

Qi Wei Zhe Qi Wan (Seven Flavors All the Qi Pills)
Shan Yao (Radix Dioscoreae), 9-15g
Shan Zhu Yu (Fructus Corni), 9-18g
Shu Di (cooked Radix Rehmanniae), 12-15g
Dan Pi (Cortex Moutan), 6-9g
Ze Xie (Rhizoma Alismatis), 6-9g
Fu Ling (Poria), 9-12g
Wu Wei Zi (Fructus Schisandrae), 9g

Acupuncture & moxibustion: *Shen Shu* (Bl 23), *Qi Hai* (CV 6), *Guan Yuan* (CV 4), *Zu San Li* (St 36), *Dan Zhong* (CV 17), *Fei Shu* (Bl 13)

Phlegm fire assailing the lungs

Main symptoms: Cough during pregnancy with expectoration of thick, sticky, yellow phlegm, a red facial complexion, a dry mouth, a somewhat red tongue with slimy, yellow fur, and a slippery, rapid pulse

Treatment principles: Clear metal and transform phlegm, stop coughing and quiet the fetus

Guiding formula:

Qing Jin Jiang Huo Tang Jia Jian
(Clear Metal & Downbear Fire Decoction with Additions & Subtractions)
Huang Qin (Radix Scutellariae), 9-12g
Xing Ren (Semen Armeniacae), 6-9g
Chuan Bei Mu (Bulbus Fritillariae Cirrhosae), 6-9g
Quan Gua Lou (Fructus Trichosanthis), 6-9g
Ju Hong (Exocarpium Citri Erythrocarpae), 6g
Jie Geng (Radix Platycodi), 6-9g
Sang Ye (Folium Mori), 9g
mix-fried *Pi Pa Ye* (Folium Eriobotryae), 9g
Qian Hu (Radix Peucedani), 6-9g

Acupuncture & moxibustion: Feng Long (St 40), *Chi Ze* (Lu 5), *He Gu* (LI 4), *Qu Chi* (LI 11), *Fei Shu* (Bl 13)

Abstract of representative Chinese research:

From "The Treatment of 56 Cases of Cough During Pregnancy with *Run Zao An Tai Tang* (Moisten Dryness & Quiet the Fetus Decoction)" by Shi Guo-ping, *Zhe Jiang Zhong Yi Za Zhi (Zhejiang Journal of Chinese Medicine)*, #1, 2002, p. 14

Cohort description:

Forty-two of the women in this study were 23-30 years old, and 14 were 31-38 years old. There were 44 primiparas and 12 multigravidas. The longest course of disease was three months and the shortest was four days. All the patients in this study suffered from an upper respiratory tract infection. This was accompanied by chronic laryngitis in 22 cases and chronic rhinitis in two cases. There was no statement of how long these women had been pregnant.

Treatment method:

Run Zao An Tai Tang was administered internally. This was composed of: *Shu Di* (cooked Radix Rehmanniae), 30g, *Sheng Di* (uncooked Radix Rehmanniae), 9g, *Yi Mu Cao* (Herba Leonuri), *Wu Wei Zi* (Fructus Schisandrae), and *E Jiao* (Gelatinum Corii Asini), 6g each, *Huang Qin* (Radix Scutellariae), 3g, *Mai Men Dong* (Tuber Ophiopogonis) and *Shan Zhu Yu* (Fructus Corni), 15g each. One packet was decocted in water two times and administered per day in two divided doses. During the time of treatment, all other medications were suspended unless there was clear-cut bacterial infection, in which case appropriate antibiotics were also administered.

Treatment outcomes:

After taking the above medicinals for 3-5 days, the cough remitted in all 56 cases. Therefore, the cure rate was 100%. If the patient's bodily condition was poor, an additional five packets were administered in order to secure the treatment effects.

Representative case history:

The patient was a 25 year-old married worker who was first examined on Jan. 12 of an undisclosed year. The patient had been pregnant for three months and had had a cough for seven days. The cough sounded phlegmy and was not crisp. There was also itching in the throat, aversion to cold, and tidal heat, chest and rib-side oppression and distention, nausea with a desire to vomit, thin, white tongue fur, and a slippery, rapid pulse. Based on these signs and symptoms, the patient's Chinese medical pattern was categorized as wind cold lodged in the lungs with phlegm and dampness internally brewing. Therefore, treatment should diffuse the lungs, course and scatter, and the following medicinals were prescribed: *Zi Su Ye* (Folium Perillae Frutescentis) and *Zi Su Gen* (Caulis Perillae Frutescentis), 6g each, *Qian Hu* (Radix Peucedani), *Huo Xiang* (Herba Pogostemonis), and *Pei Lan* (Herba Eupatorii Fortunei), 4.5g each, *Chen Pi* (Pericarpium Citri Reticulatae), 6g, processed *Ban Xia* (Rhizoma Pinelliae), 6g, ginger-processed *Zhu Ru* (Caulis Bambusae In Taeniis), 9g, *Bai Zhu* (Rhizoma Atractylodis Macrocephalae), 6g, mix-fried *Kuan Dong Hua* (Flos Farfarae), 9g, *Jie Geng* (Radix Platycodi), 6g, *Gan Cao* (Radix Glycyrrhizae) and *Zhe Bei Mu* (Bulbus Frtillariae Thunbergii), 3g each.

The second examination occurred on Jan. 15. After taking the above medicinals, the patient reported that the cold and heat had abated and her cough was now crisp. However, her eating and drinking were devitalized and she had slight low back pain. In order to prevent the previous formula from damaging the fetus and to quiet the fetus, the following medicinals were prescribed: scorched *Bai Zhu* (Rhizoma Atractylodis Macrocephalae), 6g, *Chen Pi* (Pericarpium Citri Reticulatae), 6g, *Jie Geng* (Radix Platycodi), 2.4g, *Sha Shen* (Radix Glehniae), 6g, mix-fried *Zi Wan* (Radix Asteris), 6g, mix-fried *Kuan Dong Hua* (Flos Farfarae), 6g, scorched *Shan Yao* (Radix Dioscoreae), 9g, *Du Zhong* (Cortex Eucommiae), 9g, *Xu Duan* (Radix Dipsaci), 9g, *Xing Ren* (Semen Armeniacae), 6g, and mix-fried *Gan Cao* (Radix Glycyrrhizae), 2.4g.

The third examination occurred on Jan. 18. The cough was cured and the phlegm had turned clear. The nausea and poor appetite were gone, but there was still low backache. Because the low back is the mansion of the kidneys, the following medicinals to secure the kidneys and nourish metal were prescribed: mix-fried *Kuan Dong Hua* (Flos Farfarae), 6g, mix-fried *Zi Wan* (Radix Asteris), 6g, *Mai Men Dong* (Tuber Ophiopogonis), 6g, *Zi Su Gen* (Caulis Perillae Frutescentis), 6g, *Bai Zhu* (Rhizoma Atractylodis Macrocephalae), 6g, *Bai Shao* (Radix Albus Paeoniae Lactiflorae), 6g, *Chen Pi* (Pericarpium Citri Reticulatae), 6g, *Tu Si Zi* (Semen

Cuscutae), 9g, *Fu Pen Zi* (Fructus Rubi), 9g, *Wu Wei Zi* (Fructus Schisandrae), 2.4g, and mix-fried *Gan Cao* (Radix Glycyrrhizae), 3g.

The fourth examination occurred on Jan. 21, after taking the previous medicinals, the patient reported that her chest oppression was gone and her cough was slight. However, she felt that the fetus was stirring restlessly and her low back was achy and uncomfortable. Therefore, the following medicinals were prescribed: *Pi Pa Ye* (Folium Eriobotryae), 6g, *Bai Bu* (Radix Stemonae), 9g, mix-fried *Zi Wan* (Radix Asteris), 6g, clam shell stir-fried *E Jiao* (Gelatinum Corii Asini), 9g, *Du Zhong* (Cortex Eucommiae), 9g, *Xu Duan* (Radix Dipsaci), 9g, *Wu Wei Zi* (Fructus Schisandrae), 2.4g, and *Zhu Ma Gen* (Radix Boehmeriae Niveae), 9g.

The fifth and final visit took place on Jan. 31. The phlegmy cough was completely stopped and there was only slight low backache. In order to secure the kidneys and quiet the fetus, the patient was prescribed the following medicinals: *Tai Zi Shen* (Radix Pseudostellariae), 4.5g, *Bai Zhu* (Rhizoma Atractylodis Macrocephalae), 6g, *Mai Men Dong* (Tuber Ophiopogonis), 6g, *Du Zhong* (Cortex Eucommiae), 9g, *Xu Duan* (Radix Dipsaci), 9g, *Tu Si Zi* (Semen Cuscutae), 9g, *Wu Wei Zi* (Fructus Schisandrae), 2.4g, *Shu Di* (cooked Radix Rehmanniae), 9g, *Fu Ling* (Poria), 9g, *Zhu Ma Gen* (Radix Boehmeriae Niveae), 9g, and *Nan Gua Di* (Pedunculus Melonis), 2 pieces.

Remarks:

Yin vacuity cough in the last trimester may be due to the physical size of the fetus pressing on the channels and vessels leading upward from the kidneys. Therefore, the upward flow of yin to the lungs is hindered and obstructed. In this case, the cough will spontaneously remit after delivery, but it may not go away during pregnancy even with correctly prescribed Chinese medicinal treatment.

17
Hoarseness During Pregnancy

Some women become hoarse during the last months of their pregnancy. Some pre-modern authors, such as Fu Qing-zhu, have felt that this condition does not require remedial treatment since it spontaneously resolves itself after parturition. Nevertheless, Han Bai-ling, a famous, now deceased contemporary Chinese gynecologist from Harbin in Heilongjiang, does give a differential diagnosis and treatments for this pathocondition.

Chinese medical disease categorization

Hoarseness during pregnancy is referred to as child aphonia or muteness while with child, *zi yin*, in Chinese medicine.

Disease causes & disease mechanisms

If this problem occurs during the 3rd-5th months of pregnancy, it may be due to external contraction of wind heat. In this case, wind heat evils disturb the lungs' function and the lungs lose their resonance. When this condition occurs during the last trimester, however, it is more often due to obstruction and exhaustion of the uterine vessels and network vessels. The uterine network vessels connect the uterus to the kidneys. The uterine vessel connects the uterus with the heart. As the fetus grows, it may put pressure on the uterine network vessels, thus occluding them. This is even more likely if kidney yin has become exhausted and, therefore, is less able to keep the uterine network vessels open and free-flowing against such pressure. In this case, kidney yin cannot travel upward to nourish the heart and lungs above. In addition, lung qi cannot travel downward to connect with and nourish the kidneys. This loss of communication between the lungs and kidneys results in loss of voice.

Patterns common to this condition

Yin vacuity
Lung qi blockage & obstruction
External contraction of wind heat

Treatment based on pattern discrimination:

Yin vacuity

Main symptoms: A tendency for the throat to be dry and scratchy, heart vexation, a dry mouth but no particular desire to drink, heat in the hands, feet, and heart, dizziness, tinnitus, tidal fever, night sweats, dry stools, red urine, red lips, a dry tongue with no or scanty fur, and a bowstring, fine, rapid pulse

Treatment principles: Nourish yin, moisten the lungs, and engender fluids

Guiding formulas:

Bai He Qing Fei Tang (Lily Clear the Lungs Decoction)
Bai He (Bulbus Lilii), 9-15g
Sheng Di (uncooked Radix Rehmanniae), 12-15g
Xuan Shen (Radix Scrophulariae), 9-15g
Zhe Bei Mu (Bulbus Fritillariae Thunbergii), 6-9g
Jie Geng (Radix Platycodi), 6-9g
Mai Men Dong (Tuber Ophiopogonis), 9-12g
Qing Guo (Semen Gingkonis Bilobae), 6-9g
Pang Da Hai (Semen Sterculiae), 9-12g
Bai Shao (Radix Albus Paeoniae Lactiflorae), 9g

Ba Xian Chang Shou Wan Jia Jian
(Eight Immortals Long Life Pills with Additions & Subtractions)
Mai Men Dong (Tuber Ophiopogonis), 9-12g
Shu Di (cooked Radix Rehmanniae), 12-15g
Sheng Di (uncooked Radix Rehmanniae), 12-15g
Shan Yao (Radix Dioscoreae), 9-15g
Sha Shen (Radix Glehniae), 9-12g
Wu Wei Zi (Fructus Schisandrae), 9g
Dan Pi (Cortex Moutan), 6-9g
Jie Geng (Radix Platycodi), 6-9g
Mu Hu Die (Semen Oroxyli), 9-15g
Ze Xie (Rhizoma Alismatis), 6-9g
Fu Ling (Poria), 9-12g

Lung qi blockage & obstruction

Main symptoms: Hoarseness or loss of voice during the last trimester, a replete body and normal facial complexion, chest oppression and discomfort, constipation, phlegm in the throat, cough which is not crisp, thin, slimy tongue fur, and a bowstring, slippery pulse

Treatment principles: Normalize the flow of qi and open the voice

Guiding formula:

Shou Tai Ta Qi San Jia Wei
(Thin the Fetus & Flog the Qi Powder with Added Flavors)
Xing Ren (Semen Armeniacae), 6-9g
Jie Geng (Radix Platycodi), 6-9g
Hou Po (Cortex Magnoliae Officinalis), 6-9g
Zhi Ke (Fructus Aurantii), 6g
Su Gen (Caulis Perillae Frutescentis), 9-12g
Gua Lou Pi (Pericarpium Trichosanthis), 6-9g
Zhe Bei Mu (Bulbus Fritillariae Thunbergii), 6-9g
Xuan Shen (Radix Scrophulariae), 9-15g
Gan Cao (Radix Glycyrrhizae), 3-9g

External contraction of wind heat

Main symptoms: Fever, vexation and agitation, throat pain, hoarseness, a bitter taste in the mouth, a dry throat, a desire for chilled drinks, dry stools, red urine, a red facial complexion, chapped lips, dry, yellow tongue fur, and a slippery, rapid pulse

Treatment principles: Clear heat and resolve the exterior

Guiding formula:

Qing Yan Jie Biao Tang
(Clear Inflammation & Resolve the Exterior Decoction)
Huang Qin (Radix Scutellariae), 9-12g
Lian Qiao (Fructus Forsythiae), 9-15g
Niu Bang Zi (Fructus Arctii), 9g
Jie Geng (Radix Platycodi), 6-9g
She Gan (Rhizoma Belamcandae), 6-9g
Xuan Shen (Radix Scrophulariae), 9-15g
Ban Lan Gen (Radix Isatidis/Baphicacanthi), 15g
Jin Yin Hua (Flos Lonicerae), 9-15g
Mai Men Dong (Tuber Ophiopogonis), 9-12g
Gan Cao (Radix Glycyrrhizae), 3-9g

Representative case history:

The patient was a 29 year-old female teacher who was in the ninth month of pregnancy. The patient's body was relatively thin. After becoming pregnant, she felt heat in the hearts of her hands and feet. Sometimes she was dizzy. In recent days, the woman felt as if her throat was dry and itchy, and sometimes she had a dry cough. After a couple of days, she developed hoarseness and she could not speak. The woman was seen as an outpatient at her local hospital where it was determined that kidney water was insufficient and unable to construct above. Hence lung metal had become dry and lost its moisture. The patient's tongue was red with scanty fur, and her pulse was fine, rapid, and slippery. Based on all this, the attending physician prescribed modified *Jia Wei Jie Geng Tang* (Added Flavors Platycodon Decoction): *Shu Di* (cooked Radix Rehmanniae), 12g, *Dan Pi* (Cortex Moutan), 6g, *Xuan Shen* (Radix Scrophulariae), 12g, *Mai Men Dong* (Tuber Ophiopogonis), 12g, *Shi Hu* (Herba Dendrobii), 9g, *Shan Yao* (Radix Dioscoreae), 9g, *Jie Geng* (Radix Platycodi), 9g, *Gan Cao* (Radix Glycyrrhizae), 6g, *Ze Xie* (Rhizoma Alismatis), 6g, and *Xi Xin* (Herba Asari), 1.5g.

After taking three packets of the above formula, the woman regained her voice. However, there was still some hoarseness. Therefore, *Xi Xin* was deleted and 12 grams of *Sha Shen* (Radix Glehniae) and six grams of *Gua Lou Pi* (Pericarpium Trichosanthis) were added and another three packets were prescribed. At the end of that time, the patient's voice was clear and unobstructed and her cough had entirely stopped.

Remarks:

I have often come across this condition in women with a long history of kidney vacuity. In more than one case, the woman has suffered from infertility and habitual miscarriage before conception. Because this condition has partly to do with physical obstruction of the connection between kidney water and lung yin, often the best that can be achieved through Chinese medicine is a modicum of relief. Typically, this condition is worse at night and can interfere with a woman's sleep. Because this condition usually signifies weak and vacuous kidneys and because kidney vacuity and deficiency are associated with malposition of the fetus, I believe this condition should most definitely be addressed — if not to completely eliminate the hoarseness, at least to keep the fetus from becoming malpositioned.

18

Diarrhea During Pregnancy

It is not uncommon for pregnant women to experience diarrhea. Since diarrhea entails a loss of body fluids and since yin fluids share a common source with the essence and blood, it is important to treat diarrhea so that it does not become chronic and thus result in lack of nourishment for both mother and child. Another way of explaining the clinical importance of treating diarrhea during pregnancy in Chinese medical terms is that the large intestine and the uterus are adjacent to each other and, therefore, diarrhea easily damages the fetal source.

Chinese medical disease categorization

Traditionally, this condition is called *zi xie*, child diarrhea or diarrhea while with child. In modern times, it is referred to as *ren shen xie xie*, diarrhea during pregnancy.

Disease causes & disease mechanisms

Diarrhea during pregnancy may be due to either external contraction, improper diet, or decline of yang. Contraction of wind cold, summerheat, and damp evils may all take advantage of the stressed condition of the mother during pregnancy. If damp evils cause depression which transforms into heat, damp heat may be engendered internally. This results in loss of harmony between the constructive and defensive. It is also possible for a predilection for chilled, uncooked foods to damage and cause detriment to the spleen and stomach. In this case, the spleen and stomach's ability to move and transform the qi of water and grains is impaired. Liquids and the finest essence of water and grains are not sent upward but pour downward undifferentiated with the turbid, thus resulting in loose stools and diarrhea. On the other hand, if, as pregnancy proceeds, the mother's kidney yang becomes insufficient, her life-gate fire may become empty and decline. Since this is the root of all warm transformation in the body, this also may result in diarrhea.

Patterns common to this condition

External contraction of damp evils
Damp heat in the stomach & intestines
Spleen-stomach vacuity weakness
Kidney yang vacuity

Treatment based on pattern discrimination:

External contraction of damp evils

Main symptoms: Abdominal pain, borborygmus, diarrhea and loose stools, inhibited urination, alternating fever and chills, hiccup, no desire to eat or drink, a somber white facial complexion, slimy, white tongue fur, and a floating, slippery, moderate (*i.e.*, relaxed, slightly slow) pulse

Treatment principles: Resolve the exterior and disinhibit urination, stop diarrhea and quiet the fetus

Guiding formula:

***Wu Ling San* (Five [Ingredients] Poria Powder)**
Gui Zhi (Ramulus Cinnamomi), 6-9g
Fu Ling (Poria), 9-12g
Ze Xie (Rhizoma Alismatis), 6-9g
Zhu Ling (Polyporus), 9-12g
Bai Zhu (Rhizoma Atractylodis Macrocephalae), 9g

If there is fever, sweating, thirst, heart vexation, diarrhea like yellow water, scorching heat around the anus, slightly yellow tongue fur, and a sodden, rapid pulse, delete *Gui Zhi* and add *Huang Lian* (Rhizoma Coptidis), *Dan Zhu Ye* (Herba Lophatheri), *Mai Men Dong* (Tuber Ophiopogonis), and *Hua Shi* (Talcum) to clear heat and disinhibit dampness.

Damp heat in the stomach & intestines

Main symptoms: Loose stools or diarrhea which is dark in color, burning and acidic feeling, and smelly, abdominal pain, possible explosive diarrhea, slimy, yellow tongue fur, and a slippery, soggy, rapid pulse

Treatment principles: Clear heat and eliminate dampness, quiet the fetus and stop diarrhea

Guiding formula:

Ge Gen Huang Qin Huang Lian Tang Jia Wei
(Pueraria, Scutellaria & Coptis Decoction with Added Flavors)
Ge Gen (Radix Puerariae), 9-18g
Huang Qin (Radix Scutellariae), 9-12g

Huang Lian (Rhizoma Coptidis), 3-9g
Tu Si Zi (Semen Cuscutae), 9g
Sang Ji Sheng (Herba Taxilli), 12-15g
Ai Ye (Folium Artemisiae Argyii), 9g
Mu Xiang (Radix Auklandiae), 6-9g
Gan Cao (Radix Glycyrrhizae), 3-9g

If fetal stirring is severe, add *Bai Shao* (Radix Albus Paeoniae Lactiflorae). If there is torpid intake due to food stagnation, add *Shen Qu* (Massa Medica Fermentata).

Spleen-stomach vacuity weakness

Main symptoms: Abdominal pain, borborygmus, diarrhea containing untransformed pieces of food, uninhibited urination, diminished intake of food and drink, vexation and oppression within the chest, generalized exhaustion and fatigue, a sallow yellow facial complexion, a pale tongue with moist, white, slimy fur, and a bowstring, moderate (*i.e.*, relaxed, slightly slow), slippery pulse

Treatment principles: Fortify the spleen and dry dampness, stop diarrhea and quiet the fetus

Guiding formulas:

Shen Ling Bai Zhu San (Ginseng, Poria & Atractylodes Powder)
Ren Shen (Radix Ginseng), 3-9g
Bai Zhu (Rhizoma Atractylodis Macrocephalae), 9g
Fu Ling (Poria), 9-12g
Bai Bian Dou (Semen Dolichoris), 9-12g
Chen Pi (Pericarpium Citri Reticulatae), 6g
Shan Yao (Radix Dioscoreae), 9-12g
Gan Cao (Radix Glycyrrhizae), 3-9g
Lian Zi (Semen Nelumbinis), 9g
Sha Ren (Fructus Amomi), 3-4.5g
Jie Geng (Radix Platycodi), 6-9g
Yi Yi Ren (Semen Coicis), 15-30g

If cold and dampness mutually gather and affect spleen yang with borborygmus, chilly pain, diarrhea like duck droppings, clear, white urination, lack of warmth in the four limbs, and a deep, moderate (*i.e.*, relaxed, slightly slow) pulse, add *He Zi* (Fructus Terminaliae) and *Wu Zhu Yu* (Fructus Evodiae) to warm the middle and stop diarrhea.

Si Jun Zi Tang (Four Gentlemen Decoction)
Ren Shen (Radix Ginseng), 3-9g
Bai Zhu (Rhizoma Atractylodis Macrocephalae), 9g
Fu Ling (Poria), 9-12g
mix-fried *Gan Cao* (Radix Glycyrrhizae), 6-9g

If there is complicating cold, add stir-fried *Gan Jiang* (dry Rhizoma Zingiberis) and *Wu Mei* (Fructus Mume). If there is heat, add *Huang Qin* (Radix Scutellariae). If there is thirst and chronic, intractable diarrhea, add *Bai Shao* (Radix Albus Paeoniae Lactiflorae), *He Zi* (Fructus Terminaliae), stir-fried *Gan Jiang* (dry Rhizoma Zingiberis), and *Wu Mei* (Fructus Mume).

Kidney yang vacuity

Main symptoms: Abdominal pain, borborygmus, loose stools and diarrhea, uninhibited urination, cockcrow diarrhea, dizziness, impaired memory, low back and knee soreness and limpness, lack of warmth in the four limbs, a dark, dusky facial complexion, a pale, moist tongue, and a deep, weak pulse

Treatment principles: Warm the kidneys and fortify the spleen, seep dampness and stop diarrhea

Guiding formula:

***Si Shen Wan Jia Wei* (Four Spirits Pills with Added Flavors)**
Bu Gu Zhi (Fructus Psoraleae), 9-12g
Wu Wei Zi (Fructus Schisandrae), 9g
Wu Zhu Yu (Fructus Evodiae), 6-9g
He Zi (Fructus Terminaliae), 9g
Fu Ling (Poria), 9-12g
Shan Yao (Radix Disocoreae), 9-15g

Abstract of representative Chinese research:

From "The Treatment of 30 Cases of Diarrhea During Pregnancy with *Ge Gen Qin Lian Tang Jia Wei* (Pueraria, Scutellaria & Coptis Decoction with Added Flavors)" by Chen Shou-mei, *Hu Bei Zhong Yi Za Zhi (Hubei Journal of Chinese Medicine)*, #5, 1995, p. 33

Cohort description:

The ages of the 30 women reported on in this article ranged from 23-27, with an average age of 24.8 years. For 26 of these women, this was their first pregnancy, and for four, it was their second. They had been pregnant 12-32 weeks, with an average duration of pregnancy of 21.5 weeks. The course of disease had lasted from 1-7 days, with an average duration of 3.2 days. All 30 women had varying degrees of abdominal pain and urgent diarrhea which was yellowish brown in color and watery in consistency. The least number of bowel movements per day was four and the most was 10. The stools were foul-smelling, and there was burning around the anus. In addition, there was possible oral thirst and vexatious heat and/or short, reddish urination. The tongue had slimy, yellow fur, and the pulse was slippery and rapid. Serological examination revealed elevated white blood cells and neutrophils. Stool examination showed pus (+-++) in 23 cases, (+++) in five cases, and (++++) in two cases. Based on all this, these women's Chinese medical pattern discrimination and diagnosis was damp heat pattern diarrhea during pregnancy.

Treatment method:

Ge Gen Huang Qin Huang Lian Tang Jia Wei consisted of: *Ge Gen* (Radix Puerariae), *Huang Qin* (Radix Scutellariae), *Huang Lian* (Rhizoma Coptidis), *Tu Si Zi* (Semen Cuscutae), *Sang Ji Sheng* (Herba Taxilli), 10g each, *Ai Ye* (Folium Artemisiae Argyii), *Mu Xiang* (Radix Auklandiae), 5g each, and *Gan Cao* (Radix Glycyrrhizae), 3g. If fetal stirring was severe, *Bai Shao* (Radix Albus Paeoniae Lactiflorae), 20g was added. If there was torpid intake, *Shen Qu* (Massa Medica Fermentata), 15g, was added. One packet was decocted in water and administered each day.

Treatment outcomes:

Complete cure consisted of disappearance of the clinical symptoms and the forming up of the stools within one day as well as normalization of the tongue and pulse. Twenty-five cases were thus cured. Diarrhea stopped after administering one packet of the above medicinals in 10 cases, after two packets in eight cases, and after three packets in seven cases. Marked effect meant that the clinical symptoms markedly improved and that the stools began to take form after one day. The tongue and pulse basically became normal. Thus four cases got a marked effect. No effect meant that the clinical symptoms and the diarrhea did not improve. Only one case got no effect. Therefore, the total amelioration rate was 96.6%.

Remarks:

In my experience, there is typically damp heat complicating most, if not all, diarrhea during pregnancy. Often there is a complex combination of liver depression and spleen vacuity and dampness and heat in the stomach and intestines. In this case one must course the liver and rectify the qi, fortify the spleen and supplement the qi, clear heat and eliminate dampness, and stop diarrhea all at the same time.

19

Dysentery During Pregnancy

In Chinese medicine, the difference between diarrhea and dysentery is the number of bowel movements per day. Loose stools of up to 10 movements per day are categorized as diarrhea, while loose stools of more than 10 movements per day are called dysentery. In Western medicine, dysentery mainly describes severe diarrhea associated with gastroenteritis due to either bacterial or amoebic infection. In addition, dysentery in Chinese medicine usually implies (but does not demand) the presence of mucus and/or blood in the stools. Therefore, in Chinese medicine, this disease category encompasses bacterial and amoebic dysentery but also includes chronic ulcerative colitis and Crohn's disease if there are more than 10 movements per day.

Chinese medical disease categorization

If a pregnant woman has red and white dysentery, this is traditionally called *zi li*, child dysentery, or, nowadays, *ren shen xie li*, dysentery during pregnancy.

Disease causes & disease mechanisms

In Chinese medicine, it is believed that this disease is mostly due to eating chilled, uncooked foods that damage and cause detriment to the spleen and stomach. In this case, the spleen becomes cold but the stomach becomes hot due to obstruction by stagnant food and fluids. Hot and cold mutually mix, resulting in damp heat and loss of normalcy of movement and transformation. It is also possible that, due to insufficiency of qi and blood and, therefore disharmony between the constructive and defensive, damp evils may invade externally. This also results in digestion losing its duty. If damp heat injures the qi aspect, this leads to white accumulation, *i.e.*, pus in the stools. If damp heat injures the blood aspect, this leads to red accumulation or the presence of blood in the stools.

Patterns common to this condition

Stomach & intestine damp heat
External contraction of summerheat & dampness

Treatment based on pattern discrimination:

Stomach & intestine damp heat

Main symptoms: Dysentery with pus and blood in the stools, abdominal pain, borborygmus, tenesmus after defecating, inhibited urination, heart vexation, belching and hiccup, no thought for food or drink, facial edema and red facial complexion, slightly yellow, slimy tongue fur, and a bowstring, slippery pulse

Treatment principles: Clear heat, abduct stagnation, and quiet the fetus

Guiding formulas:

Dang Gui Shao Yao Tang **(Dang Gui & Peony Decoction)**
Dang Gui (Radix Angelicae Sinensis), 9g
Bai Shao (Radix Albus Paeoniae Lactiflorae), 9-18g
Huang Qin (Radix Scutellariae), 9-12g
Huang Lian (Rhizoma Coptidis), 3-9g
Zhi Ke (Fructus Aurantii), 6g
Ze Xie (Rhizoma Alismatis), 6-9g
Mu Xiang (Radix Auklandiae), 6-9g
Bing Lang (Semen Arecae), 6-9g
scorched *Shan Zha* (Fructus Crataegi), 9g
Hou Po (Cortex Magnoliae Officinalis), 6-9g
Gan Cao (Radix Glycyrrhizae), 3-6g

Jiang Lian Wan **(Ginger & Coptis Pills)**
Huang Lian (Rhizoma Coptidis), 3-9g
Bai Zhu (Rhizoma Atractylodis Macrocephalae), 9g
Sha Ren (Fructus Amomi), 3-4.5g
E Jiao (Gelatinum Corii Asini), 9g
Pao Jiang (blast-fried Rhizoma Zingiberis), 6g
Chuan Xiong (Radix Ligustici Wallichii), 6-12g
stir-fried *Zhi Ke* (Fructus Aurantii), 6g
Mu Xiang (Radix Auklandiae), 6-9g

If there is white dysentery, take with ginger soup. If there is red dysentery, take with licorice soup. If there is red and white dysentery, take with both licorice and ginger soup.

Xiang Lian Hua Zhi Wan **(Coptis & Auklandia Transform Stagnation Pills)**
Chuan Lian (Rhizoma Coptidis), 3-9g
Huang Qin (Radix Scutellariae), 9-12g

Bai Shao (Radix Albus Paeoniae Lactiflorae), 9-12g
ginger stir-fried *Hou Po* (Cortex Magnoliae Officinalis), 9g
stir-fried *Zhi Ke* (Fructus Aurantii), 3-4.5g
Qing Pi (Pericarpium Citri Reticulatae Viride), 6g
Chen Pi (Pericarpium Citri Reticulatae), 6g
Dang Gui (Radix Angelicae Sinensis), 9g
Shan Zha (Fructus Crataegi), 9g
Gan Cao (uncooked Radix Glycyrrhizae), 3-6g
Mu Xiang (Radix Auklandiae), 6-9g

External contraction of summerheat & dampness

Main symptoms: Dysentery with yellow, watery stools, abdominal pain, borborygmus, inhibited urination, heart vexation, oral thirst, fever, aversion to cold, a red facial complexion, a dry tongue with thin, white fur, and a slippery, moderate (*i.e.*, relaxed, slightly slow), bowstring pulse

Treatment principles: Clear heat and resolve the exterior, quiet the fetus and stop dysentery

Guiding formula:

Qing Re Zhi Li Tang (Clear Heat & Stop Dysentery Decoction)
Huang Lian (Rhizoma Coptidis), 3-9g
Bai Shao (Radix Albus Paeoniae Lactiflorae), 9g
Fu Ling (Poria), 9-12g
Bai Zhu (Rhizoma Atractylodis Macrocephalae), 9g
Hua Shi (Talcum), 9-12g
Bai Bian Dou (Semen Dolichoris), 9-12g
Huo Xiang (Herba Pogostemonis), 6-9g
Huang Qin (Radix Scutellariae), 9-12g
Che Qian Zi (Semen Plantaginis), 9g
Gan Cao (Radix Glycyrrhizae), 3-9g

Remarks:

1. If there is blood in the stools, this can be due either to qi vacuity failing to contain the blood or damp heat causing the blood to move frenetically outside its pathways. In bacterial and amoebic dysentery, blood in the stools is mostly due to damp heat evils. In chronic ulcerative colitis, it may be due to either or both qi vacuity or damp heat. If there is bleeding due to qi vacuity, consider adding *Xian He Cao* (Herba Agrimoniae), *E Jiao* (Gelatinum Corii Asini), and/or *Ai Ye* (Folium Artemisiae Argyii). If there is bleeding due to damp heat, consider adding heat-clearing, bleeding-stopping medicinals such as *Dan Pi* (Cortex Moutan), *Chi Shao* (Radix Rubrus Paeoniae Lactiflorae), *Sheng Di* (uncooked Radix Rehmanniae), and *Di Yu* (Radix Sanguisorbae).

2. If there is mucus in the stools, this is an indication of profuse dampness and phlegm. In this case, consider adding *Che Qian Zi* (Semen Plantaginis), *Ze Xie* (Rhizoma Alismatis), *Cang Zhu* (Rhizoma Atractylodis), *Bai Zhu* (Rhizoma Atractylodis Macrocephalae), and/or *Yi Yi Ren* (Semen Coicis).

3. If liver depression qi stagnation complicates any of the above patterns and there is concomitant spleen vacuity, consider choosing *Xiao Chai Hu Tang* (Minor Bupleurum Decoction) or *Ban Xia Xie Xin Tang* (Pinellia Drain the Heart Decoction) and modifying these to fit the patient's presentation. This combination of patterns is more likely in the case of chronic ulcerative colitis than in dysentery per se.

20

Hemafecia
During Pregnancy

In Western medicine, hemafecia is not a disease in its own right but is rather regarded as a symptom of a number of other possible diseases. In Chinese medicine, hemafecia is regarded as a disease category of its own, and some Chinese gynecology texts include hemafecia during pregnancy as a separate obstetrical condition. In this case, hemafecia during pregnancy only refers to blood in the stools associated with the spleen qi failure to contain the blood. Hemafecia associated with dysentery or chronic ulcerative colitis have been dealt with in the preceding chapter.

Chinese medical disease categorization

Hemafecia during pregnancy is referred to in Chinese as *ren shen bian xue*.

Disease causes & disease mechanisms

If there is habitual bodily spleen vacuity, the spleen may lose its restraining and containing. The blood does not abide in the channels but seeps out into the intestines. This then produces hemafecia.

Treatment based on pattern discrimination:

Spleen vacuity not containing the blood

Main symptoms: Hemafecia during pregnancy colored fresh red, no abdominal pain or diarrhea, scanty luster to the facial complexion, lassitude of the spirit, lack of strength, no flavor when eating grains, a somewhat pale tongue with thin, slimy fur, and a fine, slippery pulse

Treatment principles: Boost the qi and contain the blood, upbear and supplement spleen yang

Guiding formula:

Bu Zhong Yi Qi Tang (Supplement the Center & Boost the Qi Decoction) plus Huai Hua San (Flos Sophorae Powder) with additions and subtractions
Huang Qi (Radix Astragali), 9-18g
Sheng Ma (Rhizoma Cimicifugae), 3-6g
Xian He Cao (Herba Agrimoniae), 9-15g
Dang Shen (Radix Codonopsitis), 9-15g
scorched *Bai Zhu* (Rhizoma Atractylodis Macrocephalae), 9g
carbonized *Huai Hua Mi* (Flos Immaturus Sophorae), 9-15g
carbonized *Di Yu* (Radix Sanguisorbae), 9g
Bai Shao (Radix Albus Paeoniae Lactiflorae), 9g
carbonized *Ce Bai Ye* (Cacumen Platyclodi), 9-12g

21
Appendicitis During Pregnancy

Although not an extremely common occurrence, it is possible for a woman to develop appendicitis during pregnancy. At least one contemporary Chinese gynecology text treats this as a separate disease category.

Chinese medical disease categorization

In Chinese medicine, appendicitis during pregnancy is referred to as *ren shen chang yong*, intestinal abscess during pregnancy.

Disease causes & disease mechanisms

If damp heat smolders and binds and *yang ming* heat is severe, the bowel qi may lose its free flow. It then smolders and steams the qi and blood and this may lead to the production of welling abscess swellings.

Treatment based on pattern discrimination:

Damp heat, stasis & stagnation

Main symptoms: Right-sided, lower abdominal aching and pain which refuses pressure, tightness of the abdomen, bending of the right hip with inhibited extension, strong fever, sweating, constipation, reddish urination, a somewhat red tongue with slimy, yellow fur, and a surging, rapid pulse

Treatment principles: Clear heat and resolve toxins, quicken the blood and scatter stasis, normalize the flow of qi and quiet the fetus

Guiding formula:

Chang Yong Huo Ming Yin Jia Wei
(Intestinal Abscess Quicken the Destiny Drink with Added Flavors)
Jin Yin Hua (Flos Lonicerae), 9-15g
Dang Gui (Radix Angelicae Sinensis), 9g
Pu Gong Ying (Herba Taraxaci), 12-30g
Mai Men Dong (Tuber Ophiopogonis), 9-12g
Xuan Shen (Radix Scrophulariae), 9-15g
Mu Xiang (Radix Auklandiae), 6-9g
Huang Qin (Radix Scutellariae), 9-12g
uncooked *Gan Cao* (Radix Glycyrrhizae), 3-6g
Tai Zi Shen (Radix Pseudostellariae), 9-12g
Zi Su Gen (Caulis Perillae Frutescentis), 9-15g
Zhu Ma Gen (Radix Boehmeriae Niveae), 9-15g

When the pain has diminished by more than half, add *Fu Ling* (Poria) and *Bai Shao* (Radix Albus Paeoniae Lactiflorae). If the aching and pain have basically disappeared but yet there is still some abdominal pain, remaining evils are not extensive but the righteous qi has suffered detriment. In that case, add *Huang Qi* (Radix Astragali).

Once the symptoms have basically remitted, one should mainly support the righteous while simultaneously clearing any remaining heat by using *Huang Qi* (Radix Astragali), *Dang Shen* (Radix Codonopsitis), *Mu Xiang* (Radix Auklandiae), *Jin Yin Hua* (Flos Lonicerae), *Dang Gui* (Radix Angelicae Sinensis), *Mai Men Dong* (Tuber Ophiopogonis), *Pu Gong Ying* (Herba Taraxaci), *Bai Shao* (Radix Albus Paeoniae Lactiflorae), *Gan Cao* (Radix Glycyrrhizae), *Bai Zhu* (Rhizoma Atractylodis Macrocephalae), and *Zhu Ma Gen* (Radix Boehmeriae Niveae).

Remarks:

1. Although I have successfully treated a number of cases of appendicitis with Chinese medicine over the last 25 years, I have never seen a case of appendicitis during pregnancy. Obviously, in such cases, extremely close monitoring would be necessary with immediate referral to Western emergency medical services if necessary. Attempting to treat appendicitis during pregnancy with Chinese medicine is not for either beginners or the faint-hearted.

2. Typically, very large doses are used when treating appendicitis with Chinese medicinals. It is not uncommon to use 30-60 grams of individual heat-clearing, toxin-resolving medicinals.

22

Urinary Tract Infection During Pregnancy

Urinary tract infections (UTIs) are the most common bacterial infections during pregnancy.[1] The incidence of UTI in pregnant women can be as high as 8%.[2,3] Urinary tract infections are common during pregnancy due to urinary stasis in turn due to hormonal dilation and urethral hypoperistalsis as well as to pressure from the pregnant uterus against the ureters.[4] Beginning in week six and peaking during weeks 22-24, approximately 90% of pregnant women develop ureteral dilation which then remains for the duration of the pregnancy. Increased bladder volume and decreased bladder and ureteral tone result in urinary stasis and ureterovesical reflux. Additionally, the physiologic increase in plasma volume during pregnancy decreases urine concentration. To make matters worse, up to 70% of pregnant women develop glycosuria which increases the growth of bacteria in the urine. Yet another factor contributing to the increased susceptibility of pregnant women to UTIs is the increase in urinary progestins and estrogens which may lead to a decreased ability of the lower urinary tract to resist invading bacteria.[5]

In terms of the organisms that cause UTIs during pregnancy, these are the same as those which cause UTIs in nonpregnant women. *Escherichia coli* is the most common bacteria accounting for UTIs and is responsible for 80-90% of such infections.[6] Other bacteria, such as Klebsiella species, Proteus species, and Enterobacter species are also common, with group B streptococcus and *Staphylococcus saprophyticus* being less common. Even less common pathogens include *Gardnerella vaginalis* and *Ureaplasma ureolyticum*.[7]

Urinary tract infections during pregnancy may be either symptomatic or asymptomatic. In addition, there may be infection of the lower urinary tract (cystitis) or the upper urinary tract (pyelonephritis). Pregnant women are more prone to pyelonephritis than nonpregnant women.[8] Patients with asymptomatic bacteriuria have no symptoms, and bacteria in their urine is usually found incidentally during routine urine analysis. Untreated asymptomatic bacteriuria is found in 10% of pregnant women. Approximately 30% of these patients go on to develop symptomatic cystitis if left untreated and 50% may go on to develop pyelonephritis.[9] The main symptom of pregnant women with symptomatic cystitis is burning pain with urination. In the case of pyelonephritis, there is typically fever (often very high), chills, nausea and vomiting, and costovertebral angle (CVA) or flank tenderness.

The Western medical diagnosis of UTIs during pregnancy is based on symptoms, physical examination, including a pelvic examination to rule out vaginitis or cervicitis, and urine analysis. When diagnosis is confirmed by the presence of bacteria in the urine, treatment consists of administration of antibiotics chosen to address the most common infecting organism. Historically, ampicillin has been the drug of choice. However, in recent years, *E. coli* has become increasingly resistant to this drug. Other choices include nitrofurantoin (Macrodantin), various cephalosporins, and fosformycin (Monurol). Sulfonamides should only be taken during the first and second trimesters, and other common antibiotics, such as fluoroquinolones and tetracyclines, should not be prescribed during pregnancy because of possible toxicity to the fetus.

Chinese medical disease categorization

In Chinese medicine, *lin zheng*, strangury condition, refers to urinary disorders characterized by dribbling and dripping. When these occur during pregnancy, they are referred to as *zi lin* or child strangury. When there is burning pain in the urethra, this is called *re lin*, heat strangury. If there is hematuria, this is referred to as *nao xue*, urinary bleeding, or *xue lin*, bloody strangury.

Disease causes & disease mechanisms

This condition is mostly due to habitual bodily vacuity and internal heat. This heat may be of two types, replete heat or vacuity heat. Replete heat may also be subdivided into two types. These are heart fire and damp heat. If heat accumulates in the heart due to depressive liver fire in turn due to emotional frustration and excessive anger, it may be passed to its paired yang bowel, the small intestine. The small intestine may likewise pass this heat to its paired *tai yang* counterpart, the urinary bladder. There, this heat scorches the fluids and humors and damages the water passageways. On the other hand, if depressive heat from the liver mixes with dampness from the spleen, this may combine to form damp heat and pour down into the lower burner, likewise disrupting the urination and causing pain and burning on urination.

Vacuity heat causing strangury typically crops up only after being pregnant for many months. If the woman is constitutionally weak, is older, has suffered from chronic disease or prolonged overtaxation, her yin may become even more exhausted by pregnancy. Since yin controls and restrains yang, if yin becomes vacuous, yang tends to become replete. Since yin vacuity originates primarily in the kidneys and since the kidneys govern urination, this vacuity heat may further damage and consume fluids and humors and cause burning and pain on urination.

Patterns common to this condition

Heart fire tending to hyperactivity
Damp heat pouring downward
Yin vacuity

Treatment based on pattern discrimination:

Heart fire tending to hyperactivity

Main symptoms: Dark yellow, choppy, painful urination during pregnancy, a red facial complexion, vexation and agitation, disquietude of the spirit, possible heart palpitations and/or insomnia, sores on the tip of the tongue, a red tongue with scanty or no fur, and a fine, slippery, rapid pulse

Treatment principles: Clear the heart and discharge fire, disinhibit urination and free the flow of strangury

Guiding formulas:

Dao Chi San Jia Wei Yi Hao
(Abduct the Red Powder with Added Flavors #1)
Sheng Di (uncooked Radix Rehmanniae), 12-15g
Mu Tong (Caulis Akebiae), 6-9g
Gan Cao (Radix Glycyrrhizae), 3-9g
Dan Zhu Ye (Herba Lophatheri), 9-15g
Xuan Shen (Radix Scrophulariae), 9-15g
Mai Men Dong (Tuber Ophiopogonis), 9-12g

Dao Chi San Jia Wei Er Hao
(Abduct the Red Powder with Added Flavors #2)
Sheng Di (uncooked Radix Rehmanniae), 12-15g
Mu Tong (Caulis Akebiae), 6-9g
Dan Zhu Ye (Herba Lophatheri), 9-15g
Gan Cao (Radix Glycyrrhizae), 3-9g
Huang Qin (Radix Scutellariae), 9-12g
Zhi Zi (Fructus Gardeniae), 6-9g

If there is hematuria, add *Xiao Ji* (Herba Cephalanoploris).

Damp heat pouring downward

Main symptoms: Short, frequent, urgent, choppy, and inhibited, yellowish red urination during pregnancy accompanied by scorching hot, piercing pain, a yellow facial complexion, dry mouth but no particular thirst, chest oppression, scanty intake, a red tongue with slimy, yellow fur, and a slippery, rapid pulse

Therapeutic principles: Clear heat, disinhibit dampness, and free the flow of strangury

Guiding formulas:

Jia Wei Wu Lin San **(Added Flavors Five [Ingredients] Strangury Powder)**
carbonized *Zhi Zi* (Fructus Gardeniae), 9g
Chi Fu Ling (Sclerotium Rubrum Poriae Cocos), 9-15g
Dang Gui (Radix Angelicae Sinensis), 9g
Bai Shao (Radix Albus Paeoniae Lactiflorae), 9g
Huang Qin (Radix Scutellariae), 9-12g
Gan Cao (Radix Glycyrrhizae), 3-9g
Sheng Di (uncooked Radix Rehmanniae), 12-15g
Ze Xie (Rhizoma Alismatis), 9g
Che Qian Zi (Semen Plantaginis), 9g
Mu Tong (Caulis Akebiae), 6-9g
Hua Shi (Talcum), 9-15g

Ba Zheng San Jia Jian **(Eight [Ingredients] Correcting Powder with Additions & Subtractions)**
Qu Mai (Herba Dianthi), 9g
Bian Xu (Herba Polygoni Avicularis), 9-15g
carbonized *Sheng Di* (uncooked Radix Rehmanniae), 12-15g
carbonized *Xiao Ji* (Herba Cephalanoploris), 9g
Han Lian Cao (Herba Ecliptae), 12-15g
scorched *Zhi Zi* (Fructus Gardeniae), 6-9g
Jin Yin Hua (Flos Lonicerae), 9-15g
scorched *Che Qian Zi* (Semen Plantaginis), 9g
Xu Duan (Radix Dipsaci), 9g
Sang Ji Sheng (Herba Taxilli), 12-15g

Yin vacuity

Main symptoms: During the advanced months of pregnancy the urine becomes frequent and strangurious. There is scorching heat and piercing pain, the volume of the urine is scanty, and it is dark yellow in color. There is bodily emaciation, flushed red cheeks, tidal fever in the afternoons and evenings, heat in the hands, feet, and heart, heart vexation, constipation, a red tongue with thin, yellow, dry fur, and a fine, slippery, rapid pulse.

Treatment principles: Enrich yin, moisten dryness, and open strangury

Guiding formulas:

Zhi Bai Di Huang Wan Jia Wei
(Anemarrhena & Phellodendron Rehmannia Pills with Added Flavors)
Shu Di (cooked Radix Rehmanniae), 12-15g
Shan Yao (Radix Dioscoreae), 9-15g
Shan Zhu Yu (Fructus Corni), 9-18g
Fu Ling (Poria), 9-12g

Dan Pi (Cortex Moutan), 6-9g
Ze Xie (Rhizoma Alismatis), 6-9g
Zhi Mu (Rhizoma Anemarrhenae), 9g
Huang Bai (Cortex Phellodendri), 9g
Mai Men Dong (Tuber Ophiopogonis), 9-12g
Wu Wei Zi (Fructus Schisandrae), 9g
Che Qian Zi (Semen Plantaginis), 9g

Zhi Bai Si Wu Tang
(Anemarrhena & Phellodendron Four Materials Decoction)
Shu Di (cooked Radix Rehmanniae), 12-15g
Dang Gui (Radix Angelicae Sinensis), 9g
Bai Shao (Radix Albus Paeoniae Lactiflorae), 9g
Chuan Xiong (Radix Ligustici Wallichii), 6-9g
Huang Qin (Radix Scutellariae), 9-12g
Zhi Mu (Rhizoma Anemarrhenae), 9g
Huang Bai (Cortex Phellodendri), 9g

Abstract of representative Chinese research:

From "The Treatment of Urinary Tract Infection During Pregnancy with *Bai Tou Weng Tang Jia Wei* (Pulsatilla Decoction with Added Flavors)" by Zhao Guang-cu, *Jiang Xi Zhong Yi Yao (Jiangxi Chinese Medicine & Medicinals)*, #6, 2000, p. 33

Cohort description:

Among the 40 patients in this study, 11 were in their first trimester, 22 were in their second trimester, and seven were in their third trimester. All had varying degrees of bladder irritation, frequent urination, urinary urgency, urinary pain, and a pressury feeling in the lower abdomen. If the condition were severe, there was also lower back pain, aversion to cold, fever, and headache. In terms of urine analysis, WBCs were scanty to +++, RBCs were +-+++, pus cells were scanty to +++, and albuminuria was scanty to +. Bacterial culture was positive in all cases.

Treatment method:

The basic formula consisted of: *Bai Tou Weng* (Radix Pulsatillae), 30g, *Qin Pi* (Cortex Fraxini), 10g, *Huang Lian* (Rhizoma Coptidis), 3g, *Huang Bai* (Cortex Phellodendri), 10g, *Pu Gong Ying* (Herba Taraxaci), 30g, *Sheng Di* (uncooked Radix Rehmanniae), 15g, tips of *Gan Cao* (Radix Glycyrrhizae), 10g, and *Dan Zhu Ye* (Herba Lopatheri), 10g. One packet of these medicinals was decocted in water three times and administered in three doses each day, with seven days equaling one course of treatment. If there was fever, *Chai Hu* (Radix Bupleuri), *Huang Qin* (Radix Scutellariae), and *Jin Yin Hua* (Flos Lonicerae) were added. If there was hematuria, *Xiao Ji* (Herba Cephalanoploris), *Da Ji* (Herba Cirsii), *E Jiao* (Gelatinum Corii Asini), and *Xue Yu Tan* (Crinis Carbonisatus) were added. If albuminuria was profuse, uncooked *Huang Qi* (Radix Astragali), uncooked *Qian Shi* (Semen Euryalis), and *Jin Ying Zi* (Fructus Rosae Laevigatae) were added. If appetite was poor, *Ji Nei*

Jin (Endothelium Corneum Gigeriae Galli), *Sha Ren* (Fructus Amomi), and scorched *San Xian* (Three Immortals: *Shan Zha* [Fructus Crataegi], *Mai Ya* [Fructus Germinatus Hordei], and *Shen Qu* [Massa Medica Fermentata]) were added. If there was nausea and vomiting, *Fu Long Gan* (Terra Flava Usta), ginger-processed *Ban Xia* (Rhizoma Pinelliae), and *Chen Pi* (Pericarpium Citri Reticulatae) were added. If there was lower abdominal distention and fullness, *Wu Yao* (Radix Linderae), processed *Xiang Fu* (Rhizoma Cyperi), and *Chuan Lian Zi* (Fructus Toosendan) were added. If there was low back pain, stir-fried *Du Zhong* (Cortex Eucommiae), *Xu Duan* (Radix Dipsaci), and *Sang Ji Sheng* (Herba Taxilli) were added. If bacteria were positive, *Zhi Zi* (Fructus Gardeniae), *Ku Shen* (Radix Sophorae Flavescentis), and *Yu Xing Cao* (Herba Houttuyniae) were added.

Treatment outcomes:

Cure was defined as disappearance of all symptoms, normal urine analysis, and negative bacterial culture. Improvement was defined as disappearance of the clinical symptoms, negative urine analysis, but still positive bacterial culture. Based on these criteria, after 1-2 courses of treatment, 32 cases were cured, six improved, and two got no effect, for a total amelioration rate of 95%.

Representative case histories:

Case 1: The patient was a 29 year-old female who was treated in 1964. This patient's body was habitually relatively weak. After she was four months pregnant, her urination became frequent, numerous, and strangurious. It was choppy, painful, and difficult to bear. Its amount was scanty and its color was dark yellow. Both of this woman's cheeks were flushed red and she had heart vexation, insomnia, constipation, a red tongue with thin, yellow, dryish fur, and a fine, rapid, slippery pulse. Based on these signs and symptoms, the woman's Chinese medical pattern was categorized as kidney water insufficiency with lifegate fire effulgence shifting heat to the urinary bladder. Therefore, the formula prescribed was *Liu Wei Di Huang Tang Jia Jian* (Six Flavors Rehmannia Decoction with Additions & Subtractions): *Sheng Di* (uncooked Radix Rehmanniae), 6g, *Shan Yao* (Radix Dioscoreae), 6g, *Dan Pi* (Cortex Moutan), 6g, *Ze Xie* (Rhizoma Alismatis), 6g, *Fu Ling* (Poria), 6g, *Dan Zhu Ye* (Herba Lophatheri), 4g, *Hua Shi* (Talcum), 4g, and *Er Chou* (Semen Pharbiditis), 3g. One packet of these medicinals was decocted in water and administered orally per day for three days.

On the second examination, the patient reported that her urinary choppiness and pain was less and that its amount was more. Its color now was pale yellow, and her heart vexation and tidal heat were improved. Her stools were now loose and her tongue and pulse were the same. Therefore, *Hua Shi* and *Er Chou* were removed from the formula and three grams of *Tong Cao* (Medulla Tetrapanacis), six grams of *Wu Wei Zi* (Fructus Schisandrae), and 1.5 grams of *Hu Po* (Succinum) were added and another two packets were prescribed.

On the third examination, the patient's urination was freely and uninhibitedly flowing. The malar flushing had disappeared, and the heart vexation and insomnia were improved. the tongue was pale red with moist, white fur, and the pulse was fine and slippery. The formula from visit #2 was continue for two more packets, after which all the woman's symptoms were eliminated and the disease was considered cured.

Case 2: The patient was a 34 year-old female who was also treated in 1964. This patient was also habitually fatigued and lacked strength, and she was five months pregnant with her third child. The patient had a feeling that her bladder was not able to empty itself, and, after urinating, there was aching and pain and dribbling and dripping that would not stop. The color of the urine was white, and sometimes it was pale yellow. The patient's tongue was pale with normal fur, and her pulse was moderate (*i.e.*, relaxed or slightly slow) and slippery. The patient's pattern was discriminated as downward falling of the central qi, and she was prescribed the following medicinals to boost the qi, upbear and lift: *Ren Shen* (Radix Ginseng), 6g, *Huang Qi* (Radix Astragali), 15g, *Fu Ling* (Poria), 6g, *Bai Zhu* (Rhizoma Atractylodis Macrocephalae), 10g, *Sheng Ma* (Rhizoma Cimicifugae), 4g, *Tu Si Zi* (Semen Cuscutae), 6g, *Wu Yao* (Radix Linderae), 6g, and *Yi Zhi Ren* (Fructus Alpiniae Oxyphyllae), 6g. Two packets were prescribed to be taken one packet per day after decocting in water.

On the second visit, the urinary dribbling and pain was decreased and the woman's breathing was smooth and freely flowing. Her tongue and pulse, however, were the same as before, so she was prescribed two more packets of the original formula. On the third visit, the woman reported that all her symptoms were cured except that, each day in the afternoon, she noticed some slight lower abdominal distention and sagging, she did not have much flavor for eating or drinking, and her mouth was dry. Therefore, she was prescribed two packets of the original formula minus *Huang Qi* and *Tu Si Zi* but plus six grams each of *Sha Ren* (Fructus Amomi) and *Mai Men Dong* (Tuber Ophiopogonis), and the woman was judged cured.

Remarks:

1. Urinary tract infections during pregnancy are a common cause of maternal and fetal morbidity. Therefore, great care should be exercised in their treatment, and all pregnant women should be routinely screened for bacteriuria. Chinese medicine, either alone or in combination with Western medicine, can effectively treat UTIs during pregnancy. However, practitioners should be ready and willing to make timely, appropriate referrals to Western medical services as the situation requires. This condition should not be treated lightly, nor should it be treated by anyone without adequate training.

2. If clearing and cooling, freeing and disinhibiting medicinals are not effective for treating this condition, then one may try using *Bu Zhong Yi Qi Tang* (Supplement the Center & Boost the Qi Decoction) plus six grams

of *Che Qian Zi* (Semen Plantaginis). When the central qi is upborne, this simultaneously opens the lower portals. Because *Che Qian Zi* disinhibits water and frees the flow of strangury, there is both upbearing and down-bearing and thus things take care of themselves. Along these same lines, it is also possible to prescribe both *Bu Zhong Yi Qi Tang* with *Zhi Bai Di Huang Wan* (Anemarrhena & Phellodendron Rehmannia Pills) with *Che Qian Zi* if there is both qi vacuity and yin vacuity with vacuity heat.

Endnotes:

[1] www.emedicine.com/emerg/topic485.htm

[2] Paterson, T.F. & Andriole, V.T., "Bacteriuria in Pregnancy," *Infectious Diseases Clinic of North America*, #1, 1987, p. 807-822

[3] Mikhail, M.S. & Anyaegbunam, A., "Lower Urinary Tract Dysfunction in Pregnancy: A Review," *Obstetrical Gynecology Survey*, #50, 1995, p. 675-683

[4] Beers, Mark H. & Berbow, Robert, *The Merck Manual, op. cit.*, p. 2041

[5] www.aafp.org/afp/20000201/713.htm

[6] *Ibid*.

[7] Barr, J. G. *et al.*, "Microaerophilic/Anearobic Bacteria as a Cause of Urinary Tract Infection in Pregnancy," *British Journal of Obstetric Gynecology*, #92, 1985, p. 506-510

[8] www.niddk.nih.gov/health/urolog/pubs/utiadult/utiadult.htm

[9] www.aafp.org, *op. cit.*

23

Urinary Retention During Pregnancy

Urinary retention during pregnancy is a relatively common condition in later pregnancy which is mostly related to changes in the position of the cervix from middle pregnancy on. It tends to occur gradually, the flow of urine becoming progressively scantier. There may be intermittent pain in the bladder area, but, unless this condition leads to cystitis, which it may, it is not accompanied by burning urination. Urinary retention may be one of the causes of an abdomen which is larger in size than weeks of gestation would normally suggest. In some cases, the bladder may be visibly distended when the woman is lying on her back. This condition often complicates abnormal position of the fetus. Its Western medical treatment consists of catheter drainage of the bladder.

Chinese medical disease categorization

Traditionally, this condition is called *zhuan bao* or rotated uterus. In the modern Chinese medical literature, it is referred to as *ren shen xiao bian bu tong*, non-freely flowing urination during pregnancy.

Disease causes & disease mechanisms

This condition is mostly due to insufficient qi to hold up the growing fetus and to move and to transport water fluids. Either the mother suffers chronically from spleen-stomach vacuity weakness with downward falling of the central qi or from kidney yang insufficiency with inability to promote the movement of water in the bladder. In either case, the uterus presses down on the bladder compressing the water passageways and prohibiting water's easy exit. Non-freely flowing urination during pregnancy may also be due to damp heat accumulating in the lower burner. This disease mechanism is the most likely one when this condition develops into an actual UTI.

Patterns common to this condition

Central qi vacuity

Kidney yang vacuity

Damp heat

Treatment based on pattern discrimination:

Central qi vacuity

Main symptoms: Non-freely flowing urination and difficulty voiding 7-8 months after conception. There is no pain in the urethra, but there is the need to constantly go to the bathroom day and night without limit, lower abdominal pain and distention, dizziness, shortness of breath, heart vexation, lassitude of the spirit, a somber white facial complexion, and a vacuous, slippery, moderate (*i.e.*, relaxed, slightly slow) pulse.

Treatment principles: Supplement the middle, boost the qi, and lift the fallen

Guiding formulas:

Bu Zhong Yi Qi Tang Jia Wei
(Supplement the Center & Boost the Qi Decoction with Added Flavors)
Huang Qi (Radix Astragali), 9-18g
Ren Shen (Radix Ginseng), 3-9g
Bai Zhu (Rhizoma Atractylodis Macrocephalae), 9g
Chen Pi (Pericarpium Citri Reticulatae), 6g
Sheng Ma (Rhizoma Cimicifugae), 3-6g
Chai Hu (Radix Bupleuri), 3-9g
Dang Gui (Radix Angelicae Sinensis), 6-9g
mix-fried *Gan Cao* (Radix Glycyrrhizae), 6-9g
Fu Ling (Poria), 9-12g

Yi Qi Dao Ni Tang **(Boost the Qi & Abduct the Urine Decoction)**
Dang Shen (Radix Codonopsitis), 9-15g
Bai Zhu (Rhizoma Atractylodis Macrocephalae) , 9g
Bai Bian Dou (Semen Dolichoris), 9-12g
Fu Ling (Poria), 9-12g
Gui Zhi (Ramulus Cinnamomi), 6-9g
Sheng Ma (Rhizoma Cimicifugae), 3-6g
Jie Geng (Radix Platycodi), 6-9g
Tong Cao (Medulla Tetrapanacis), 9g
Wu Yao (Radix Linderae), 6-9g

Shen Zhu Er Chen Tang
(Ginseng & Atractylodes Two Aged [Ingredients] Decoction)
Ren Shen (Radix Ginseng), 3-9g

stir-fried *Bai Zhu* (Rhizoma Atractylodis Macrocephalae), 9g
Dang Gui (Radix Angelicae Sinensis), 6-9g
Bai Shao (Radix Albus Paeoniae Lactiflorae), 9g
Chen Pi (Pericarpium Citri Reticulatae), 6g
ginger-processed *Ban Xia* (Rhizoma Pinelliae), 9g
mix-fried *Gan Cao* (Radix Glycyrrhizae), 6-9g

Acupuncture & moxibustion: *Qi Hai* (CV 6), *Yin Ling Quan* (Sp 9), *Pang Guang Shu* (Bl 28), *Zu San Li* (St 36)

Kidney yang vacuity

Main symptoms: After conception urination becomes frequent and repeated. There is some difficulty voiding, lower abdominal distention and pain, heart vexation, low back and knee soreness and limpness, fear of cold, lack of warmth of the four limbs, dizziness, tinnitus, a dark, dusky facial complexion, pale, moist lips and tongue with white, glossy fur, and a deep, weak pulse.

Treatment principles: Supplement the kidneys, warm yang, and move water

Guiding formulas:
Shen Qi Wan Jia Wei (Kidney Qi Pills with Added Flavors)
Shu Di (cooked Radix Rehmanniae), 12-15g
Shan Yao (Radix Dioscoreae), 9-15g
Shan Zhu Yu (Fructus Corni), 9-18g
Fu Ling (Poria), 9-12g
Ze Xie (Rhizoma Alismatis), 9g
Dan Pi (Cortex Moutan), 6-9g
Rou Gui (Cortex Cinnamomi), 6-9g
Zhi Fu Zi (Radix Lateralis Praeparatus Aconiti Carmichaeli), 3-9g
Tu Si Zi (Semen Cuscutae), 9g
Ba Ji Tian (Radix Morindae), 9g
Gui Zhi (Ramulus Cinnamomi), 6-9g

Acupuncture & moxibustion: Same as above plus moxa at *Guan Yuan* (CV 4) and *Da Zhui* (GV 14).

Damp heat

Main symptoms: Not smoothly flowing urination, dry stools, epigastric and abdominal glomus and fullness, slimy, thin tongue fur, and slippery, rapid pulse

Treatment principles: Clear heat and disinhibit dampness

Guiding formula:
Unnamed experiential formula
Fan Xie Ye (Folium Sennae), 6-9g
uncooked *Gan Cao* (Radix Glycyrrhizae), 3-9g

Soak for 1/2 hour. Then drink.

Note: *Fan Xie Ye* is a forbidden medicinal during pregnancy. However, it is able to free the flow of the viscera and bowels and dispel evils without hindering the fetus. It frees the stools but does not cause abdominal diarrhea. Thus it is permitted to be used boldly as long as it is based on pattern discrimination.

Representative case histories:

Case 1: The patient was a 38 year-old, married female who was initially seen in June 1960. This woman was constitutionally vacuous and weak and she had also had a number of children. At present, she was four months pregnant. She had torpid intake and low backache, and her urination was not freely flowing. There was lower abdominal distention and sagging which were severe, her tongue fur was thin and white, and her pulse was fine and slippery. Therefore, the woman was diagnosed with rotated uterus and her pattern was categorized as kidney qi insufficiency. The formula this woman was initially prescribed consisted of: *Sheng Ma* (Rhizoma Cimicifugae), 2.4g, *Wu Wei Zi* (Fructus Schisandrae), 4.5g, *Du Zhong* (Cortex Eucommiae), 9g, *Xu Duan* (Radix Dipsaci), 9g, *Tu Si Zi* (Semen Cuscutae), 9g, *Shan Yao* (Radix Dioscoreae), 9g, *Bai Zhu* (Rhizoma Atractylodis Macrocephalae), 6g, *Fu Ling* (Poria), 9g, and *Chen Pi* (Pericarpium Citri Reticulatae), 6g.

After taking one packet of the above medicinals, the woman's urination was still not freely flowing. However, the abdominal distention was better and the low back ache had improved. Now there was slight tinnitus and blurred vision, for which the woman was prescribed: *Sheng Ma* (Rhizoma Cimicifugae), 2.4g, *Wu Wei Zi* (Fructus Schisandrae), 4.5g, *Huang Qi* (Radix Astragali), 9g, *Tai Zi Shen* (Radix Pseudostellariae), 4.5g, *Gou Ji* (Rhizoma Cibotii), 9g, *Tu Si Zi* (Semen Cuscutae), 9g, *Shan Yao* (Radix Dioscoreae), 9g, stir-fried *Zhi Ke* (Fructus Aurantii), 4.5g, *Fu Pen Zi* (Fructus Rubi), 9g, *Bai Zhu* (Rhizoma Atractylodis Macrocephalae), 6g, and *Fu Ling* (Poria), 9g. At this point the patient was deemed cured.

Case 2: The patient was a 26 year-old female who was initially examined in June 1965. This woman was a primigravida who was eight months pregnant and whose urine was not freely flowing. There was lower abdominal distention and pain, vexation, and insomnia but normal eating and drinking. Her pulse was deep and fine and her tongue fur was thin and moist. Based on these findings, the woman's Chinese medical pattern was categorized as qi stagnation and she was prescribed: stir-fried *Zhi Ke* (Fructus Aurantii), 9g, *Su Gen* (Caulis Perillae Frutescentis), 5g, *Jie Geng* (Radix Platycodi), 5g, *Fu Ling* (Poria), 10g, *Chen Pi* (Pericarpium Citri Reticulatae), 4g, *Da Fu Pi* (Pericarpium Arecae), 4g, scorched *Zhi Zi* (Fructus Gardeniae), 9g, *Chai Hu* (Radix Bupleuri), 5g, and stir-fried *Bai Shao* (Radix Albus Paeoniae Lactiflorae), 10g.

After taking six packets of this formula, the patient's urination was relatively smooth and easily flowing. Her lower abdominal distention and pain were no longer uncomfortable and she was able to lie down quietly to sleep. Therefore, *Qian Hu* was removed from the previous formula and another five packets were prescribed. At that point, all the patient's symptoms were eliminated, the fetus was also quiet, and she was judged cured.

Remarks:

1. Urinary retention during pregnancy includes not only scanty urination but complete anuria. This is an emergency condition which can lead to uremic poisoning.

2. Urination during pregnancy is commonly associated with malposition of the fetus. Therefore the name, "rotated uterus."

3. Because this is an emergency condition, acupuncture in addition to internally administered Chinese medicinals is indicated if catheterization is not for any reason possible. In that case, retain the needles 15-20 minutes. Every 1-2 minutes, twirl and rotate the needles again. After the needles are withdrawn, one may also use either pole moxa or moxa cones.

4. In case of spleen-kidney dual vacuity, combine *Bu Zhong Yi Qi Tang* (Supplement the Center & Boost the Qi Decoction) with *Shen Qi Wan* (Kidney Qi Pills).

24

Urinary Incontinence During Pregnancy

Urinary incontinence during pregnancy refers to the involuntary loss of urine during pregnancy, and nearly half of all pregnant women complain of this condition.[1] During pregnancy, high levels of the hormone relaxin are secreted which soften the ligaments and muscles of the pelvic floor so that the baby can be pushed out more easily during childbirth. However, this same hormone also relaxes the sphincter muscles. This condition is typically transient and usually disappears spontaneously 4-6 weeks postpartum.

Chinese medical disease categorization

This condition is referred to as *ren shen shi sou*, loss of urine during pregnancy.

Disease causes & disease mechanisms

This condition is mostly due to kidney qi insufficiency. The kidney qi is too weak to secure. Thus the bladder loses its restraint, and the urine exits involuntarily.

Treatment based on pattern discrimination:

Kidney qi vacuity

Main symptoms: Frequent urination, incontinence, low back ache, weak limbs, lower abdominal heaviness and sagging, lassitude of the spirit, torpid intake, a pale tongue with a thin coating, and a fine, slippery pulse

Treatment principles: Supplement the qi and nourish the blood, secure the kidneys and quiet the fetus

Guiding formulas:

Gu Jing Wan (Secure the Menses Pills)
Tu Si Zi (Semen Cuscutae), 9g

Xiao Hui Xiang (Fructus Foeniculi), 6-9g
Sang Piao Xiao (Ootheca Mantidis), 9g
processed *Xiang Fu* (Rhizoma Cyperi), 6-9g
uncooked *Mu Li* (Concha Ostreae), 9-15g
Yan (salt), a small amount

Suo Quan Wan (Withdraw the Spring Pills) plus *Ju Yuan Jian Tang* (Raise the Source Decoction) with additions and subtractions
Dang Shen (Radix Codonopsitis), 9-15g
Huang Qi (Radix Astragali), 9-18g
Bai Zhu (Rhizoma Atractylodis Macrocephalae), 9g
mix-fried *Gan Cao* (Radix Glycyrrhizae), 6-9g
Sheng Ma (Rhizoma Cimicifugae), 3-6g
Xu Duan (Radix Dipsaci), 9g
Sang Ji Sheng (Herba Taxilli), 12-15g
Du Zhong (Cortex Eucommiae), 9-15g
Tu Si Zi (Semen Cuscutae), 9g
Sang Piao Xiao (Ootheca Mantidis), 9-15g
Yi Zhi Ren (Fructus Alpiniae Oxyphyllae), 9-15g
Jin Ying Zi (Fructus Rosae Laevigatae), 9g

This formula treats a spleen-kidney dual vacuity pattern, whereas the first formula mostly just secures and astringes the kidney qi.

Remarks:

Kegel exercises may help in the overall treatment of urinary incontinence during pregnancy.

Endnote:

1 www.gynaesurgeon.co.uk/incontinence/incontinence3.htm

25

Emotional Dysphoria During Pregnancy

Although emotional dysphoria during pregnancy is common enough to be a cultural cliché, interestingly, there is no named disorder describing psychoemotional disease during pregnancy in the fourth edition of the American Psychiatric Association's *Diagnosis & Statistical Manual* (*DSM-IV*), unless such conditions are specified under mental disorders due to a general medical condition. Nevertheless, psychoemotional disorders and discomfort during pregnancy are relatively common and are recognized as obstetrical disorders in Chinese gynecology.

Chinese medical disease categorization

Emotional dysphoria during pregnancy is covered by several different traditional obstetrical diseases in Chinese medicine. *Zi xuan* or child suspension is characterized by anxiety and a full, aching feeling below the heart. It typically presents after 4-5 months of pregnancy. *Zi fan* or child vexation typically presents after 5-6 months of pregnancy. It is characterized by fear and fright, vexation and restlessness. In *zi kuang*, child mania, the woman's mind runs unchecked and there are thirst and sweating. The vexation and agitation are so bad that the woman is described as insane. Although premodern Chinese gynecology texts discuss these as separate topics, because their disease mechanisms are related, modern TCM authors tend to discuss these categories simultaneously.

Disease causes & disease mechanisms

It is kidney essence and blood that nourish the fetus impelled by both sovereign and ministerial fires. As the fetus grows, yin essence, blood, and fluids and humors may become insufficient for the mother since what there is of these tends to be focused on the fetus. At the same time, because sovereign and ministerial fires are both "cooking" the fetus, these may easily become hyperactive and stir frenetically out of control. This can give rise to liver yin vacuity below with harassing of liver yang above, accumulation of phlegm fire in the heart, and heart-gallbladder insufficiency. It is flushing up of yang qi into the chest under the heart which causes fullness and distention in the chest and rib-sides and inability to lie down. This scenario may be complicated by the liver's assailing the spleen and the spleen losing its ability to promote the movement of water fluids and the engenderment and transformation of the blood. In the former case, dampness may congeal into phlegm which congests in the chest, confounding the orifices of the heart. In the latter case, there is insufficient blood to construct and nourish the spirit within the heart.

In the case of *zi kuang* or child mania, stomach fire flares, stagnates, and accumulates. This boils and stews the uterine and fetal juices and results in these drying up. The fetus loses its nourishment and so moves upward in the abdomen toward the heart as if looking for nourishment from heart blood. Therefore, although insanity is mostly thought of in the premodern texts as flaring of stomach fire, during pregnancy, *zi kuang* is described as being due to fire in the heart and spleen channels.

Patterns common to this condition

Liver assailing the spleen with malnourishment of the heart spirit
Yin vacuity with liver yang harassing above
Phlegm fire

Treatment based on pattern discrimination:

Liver assailing the spleen with malnourishment of the heart spirit

Main symptoms: Chest oppression, rib-side distention, stomach duct distention and fullness, easy anger, heart palpitations, fatigue, disquietude of the spirit, a pale tongue with thin, white fur, and a bowstring, fine pulse

Treatment principles: Harmonize the liver and spleen, nourish the blood and quiet the spirit

Guiding formulas:

Zi Su Yin (Perilla Beverage)
Da Fu Pi (Pericarpium Arecae), 6-9g
Chuan Xiong (Radix Ligustici Wallichii), 6-9g
Chen Pi (Pericarpium Citri Reticulatae), 6g
wine stir-fried *Bai Shao* (Radix Albus Paeoniae Lactiflorae), 9-18g
Zi Su Ye (Folium Perillae Frutescentis), 9-12g
Dang Gui (Radix Angelicae Sinensis), 9g
Ren Shen (Radix Ginseng), 3-9g
Gan Cao (Radix Glycyrrhizae), 3-9g
Sheng Jiang (uncooked Rhizoma Zingiberis), 6g

Cong Bai (Herba Allii Fistulosi), 6-9g

If the tongue coating is thin and yellow, add Radix Scutellariae (*Huang Qin*).

Zi Xuan Tang (Child Suspension Decoction)
Ren Shen (Radix Ginseng), 3-9g
Dang Gui (Radix Angelicae Sinensis), 9g
Bai Shao (Radix Albus Paeoniae Lactiflorae), 9-18g
Huang Qin (Radix Scutellariae, 9-12g
Dan Shen (Radix Salviae Miltiorrhizae), 9-15g
Zi Su Ye (Folium Perillae Frutescentis), 9-12g
Chen Pi (Pericarpium Citri Reticulatae), 6g
Sha Ren (Fructus Amomi), 3-4.5g
processed *Xiang Fu* (Rhizoma Cyperi), 9g
Sheng Jiang (uncooked Rhizoma Zingiberis), 6g
Cong Bai (Herba Allii Fistulosi), 6-9g

Jia Wei Gui Pi Tang (Added Flavors Restore the Spleen Decoction)
Ren Shen (Radix Ginseng), 3-9g
Huang Qi (Radix Astragali), 9-18g
Bai Zhu (Rhizoma Atractylodis Macrocephalae), 9g
Fu Ling (Poria), 9-12g
Suan Zao Ren (Semen Zizyphi Spinosae), 12-15g
processed *Yuan Zhi* (Radix Polygalae), 6-9g
Dang Gui (Radix Angelicae Sinensis), 9g
Chai Hu (Radix Bupleuri), 3-9g
Zhi Zi (Fructus Gardeniae), 6-9g
stir-fried *Zhi Ke* (Fructus Aurantii), 6g
Mu Xiang (Radix Auklandiae), 6-9g
mix-fried *Gan Cao* (Radix Glycyrrhizae), 6-9g
Long Yan Rou (Arillus Euphoriae Longanae), 9-12g

Yin vacuity with liver yang harassing above

Main symptoms: Heart vexation, restless when sitting or lying down, chest and rib-side distention and fullness, belching, wheezing when lying down, a bitter taste in the mouth, a dry throat, heat in the hands and feet, tidal fever, night sweats, a red facial complexion, chapped lips, constipation, short, red urination, a red, dry tongue with no or scanty, yellow fur, and a bowstring, fine, rapid pulse

Treatment principles: Clear the liver and nourish yin, downbear counterflow and eliminate vexation

Guiding formulas:

Yang Yin Chu Fan Tang (Nourish Yin & Eliminate Vexation Decoction)
Zhi Mu (Rhizoma Anemarrhenae), 9g
Mai Men Dong (Tuber Ophiopogonis), 9-12g
Huang Qin (Radix Scutellariae), 9-12g

Sheng Di (uncooked Radix Rehmanniae), 12-15g
Bai Shao (Radix Albus Paeoniae Lactiflorae), 9g
Fu Ling (Poria), 9-12g
Zhu Ru (Caulis Bambusae In Taeniis), 6-9g
Dan Dou Chi (Semen Praeparatus Sojae), 9-15g
Shi Chang Pu (Rhizoma Acori Tatarinowii), 6-9g

Bai Zi Yang Xin Tang (Semen Biotae Nourish the Heart Decoction)
Sheng Di (uncooked Radix Rehmanniae), 12-15g
Mai Men Dong (Tuber Ophiopogonis), 9-12g
Suan Zao Ren (Semen Zizyphi Spinosae), 12-15g
Ren Shen (Radix Ginseng), 3-9g
Bai Zi Ren (Semen Platycladi), 9-15g
Fu Shen (Sclerotium Pararadicis Poriae Cocos), 12-15g
Chuan Xiong (Radix Ligustici Wallichii), 6-9g
Yuan Zhi (Radix Polygalae), 6-9g
Dang Gui (Radix Angelicae Sinensis), 9g
Wu Wei Zi (Fructus Schisandrae), 9g
mix-fried *Gan Cao* (Radix Glycyrrhizae), 6-9g
Sheng Jiang (uncooked Rhizoma Zingiberis), 6g

Phlegm fire

Main symptoms: Dizziness, heart vexation, easy fright, chest and rib-side distention and fullness, belching, vomiting of phlegmy saliva, unsatisfying defecation, turbid, cloudy urination, slimy, yellow tongue fur, and a bowstring, slippery, rapid pulse

Treatment principles: Fortify the spleen, clear heat, and wash away phlegm

Guiding formula:

Qing Re Chu Fan Tang (Clear Heat & Eliminate Vexation Decoction)
Zhu Ru (Caulis Bambusae In Taeniis), 6-9g
Chen Pi (Pericarpium Citri Reticulatae), 6g
Zhi Shi (Fructus Immaturus Aurantii), 6g
Fu Ling (Poria), 9-12g
Mai Men Dong (Tuber Ophiopogonis), 9-12g
Zhu Li (Succus Bambusae), 30-60g
Huang Qin (Radix Scutellariae), 9-12g
Zhi Mu (Rhizoma Anemarrhenae), 9g
Shi Chang Pu (Rhizoma Acori Tatarinowii), 6-9g

Ren Shen Mai Dong San (Ginseng & Ophiopogon Powder)
Ren Shen (Radix Ginseng), 3-9g
Fu Ling (Poria), 9-12g
Huang Qin (Radix Scutellariae), 9-12g
Mai Men Dong (Tuber Ophiopogonis), 9-12g

Zhi Mu (Rhizoma Anemarrhenae), 9g
mix-fried *Gan Cao* (Radix Glycyrrhizae), 6-9g
Sheng Di (uncooked Radix Rehmanniae), 12-15g
Zhu Ru (Caulis Bambusae In Taeniis), 6-9g

This formula addresses elements of spleen vacuity, phlegm, fire, and yin vacuity.

Representative case history:

The patient was a 27 year-old female who was initially seen on March 25, 1973. The patient was six months pregnant and complained of vexation and agitation and heart palpitations. Her tongue was pale red, and her pulse was slightly slippery. Based on a Chinese medical pattern discrimination of liver depression transforming heat, the patient was prescribed three packets of the following medicinals: *Zhu Ru* (Caulis Bambusae In Taeniis), 9g, *Bai Shao* (Radix Albus Paeoniae Lactiflorae), 9g, *Sang Ye* (Folium Mori), 9g, *Chuan Bei Mu* (Bulbus Fritillariae Cirrhosae), 6g, *Sha Ren* (Fructus Amomi), 3g, and *Shan Zha Hua* (Flos Crataegi), 6g. One packet of these medicinals was decocted in water per day and administered orally. After three days, the patient was considered cured.

Remarks:

In my experience, Chinese medicine treats emotional dysphoria during pregnancy quite well. I have treated a number of pregnant women with otherwise various ill-defined emotional discomforts successfully using Chinese medicinals.

26

Heart Palpitations During Pregnancy

Maternal heart palpitations are common in pregnancy, although sustained dys-rhythmias are relatively rare. Of the dysrhythmias that do occur in pregnancy, almost all are supraventricular. Usually heart palpitations during pregnancy are the subjective experience of premature ventricular contractions (PVCs). They are more likely during pregnancy due to increased blood volume which peaks at 28-32 weeks at 40-50% above normal, nonpregnant volume. Because of this, the stroke volume of the heart increases. That plus the influence of progestrone may make the heart beat irregularly on occasion. In a lesser number of cases, heart palpitations during pregnancy may be associated with severe, life-threatening heart disease. Mitral valve prolapse (MVP) is another cause of heart palpitations in general. However, the signs and symptoms of MVP are usually stable or improved during pregnancy since decreased systemic vascular resistance reduces the afterload of the left ventricle and improves the forward flow of blood.[1] Western medical treatment for heart arrhythmias during pregnancy can vary from observation to implanted devices or aggressive drug therapy. Drugs should be considered carefully because of risk of transmission to the fetus in the uterus or through breast milk after birth. Digoxin, quinidine, procainamide, propanolol, and verapamil are the common drugs of choice for the treatment of dysrrhythmia during pregnancy. Those dysrrhythmias which are reclacitrant to medical treatment may be treated with direct current cardioversion. Because patients with atrial fibrillation are at high risk for thrombus formation, such patients are commonly treated with heparin which does not cross the placenta and is not recognized as a teratogen. However, prolonged administration of heparin is associated with maternal osteopenia.

Chinese medical disease categorization

Heart palpitations during pregnancy are referred to as *ren shen xin ji* in Chinese medicine.

Disease causes & disease mechanisms

After a woman becomes pregnant, blood gathers to nourish the fetus. Thus the heart blood may lose nourishment and the heart qi may become insufficient. This then may result in heart palpitations.

Treatment based on pattern discrimination:

Heart qi & blood vacuity

Main symptoms: Heart palpitations and rapid breathing during pregnancy accompanied by chest oppression and discomfort which worsens on stirring, superficial edema of the face and eyes, restless sleep at night, a somewhat pale tongue with thin, slimy fur, and a fine, slippery or bound, regularly interrupted pulse

Treatment principles: Boost the qi and nourish the blood, calm the heart and quiet the spirit

Guiding formula:

Sheng Mai Yin (Engender the Pulse Beverage) plus *Zhi Gan Cao Tang* (Mix-fried Licorice Decoction) with added flavors
Dang Shen (Radix Codonopsitis), 9-15g
Mai Men Dong (Tuber Ophiopogonis), 9-12g
Wu Wei Zi (Fructus Schisandrae), 9g
mix-fried *Gan Cao* (Radix Glycyrrhizae), 6-9g
Fu Ling (Poria), 9-12g
Bai Shao (Radix Albus Paeoniae Lactiflorae), 9-18g
Bai Zi Ren (Semen Platycladi), 9-15g
Gua Lou (Fructus Trichosanthis), 6-9g
Dan Shen (Radix Salviae Miltiorrhizae), 9-15g

Remarks:

If there is dizziness or shortness of breath, the patient should be referred to their Western physician for immediate examination and assessment. Serious heart arrhythmias may present a serious risk to the mother and/or the fetus.

Endnote:

[1] Jackson, G. Marc & Clark, Steven L., "Cardiac and Pulmonary Disorders and Pregnancy," *Gynecology & Obstetrics: A Longitudinal Approach, op. cit.*, p. 289

27

Preeclampsia & Eclampsia

Preeclampsia refers to the development of hypertension during pregnancy with albuminuria and/or edema between the 20th week of pregnancy and the end of the first week postpartum. Eclampsia refers to convulsive seizures or coma without other etiology occurring during the same time period. Preeclampsia and eclampsia may affect both the mother and the unborn baby, and the evolution from preeclampsia to eclampsia may develop rapidly, with some women with rapidly progressing disease presenting few symptoms.[1] The etiology of preeclampsia and eclampsia is unknown. The incidence of preeclampsia is 5% and usually occurs in primigravidas and women with pre-existing hypertension, kidney, or vascular disease.[2] Its incidence is also higher in women carrying multiple babies, teenage mothers, mothers over 40 years of age, and women whose mothers or sisters have had preeclampsia. Mild preeclampsia is characterized by borderline hypertension (140/90mm/Hg), edema, and albuminuria. Severe preeclampsia is characterized by blood pressure of 150/110mm/Hg or above, severe edema, and albuminuria. If these conditions are not checked, then the patient may develop full-fledged eclampsia with coma and convulsive seizures.

The primary Western medical treatment for both preeclampsia and eclampsia is induced delivery. Mild preeclampsia may be treated by strict bed rest, normal salt intake, and increased water intake. Severe preeclampsia is treated as a hospital in-patient with IV infusion of Ringer's solution and magnesium sulfate. As soon as the patient is stabilized, delivery is accomplished. Established eclampsia is treated essentially the same way. All patients, regardless of the severity of their condition, should be monitored for headaches, blurred vision, confusion, abdominal pain, vaginal bleeding, and loss of fetal heart sounds, with observations being recorded every 15 minutes. Eclampsia, if left untreated, is usually fatal. It is the leading cause of maternal and infant illness and death in the world and is responsible for not less than 76,000 deaths per year.[3] Preeclampsia should begin to resolve spontaneously within 4-6 hours after delivery.

Chinese medical disease categorization

The traditional Chinese term *zi xian* literally means child epilepsy or epilepsy while with child. Other traditional names for this condition are *zi yun*, child dizziness, and *zi jing*, child convulsions. In modern Chinese medicine, hypertension during pregnancy is referred to as *ren shen gao xue ya*, albuminuria is *dan bai niao*, and preeclampsia is *xian bei zi xian* or pre-child epilepsy

Disease causes & disease mechanisms

According to Chinese medical theory, excessive eating of chilled, uncooked foods, habitual depression and emotional disease, or failure of yin to control and support yang's extension and spreading may give rise to conditions which obstruct and hinder the *qi* transformation and the movement of water. This may then give rise to water dampness gathering and accumulating in the body and limbs and, therefore, swelling and distention. It may also give rise to the finest essence of foods and liquids being discharged downward and, thus, albuminuria.

Failure of yin to control and support yang tends to develop in the later months of pregnancy since kidney yin is used to nourish the fetus. Besides yin providing the basis for the smooth extension and spreading of kidney yang, if yin becomes vacuous and insufficient, heart and liver yang may become hyperactive. If heart fire flares upward, this may cause vexation and hypertension. If liver yang flares upward, this may cause dizziness and hypertension. If kidney yin becomes even more withered, the fetal source loses its nourishment and fetal fire will become effulgent. Since heat engenders wind and stews the juices into phlegm, this may cause twitching, spasm, and convulsions due to internal stirring of wind and phlegm obstructing the channels and network vessels. If heart and liver yang become hyperactive and effulgent, they may lose restraint and flush upward with phlegm obstructing the portals of the heart. In this case, there may be unconsciousness and confused spirit.

Thus it can be seen that preeclampsia and eclampsia are due to a combination of spleen and stomach dysfunction *vis à vis* the transportation and transformation of water, liver depression qi stagnation, and kidney yin vacuity leading to hyperactivity of the heart and liver. As Ye Heng-yin says, "[Child epilepsy] is due to wind heat in the two channels of the liver and heart."

Treatment based on pattern discrimination

Mild Preeclampsia

Liver-kidney yin vacuity with liver yang exuberance

> **Main symptoms:** Repeated attacks of headaches during the last trimester, dizziness, blurred vision, tinnitus, heart vexation, a flushed red facial complexion, slight edema in the lower limbs, a red tongue tip, and a bowstring, slippery pulse

> **Treatment principles:** Enrich yin and subdue yang assisted by levelling the liver

Guiding formula:

Qi Ju Di Huang Tang Jia Jian (Lycium & Chrysanthemun Rehmannia Decoction with Additions & Subtractions)
Sheng Di (uncooked Radix Rehmanniae), 12g
Shan Zhu Yu (Fructus Corni), 9g
Nu Zhen Zi (Fructus Ligustri Lucidi), 12g
Gou Qi Zi (Fructus Lycii), 9g
Fu Ling (Poria), 9g
Dan Pi (Cortex Moutan), 9g
Ze Xie (Rhizoma Alismatis), 9g
Long Gu (Os Draconis), 12-15g
Mu Li (Concha Ostreae), 12-15g
Shi Jue Ming (Concha Haliotidis), 12-15g
Gou Teng (Ramulus Uncariae Cum Uncis), 9-15g
Huang Qin (Radix Scutellariae), 9g
Bai Shao (Radix Alba Paeoniae), 9g
Ju Hua (Flos Chrysanthemi), 9g

Yi Guan Jian Jia Wei (One Link Decoction with Added Flavors)
Sha Shen (Radix Glehniae), 12-15g
Sheng Di (uncooked Radix Rehmanniae), 12-15g
Mai Men Dong (Tuber Ophiopogonis), 9-15g
Gou Qi Zi (Fructus Lycii), 9g
Dang Gui (Radix Angelicae Sinensis), 9g
Chuan Lian Zi (Fructus Toosendan), 9g
Shi Jue Ming (Concha Haliotidis), 12-15g
Gou Teng (Ramulus Uncariae Cum Uncis), 9-15g
Huang Qin (Radix Scutellariae), 9g

Mu Li Long Chi Tang (Oyster Shell & Dragon's Teeth Decoction)
Mu Li (Concha Ostreae), 12-15g
Long Chi (Dens Draconis), 12-15g
Shi Jue Ming (Concha Haliotidis), 12-15g
Xia Ku Cao (Spica Prunellae), 9-15g
Sang Ji Sheng (Herba Taxilli), 12-15g
Fu Ling (Poria), 9g
Ze Xie (Rhizoma Alismatis), 9g

If there is water swelling, add *Che Qian Zi* (Semen Plantaginis), *Chi Xiao Dou* (Semen Phaseoli Calcarati), and *Zhu Ling* (Polyporus). If there is harboring of phlegm, add *Zhu Li* (Succus Bambusae), *Ban Xia* (Rhizoma Pinelliae), *Dan Nan Xing* (bile-processed Rhizoma Arisaematis), *Shi Chang Pu* (Rhizoma Acori Tatarinowii), and *Xuan Fu Hua* (Flos Inulae).

Liver-gallbladder replete fire

Main symptoms: Dizziness, red eyes, heart vexation, rib-side pain, a bitter taste in the mouth, dry throat, scanty, yellow urine, a red tongue with yellow fur, and a bowstring, rapid pulse

Treatment principles: Clear the liver and discharge fire

Guiding formula:

Long Dan Xie Gan Tang Jia Jian (Gentiana Drain the Liver Decoction with Additions & Subtractions)

Long Dan Cao (Radix Gentianae), 9g
Sheng Di (uncooked Radix Rehmanniae), 12-15g
Huang Qin (Radix Scutellariae), 9-15g
Gan Cao (Radix Glycyrrhizae), 9-15g
Zhi Zi (Fructus Gardeniae), 9g
Ju Hua (Flos Chrysanthemi), 9g
Shi Jue Ming (Concha Haliotidis), 12-15g

Liver effulgence-spleen vacuity

Main symptoms: Edema during the last trimester, a yellowish white facial complexion, facial edema, scanty urination, dizziness, blurred vision, nausea, vomiting, heart vexation, diminished intake of food and drink, chest and rib-side aching and pain, diarrhea, constipation, or stringy stools followed by diarrhea, slimy, slightly yellow tongue fur, and deep, slippery pulse

Treatment principles: Fortify the spleen and move water, level the liver and subdue yang

Guiding formula:

Bai Zhu San Jia Wei (Atractylodes Powder with Added Flavors)

Bai Zhu (Rhizoma Atractylodis Macrocephalae), 9-15g
Fu Ling (Poria), 9g
Sang Bai Pi (Cortex Mori), 9-15g
Da Fu Pi (Pericarpium Arecae), 6-9g
Chen Pi (Pericarpium Citri Reticulatae), 6g
Jiang Pi (Cortex Rhizomatis Zingiberis), 9g
Mu Xiang (Radix Auklandiae), 9g
Shi Jue Ming (Concha Haliotidis), 12-15g
Dang Gui (Radix Angelicae Sinensis), 9g
Bai Shao (Radix Alba Paeoniae), 9g

Serious Preeclampsia

Yin vacuity-yang effulgence

Main symptoms: Frequent attacks of headache and dizziness in the last trimester, blurred vision, nausea, rib-side distention and stomach duct oppression, emission heat from the hands and feet, dry mouth, heart vexation, a red facial complexion, a red tongue with scanty fur, and a bowstring, rapid pulse

Treatment principles: Nourish yin, level the liver, and boost the kidneys

Guiding formulas:

Ling Yang Gou Teng Tang Jia Wei (Antelope Horn & Uncaria Decoction with Added Flavors)
Shan Yang Jiao (Cornu Caprae), 12-18g
Gou Teng (Ramulus Uncariae Cum Uncis), 9-15g
Sang Ye (Folium Mori), 9-15g
Chuan Bei Mu (Bulbus Fritillariae Cirrhosae), 9g
Sheng Di (uncooked Radix Rehmanniae), 12-15g
Ju Hua (Flos Chrysanthemi), 9-12g
Bai Shao (Radix Alba Paeoniae), 9g
Fu Ling (Poria), 9-18g
Zhu Ru (Caulis Bambusae In Taeniis), 9-15g
Gan Cao (Radix Glycyrrhizae), 6-9g
Gui Ban (Plastrum Testudinis), 12-15g
Du Zhong (Cortex Eucommiae), 9-15g
Sang Ji Sheng (Herba Taxilli), 12-15g

San Jia Fu Mai Tang (Three Nails Restore the Vessels Decoction)
Gou Teng (Ramulus Uncariae Cum Uncis), 9-15g
Dang Gui (Radix Angelicae Sinensis), 9g
Fu Shen (Sclerotium Pararadicis Poriae), 9-18g
Sang Ji Sheng (Herba Taxilli), 12-15g
Jie Geng (Radix Platycodi), 9g
Gui Ban (Plastrum Testudinis), 12-15g
Mu Li (Concha Ostreae), 12-18g
Bie Jia (Carapax Trionycis), 12-15g
Long Chi (Dens Draconis), 12-18g
Sheng Di (uncooked Radix Rehmanniae), 12-15g
Sha Shen (Radix Glehniae), 9-12g
Mai Men Dong (Tuber Ophiopogonis), 9-12g
E Jiao (Gelatinum Corii Asini), 9-12g
Shan Yang Jiao (Cornu Caprae), 12-18g
Bai Shao (Radix Alba Paeoniae), 9g

Liver effulgence-spleen vacuity

Main symptoms: The same as above under mild preeclampsia only worse

Treatment principles: The same as above

Guiding formula:

Quan Sheng Bai Zhu San Jia Wei (Whole Life Atractylodes Powder with Added Flavors)
Bai Zhu (Rhizoma Atractylodis Macrocephalae), 9g
Fu Ling (Poria), 9-12g
Da Fu Pi (Pericarpium Arecae), 9-12g
Jiang Pi (Cortex Rhizomatis Zingiberis), 9g
Chen Pi (Pericarpium Citri Reticulatae), 6-9g
Gou Teng (Ramulus Uncariae Cum Uncis), 9-15g
Shi Jue Ming (Concha Haliotidis), 12-15g
Gui Ban (Plastrum Testudinis), 12-15g
Dang Shen (Radix Codonopsis), 9-15g
Ju Hua (Flos Chrysanthemi), 9-12g

Eclampsia

Liver wind internally stirring

Main symptoms: Vertigo, dizziness, vexation and agitation, a flushed, red facial complexion, heart palpitations, loss of consciousness, inability to speak, spasms and convulsions, a red tongue with thin, yellow fur, and a bowstring, slippery, rapid pulse

Treatment principles: Settle the liver and extinguish wind

Guiding formula:

Zhen Gan Xi Feng Tang (Settle the Liver & Extinguish Wind Decoction)
Gou Teng (Ramulus Uncariae Cum Uncis), 9-15g
Ju Hua (Flos Chrysanthemi), 9-12g
Sheng Di (uncooked Radix Rehmanniae), 12-15g
Quan Xie (Scorpio), 9g
Huang Lian (Rhizoma Coptidis), 3-9g
Da Qing Ye (Folium Daqingye), 9-15g
Yu Jin (Tuber Curcumae), 9g
Shi Chang Pu (Rhizoma Acori Tatarinowii), 9g
Gui Ban (Plastrum Testudinis), 12-15g
Bai Shao (Radix Alba Paeoniae), 9g
Zi Bei Chi (Concha Cypraeae Maculae), 9-15g

Gou Teng Tang (Uncaria Decoction)
Gou Teng (Ramulus Uncariae Cum Uncis), 9-15g
Dang Gui (Radix Angelicae Sinensis), 9g
Fu Shen (Sclerotium Pararadicis Poriae), 9-18g
Ren Shen (Radix Ginseng), 6-9g
Jie Geng (Radix Platycodi), 6-9g
Sang Ji Sheng (Herba Taxilli), 12-15g

Ling Yang Jiao San (Antelope Horn Powder)
Shan Yang Jiao (Cornu Caprae), 12-18g
Du Huo (Radix Angelicae Pubescentis), 9g
Suan Zao Ren (Semen Zizyphi Spinosae), 9-15g
Wu Jia Pi (Cortex Acanthopanacis), 9g
Yi Yi Ren (Semen Coicis), 15-30g
Fang Feng (Radix Sapashnikoviae), 9g
Dang Gui (Radix Angelicae Sinensis), 9g
Chuan Xiong (Rhizoma Chuanxiong), 9-15g
Fu Shen (Sclerotium Pararadicis Poriae), 9-18g
Xing Ren (Semen Armeniacae), 9g
Mu Xiang (Radix Auklandiae), 6-9g
Gan Cao (Radix Glycyrrhizae), 6-9g

Ling Yang Gou Teng Tang Jia Wei (Antelope Horn & Uncaria Decoction with Added Flavors)
Gou Teng (Ramulus Uncariae Cum Uncis), 9-15g
Shan Yang Jiao (Cornu Caprae), 12-18g
Fu Shen (Sclerotium Pararadicis Poriae), 9-18g
Dang Gui (Radix Angelicae Sinensis), 9g
Suan Zao Ren (Semen Zizyphi Spinosae), 9-15g
Sang Ye (Folium Mori), 9-15g
Chuan Bei Mu (Bulbus Fritillariae Cirrhosae), 9g
Sheng Di (uncooked Radix Rehmanniae), 12-15g
Ju Hua (Flos Chrysanthemi), 9-12g
Bai Shao (Radix Alba Paeoniae), 9g
Zhu Ru (Caulis Bambusae In Taeniis), 6-9g
Gui Ban (Plastrum Testudinis), 12-15g
Sang Ji Sheng (Herba Taxilli), 12-15g
Gan Cao (Radix Glycyrrhizae), 6-9g

Phlegm fire harassing above

Main symptoms: Loss of consciousness, spasms and convulsions of the four limbs, obstructed breathing and the sound of phlegm in the throat, a red tongue with yellow, slimy fur, and a bowstring, slippery pulse

Treatment principles: Clear heat, break apart phlegm, and open the orifices

Guiding formulas:

Niu Huang Qing Xin Wan Jia Zhu Li (Bezoar Clear the Heart Pills with Bamboo Juice)
Niu Huang (Calculus Bovis), 3-9g
Zhu Sha (Cinnabar), 1.5-3g
Huang Lian (Rhizoma Coptidis), 3-9g
Huang Qin (Radix Scutellariae), 9-15g

Zhi Zi (Fructus Gardeniae), 9g
Yu Jin (Tuber Curcumae), 9g
Zhu Li (Succus Bambusae), 9g

Qing Re Chu Fan Tang Jia Wei (Clear Heat & Eliminate Vexation Decoction with Added Flavors)
Zhu Ru (Caulis Bambusae In Taeniis), 9g
Chen Pi (Pericarpium Citri Reticulatae), 6-9g
Zhi Shi (Fructus Immaturus Aurantii), 6-9g
Fu Ling (Poria), 9g
Mai Men Dong (Tuber Ophiopogonis), 12-15g
Zhu Li (Succus Bambusae), 9g
Huang Qin (Radix Scutellariae), 9-15g
Zhi Mu (Rhizoma Anemarrhenae), 9g
Shi Chang Pu (Rhizoma Acori Tatarinowii), 6-9g
Da Huang (Radix Et Rhizoma Rhei), 3-9g
Shi Jue Ming (Concha Haliotidis), 12-15g

Acupuncture & moxibustion: For eclampsia, needle *Bai Hui* (GV 20), *Yin Tang* (M-HN-3), *Ren Zhong* (GV 26), *Nei Guan* (Per 6), *Feng Chi* (GB 20), *Xing Jian* (Liv 2), *Tai Chong* (Liv 3), *Tai Xi* (Ki 3), and *San Yin Jiao* (Sp 6).

If the teeth are clenched, add *Jia Che* (St 6) and *Xia Guan* (St 7). If there are whole body convulsions with ophisthotonus, add *Da Zhui* (GV 14), *Hou Xi* (SI 3), and *Yang Ling Quan* (GB 34).

Another formula is to needle *Feng Chi* (GB 20), *Ren Zhong* (GV 26), *Feng Long* (St 40), *Da Dun* (Liv 1), and *Xing Jian* (Liv 2).

Abstract of representative Chinese research

From *"A Survey of the Therapeutic Efficacy of Acupuncture in the Treatment of 36 Cases of Hypertension During Pregnancy"* by Qin Xiao-guang *et al., Shan Xi Zhong Yi (Shanxi Chinese Medicine)*, #6, 2001, p. 31

Cohort description:

All 36 women in this study were seen as out-patients. The youngest was 21 and the oldest was 37, with an average age of 28.3 years. The shortest duration of pregnancy was 17 weeks and the longest was 31 weeks, with an average duration of 22.6 weeks. Twenty-eight women had a systolic pressure of 17.3-21.3kPa and a diastolic pressure of 14.0-15.3kPa. Twenty-three cases presented with edema and 18 with albuminuria. Six cases had 24 hour excretion of albuminuria equal to or in excess of 0.5g. All these patients had accompanying dizziness, headache, and heart palpitations.

In terms of pattern discrimination, 21 cases were categorized as presenting a yin vacuity-liver effulgence pattern as evidenced by dizziness, vertigo, headache, head distention, tinnitus, low back soreness, dry mouth and throat, vexation, agitation, and restlessness, numbness of the fingers, scanty urination, constipation, a red, fissured tongue, and a bowstring, slippery, rapid pulse. Fifteen cases were categorized as presenting a spleen vacuity-liver effulgence pattern. Their symptoms included generalized and/or facial edema, dizziness and vertigo or headache and numbness, chest oppression, nausea, torpid intake, lassitude of the spirit, lack of strength, unreplete stools, a fat tongue body, and a bowstring, slippery pulse.

Treatment method:

The main points consisted of: bilateral *Feng Chi* (GB 20), *Tai Chong* (Liv 3), *He Gu* (LI 4), *San Yin Jiao* (Sp 6), and *Bai Hui* (GV 20). If there was yin vacuity with liver effulgence, *Tai Xi* (Ki 3) was added. If there was spleen vacuity and liver effulgence, *Nei Guan* (Per 6) and *Tai Bai* (Sp 3) were added. These points were needled with one *cun*, 30 gauge needles. *Feng Chi* and *Tai Chong* were needled with draining technique. *He Gu, San Yin Jiao,* and *Nei Guan* were needled with even supplementing-even draining technique and mild stimulation. *Bai Hui, Tai Xi,* and *Tai Bai* were needled with supplementing technique. Needling was done for 30 minutes each time, once per day, with the needles stimulated every five minutes. Five such treatments equaled one course of treatment, and a two day rest was allowed between successive courses.

Treatment outcomes:

Marked effect was defined as reduction of the blood pressure to normal or, if the blood pressure was not able to be returned to normal, at least there was a reduction of more than 5.3kPa in the systolic pressure. Some effect was defined as a reduction in blood pressure of 2.7-5.3kPa in systolic pressure and 1.3-2.7kPa in diastolic pressure. No effect meant that any changes in the blood pressure did not met these criteria. Based on these criteria, 19 cases (52.85) got a marked effect, 13 cases (36.1%) got some effect, and four cases (11.1%) got no effect, for a total amelioration rate of 88.9%. The longest duration of treatment was five courses and the shortest was two courses.

From *"The Treatment of 60 Cases of Hypertension During Pregnancy* with *Zi Cao Jue Ming Tang* (Lithospermum & Abalone Shell Decoction)" by Wang Luying, *Zhe Jiang Zhong Yi Za Zhi (Zhejiang Journal of Chinese Medicine)*, #7, 1998, p. 303

Cohort description:

Altogether, 90 women were included in this study. The oldest was 35 and the youngest was 23 years old, with a median age of 27. Seventy-six were primagravidas and 14 had already given birth before. Five cases were within their first 24 weeks of pregnancy, 35 cases were 25-34 weeks, and 50 cases were over 35 weeks. Their clinical symptoms mainly included dizziness, vertigo, tinnitus, heart palpitations, racing heart, tidal redness of the cheeks of the face, lower limb superficial edema, a red or possibly crimson tongue with purple-colored tortuously distended veins sublingually, and a bowstring, fine, slippery, and/or rapid pulse. None of the patients had any history of high blood pressure, albuminuria, or edema before becoming pregnant. These 90 women were then divided into a group of 60, labeled the treatment group, and another group of 30, the comparison group. There was no marked difference in ages, history of pregnancy and birth, and disease nature between these two groups.

Treatment method:

The treatment group was administered self-composed *Zi Cao Jue Ming Tang*: *Zi Cao* (Radix Arnebiae/Lithospermi) and *Shi Jue Ming* (Concha Haliotidis), 30g each, *Gou Teng* (Ramulus Uncariae Cum Uncis), *Sheng Di* (uncooked Radix Rehmanniae), *Dan Shen* (Radix Salviae Miltiorrhizae), and *Dan Pi* (Cortex Moutan), 15g each, and *Ju Hua* (Flos Chrysanthemi), *Zhi Zi* (Fructus Gardeniae), and *Shan Zhu Yu* (Fructus Corni), 10g each. If phlegm heat was exuberant, aged *Dan Nan Xing* (bile-processed Rhizoma Arisaematis) and *Tian Zhu Huang* (Concretio Silicea Bambusae) were added. If edema was severe, *Che Qian Zi* (Semen Plantaginis) was added. If there were signs of stirring of wind, powdered *Ling Yang Jiao* (Cornu Antelopis Saiga-tatarici) was added and the dose of *Gou Teng* was doubled. One packet was administered per day, decocted in water and given in two divided doses. Seven days equaled one course of treatment. After two courses, treatment efficacy was examined. The comparison group was administered *Tian Ma Gou Teng Yin* (Gastrodia & Uncaria Beverage). The administration method and duration of treatment was the same as above.

Treatment outcomes:

Marked effect meant that blood pressure was below 17/12kPa and that albuminuria had disappeared. Improvement meant that blood pressure was decreased from before treatment equal to or below 17/12kPa, albuminuria was ", and all the symptoms had markedly decreased. No effect meant that blood pressure was still high, albuminuria was still positive, and there was no marked change in the symptoms. Based on these criteria, 39 cases in the treatment group were judged to have gotten a marked effect, 16 were improved, and five got no effect. In the comparison group, 13 were said to have gotten a marked effect, nine improved, and eight got no effect. Thus the total amelioration rate in the treatment group was 91.7%, while that of the comparison group was only 73.3%. Therefore, there was a significant statistical difference in outcomes between these two groups (P + 0.05).

Representative case histories

Case 1: The patient was a 29 year old female who was initially examined on January 28, 1964. The patient had gotten married when she was 26 years old. After being married for six months, she delivered prematurely for the first time. She then delivered prematurely a second time after seven months of pregnancy. Now she was in the fourth month of pregnancy and was experiencing generalized edema which was especially severe in her abdominal region. The patient saw several doctors and was prescribed 40 packets of Chinese medicinals without effect. Besides the abdominal distention and superficial edema of the four extremities, there was shortness of breath, heart palpitations, scanty eating and drinking, low back pain and heaviness of the lower legs, a a profuse white vaginal discharge. In terms of Western medical examination, there was marked pitting edema of the lower extremities, blood pressure was 160/100mm/Hg, and albuminuria was (+++). Therefore, the patient was diagnosed with toxemia of pregnancy. Blood pressure was lowered by disinhibiting urination, and the blood pressure returned to normal. However, the patient's appetite was still poor and her abdomen was still enlarged.

In terms of the four examinations of Chinese medicine, the patient's facial complexion was yellowish white and her affect was bitter and oppressed. There was lassitude of the spirit and fatigue, disinclination to speak and weak voice, cough, slight hasty breathing, superficial edema of the four extremities, pale lips, a pale red tongue with glossy, white fur, and a bowstring, slippery, forceless pulse. Based on these signs and symptoms, the patient's Chinese medical pattern was categorized as spleen vacuity unable to control water. Therefore, she was prescribed *Fu Ling Dao Shui Tang Jia Jian* (Poria Abduct Water Decoction with Additions & Subtractions): *Fu Ling* (Poria), 15g, *Bai Zhu* (Rhizoma Atractylodis Macrocephalae), 15g, *Zhu Ling* (Polyporus), 15g, *Ze Xie* (Rhizoma Alismatis), 5g, *Bing Lang* (Semen Arecae), 5g, *Sha Ren* (Fructus Amomi), 7.5g, *Mu Xiang* (Radix Auklandiae), 3.5g, *Chen Pi* (Pericarpium Citri Reticulatae), 10g, *Da Fu Pi* (Pericarpium Arecae), 15g, *Su Geng* (Caulis Perillae), 10g, *Dang Gui* (Radix Angelicae Sinensis), 10g, and *Bai Shao* (Radix Alba Paeoniae), 7.5g.

At the second examination, the patient reported chest oppression, nausea, shortness of breath, and heart palpitations. therefore, 10 grams each of *Yuan Zhi* (Radix Polygalae) and *Zhu Ru* (Caulis Bambusae In Taeniis) were added to the formula. At the third examination, all the patient's symptoms were decreased and there was no nausea. There was still some heart palpitations and shortness of breath as well as generalized lack of strength. Therefore, *Zhu Ru* was removed from the formula and 30 grams of *Huang Qi* (Radix Astragali) were added. At the fourth examination, the distention and edema had disappeared, but there was still some low back soreness and abdominal pain and sagging. Thus, 15 grams of *Du Zhong* (Cortex Eucommiae) and 10 grams of *Wu Yao* (Radix Linderae) were added to the formula. At the fifth examination, there were no changes made to the formula. the sixth examination was held on Feb. 15 when all the symptoms were basically cured. The edema and pain were decreased and, despite, slight weakness of the body, there was no low back or abdominal discomfort. Therefore, the woman was prescribed *Dang Gui San* (Dang Gui Powder) to nourish the blood and quiet the fetus and eventually was fine afterwards. On follow-up, it was learned that the woman had given birth at full term to a healthy child and that her health was also good.

Case 2: The patient was a 31 year old female who was seven months pregnant and complained of dizziness, tinnitus, lower extremity edema, dry, bound stools, and qi counterflow when stirring. Her tongue was slightly crimson red, and her pulse was bowstring, small, and slippery. Her blood pressure was 148/104mm/Hg, and her Western medical diagnosis was toxemia during pregnancy. Her Chinese medical pattern discrimination was yin fluid depletion and detriment with liver wind internally stirring. For this, she was prescribed: *Sheng Di* (uncooked Radix Rehmanniae), 30g, *Shi Hu* (Herba Dendrobii), 9g, *Nu Zhen Zi* (Fructus Ligustri Lucidi), 15g, *Huang Jing* (Rhizoma Polygonati), 12g, stir-fried *Huai Hua Mi* (Fructus Immaturus Sophorae), 30g, calcined *Shi Jue Ming* (Concha Haliotidis), 30g, *Jue Ming Zi* (Semen Cassiae), 30g, *Ci Shi* (Magnetitum), 30g, *Huang Qin* (Radix Scutellariae), 9g, and *Sang Ji Sheng* (Herba Taxilli), 9g.

After taking three packets of this prescription, the patient's dizziness was somewhat less and her stools were more moist. Also, the qi counterflow was leveled. Therefore, she was prescribed: *Sheng Di* (uncooked Radix Rehmanniae), 30g, *Nu Zhen Zi* (Fructus Ligustri Lucidi), 15g, *Huang Jing* (Rhizoma Polygonati), 12g, stir-fried *Huai Hua Mi* (Fructus Immaturus Sophorae), 30g, calcined *Mu Li* (Concha Ostreae), 30g, *Jue Ming Zi* (Semen Cassiae), 30g, *Ci Shi* (Magnetitum), 30g, *Huang Qin* (Radix Scutellariae), 9g, *Sang Ji Sheng* (Herba Taxilli), 9g, *Bai Shao* (Radix Alba Paeoniae), 9g, and calcined *Shi Jue Ming* (Concha Haliotidis), 30g. Five packets of this formula and the patient was judged cured.

Case 3: The patient was a 36 year old female who was first seen on April 20, 1967 and who was in her sixth month of pregnancy. The patient presented with convulsion, coma, clenched jaws, and the sound of phlegm in her throat. Before this, the patient had complained of an uncomfortable sensation, heart vexation, a bitter taste in the mouth, insomnia, and dizziness. Previous treatment for these complaints had been ineffective. The patient's pulse was bowstring, slippery, and rapid, while her tongue was red with yellow fur. These symptoms were due to liver yang counterflowing upward mixed with phlegm obstructing and blocking the clear orifices. Therefore, in order to level the liver, nourish the blood, and dispel phlegm, the following medicinals were prescribed: *Gou Teng* (Ramulus Uncariae Cum Uncis), 15g, *Sheng Di* (uncooked Radix Rehmanniae), 15g, *Chuan Bei Mu* (Bulbus Frtillariae Cirrhosae), 9g, uncooked *Mu Li* (Concha Ostreae), 15g, *Zhu Ru* (Caulis Bambusae In Taeniis), 9g, *Shi Jue Ming* (Concha Haliotidis), 12g, *Bai Shao* (Radix Alba Paeoniae), 12g, *Huang Qin* (Radix Scutellariae), 10g, and *Gan Cao* (Radix Glycyrrhizae), 3g.

The second examination occurred on April 28 after the woman had taken three packets of medicinals. The convulsions had stopped and her mind was clear and conscious. Therefore, another three packets were prescribed. The patient was seen again on May 2, at which time all her symptoms had disappeared. In order to hasten delivery, she was then prescribed three packets of *Cui Sheng Wu You Tang* (Hasten Birth No Worries Decoction) and the patient was judged cured.

Remarks

Obviously, eclampsia is a life-threatening, dangerous disease. However, my experience is that Chinese medicine can be effective for treating preeclampsia and can prevent a woman's condition from worsening to the point of eclampsia. If one chooses to treat preeclampsia, this requires extremely close monitoring of the patient, and both practitioner and patient should be prepared to go to the emergency room should the Chinese medical therapy not halt the progression of the disease and regress the symptoms. In fact, the woman has probably already been hospitalized under close observation as soon as her Western phsyician diagnosed pre-eclampsia. Since the first Western response is to simply monitor the mother's condition, some MDs may be willing to allow acupuncture and/or Chinese herbal medicine during this time. At least, that has been my experience.

Endnotes

[1] www.preeclampsia.org/about.asp

[2] Beers, Mark H. & Berkow, Robert, *The Merck Manual of Diagnosis & Therapy, 17th edition*, Merck Research Laboratories, Whitehouse Station, NJ, 1999, p. 2058

[3] www.preeclampsia.org, op. cit.

28
Gestational Diabetes

Gestational diabetes mellitus (GDM) is defined as any degree of glucose intolerance with onset or first recognition during pregnancy.[1] This definition is applicable whether or not insulin is used for treatment and whether or not the condition persists after pregnancy. It does not exclude the possibility that an unrecognized glucose intolerance may have antedated or begun concomitantly with pregnancy. Three to five percent of all pregnant women in the United States are diagnosed as having GDM resulting in approximately 185,000 cases per year.[2] The actual prevalence of GDM may be as high as 14% of all pregnancies depending on the population studied and the diagnostic tests employed.[3] Gestational diabetes usually develops because of a faulty physical interaction between the mother and baby. During the second trimester, somewhere between 24-28 weeks, the placenta begins producing many hormones. One of these hormones may block the action of insulin in the mother, thus creating insulin resistance. If the mother cannot produce enough extra insulin to overcome this resistance, her blood sugar will rise. The mother's high blood sugar then stimulates the baby to make more insulin and move more sugar into his or her cells, causing him or her to gain extra weight. If left unregulated, these changes can have serious harmful effects on both the mother and child.

While any woman may develop GDM, some of the risk factors are a previous diagnosis of GDM, severe physical or emotional stress if prone to GDM, obesity, a family history of diabetes, a history of miscarriage, having previously given birth to a very large infant (*i.e.*, greater than nine pounds), stillbirth, or a child with a birth defect, or having too much amniotic fluid (polyhydraminos). Women over 25 years of age are also at greater risk than those under 25.[4] Western medical screening for GDM is routinely performed (unless otherwise indicated) between weeks 24-28 of gestation in women meeting one of more of the following criteria:

1. Twenty-five years of age or older

2. Less than 25 years of age and obese (*i.e.*, 20% or more over desired body weight or a body mass index (BMI) equal to or over 27kg/m$^{2)}$

3. A family history of diabetes in a first degree relative

4. Member of an ethnic/racial group with a high prevalence of diabetes, *e.g.*, Hispanic-American, Native-American, Asian-American, African-American, or Pacific Islander.

Such screening tests consist of a 50g oral glucose load followed by plasma glucose determination one hour later. A value equal to or greater than 140mg/dL (7.8mmol/L) one hour after a 50g load indicates the need for a full diagnostic 100g three-hour oral glucose tolerance test (OGTT) performed in the fasting state. A Western medical diagnosis of gestational diabetes is made if two or more of the following blood sugar levels are higher than the following criteria:

1. Fasting blood glucose ≥ 105mg/dL

2. One-hour blood glucose ≥ 190mg/dL

3. Two-hour blood glucose ≥ 165mg/dL

4. Three-hour blood glucose ≥ 145mg/dL

The Western medical treatment of gestational diabetes consists of immediate dietary modification in order to regulate blood sugar levels. If dietary modification alone is not able to control blood glucose, insulin injections may be necessary. In order to determine blood glucose levels, women with GDM must self-monitor their blood glucose up to four times per day as well as test for ketones in their urine 1-2 times per week. For some women, exercising, such as walking after meals or at specific times of the day, helps to keep blood sugar in better control.[5]

Risks to the mother if GDM is not controlled include the possibility of delivery by cesarean section due to the baby's large size or the development of toxemia (a.k.a. eclampsia), increased urinary tract infections, and development of pregnancy-induced high blood pressure. About 5% of women with GDM develop toxemia during pregnancy.[6] Approximately 40% of women diagnosed with GDM develop type 2 diabetes later in life.[7] In one large study, more than half of all women with GDM developed overt type 2 diabetes within 15 years of pregnancy.[8] The risks to the infant include macrosomia (*i.e.*, a large, fat baby), shoulder dystocia, neonatal hypoglycemia, increased risk for obesity and diabetes, prolonged neonatal jaundice, low blood calcemia, and respiratory distress syndrome. In the majority of cases, GDM disappears automatically after delivery.

Chinese medical disease categorization

The traditional Chinese disease categories which correspond to gestational diabetes or its complications include *ren shen fan re*, vexatious heat during pregnancy, *ren shen fan ke*, vexatious thirst during pregnancy, *ren shen xuan yun*, dizziness and vertigo during pregnancy, *ren shen tou zhang tong*, head distention and pain during pregnancy, *ren shen xian zheng*, epilepsy during pregnancy, *ren shen xiao bian lin tong*, urinary strangury and pain during pregnancy, and *ren shen duo niao*, polyuria during pregnancy.

Disease causes & disease mechanisms

During pregnancy, yin, essence, blood, and fluids are transported downward to the uterus in order to foster and nourish the fetus. Due to natural endowment insufficiency or habitual bodily yin vacuity, this may leave yin and blood within the mother's body depleted and vacuous. Thus yin vacuity may engender heat internally, and this heat may further damage and consume yin fluids, leading to the easy engenderment of wasting and thirsting disease. It is also possible for habitual depression to cause the liver to lose its spreading. Because the fetus already obstructs the mother's qi mechanism as it grows in size towards the end of the pregnancy, qi stagnation often becomes more severe during the last trimester, and enduring or aggravated depression may transform fire which may also damage and consume yin fluids. Further, habitual addiction to sweets and fats may also cause accumulation of heat brewing internally. If, during the later half of pregnancy when yin and blood tend to become vacuous and insufficient and yang qi tends to become exuberant, such exuberant yang qi may join with these heat evils, thus exacerbating each other. Hence, there is yin vacuity with heat exuberance which is also able to give rise to wasting and thirsting disease.

Patterns common to this condition

Yin vacuity with heat exuberance
Qi & yin vacuity
Liver-kidney yin vacuity

Treatment based on pattern discrimination:

Yin vacuity with heat exuberance

Main symptoms: Dry mouth and parched throat, vexatious thirst, polydipsia, frequent, numerous, excessive urination, polyphagia, rapid hungering, dry, bound stools, a red tongue with scanty fluids, and a slippery, rapid pulse

Treatment principles: Enrich yin and clear heat

Guiding formula:

Zheng Ye Tang (Increase Humors Decoction) plus Bai Hu Tang (White Tiger Decoction) with additions and subtractions
uncooked *Shi Gao* (Gypsum Fibrosum), 9-21g
Sheng Di (uncooked Radix Rehmanniae), 12-15g

Xuan Shen (Radix Scrophulariae), 9-15g
Sha Shen (Radix Glehniae), 9-12g
Mai Men Dong (Tuber Ophiopogonis), 9-12g
Zhi Mu (Rhizoma Anemarrhenae), 9g
Huang Qin (Radix Scutellariae), 9-12g

If there are dry, bound stools, one can increase the doses of *Sheng Di* and *Xuan Shen* in order to enrich yin and increase humors, moisten the intestines and free the flow of the stools. If there is simultaneous obstruction and stagnation of the qi mechanism with chest and rib-side distention and oppression, add nine grams each of *Qing Pi* (Pericarpium Citri Reticulatae Viride), *Chuan Lian Zi* (Fructus Toosendan), and *Zhi Ke* (Fructus Aurantii) to course the liver and rectify the qi. If oral thirst is severe, add nine grams each of *Shi Hu* (Herba Dendrobii), *Lu Gen* (Rhizoma Phragmitis), and *Wu Mei* (Fructus Mume) to engender fluids and stop thirst.

Acupuncture & moxibustion: *Tai Xi* (Ki 3), *Zhao Hai* (Ki 6), *Nei Ting* (St 44)

If oral thirst is severe, add supplementing *Cheng Jiang* (CV 24) and *Lie Que* (Lu 7). If there is concomitant liver depression qi stagnation, add draining *Tai Chong* (Liv 3).

Qi & yin vacuity

Main symptoms: Shortness of breath, lack of strength, dry mouth and a desire to drink, dry, bound stools, frequent, numerous, excessive urination, a fat tongue with white fur, and a deep, fine, slippery pulse

Treatment principles: Boost the qi and nourish yin

Guiding formula:

Sheng Mai San (Engender the Pulse Powder) plus *Zeng Ye Tang* (Increase Humors Decoction) with additions and subtractions
Huang Jing (Rhizoma Polygonati), 9-15g
Tai Zi Shen (Radix Pseudostellariae), 9g
Sha Shen (Radix Glehniae), 9-12g
Sheng Di (uncooked Radix Rehmanniae), 12-15g
Xuan Shen (Radix Scrophulariae), 9-15g
Mai Men Dong (Tuber Ophiopogonis), 9-12g
Tian Men Dong (Tuber Asparagi), 9-12g
Wu Wei Zi (Fructus Schisandrae), 9g
Gou Qi Zi (Fructus Lycii), 9g
Shan Zhu Yu (Fructus Corni), 9g

If there is lassitude of the spirit, lack of strength, and other such obvious qi vacuity symptoms, add *Huang Qi* (Radix Astragali) and *Dang Shen* (Radix Codonopositis). If there is dry mouth and polydipsia due to yin vacuity and internal heat, add *Zhi Mu* (Rhizoma Anemarrhenae), *Wu Mei* (Fructus Mume), and

Shi Hu (Herba Dendrobii) to clear heat, enrich yin, and engender fluids. If there is dizziness or vertigo due to liver-kidney yin vacuity, add *Ju Hua* (Flos Chrysanthemi) and *Gou Teng* (Ramulus Uncariae Cum Uncis). If there is polyphagia and rapid hungering, add *Shu Di* (cooked Radix Rehmanniae) and *Yu Zhu* (Rhizoma Polygonati Odorati).

Acupuncture & moxibustion: *Tai Xi* (Ki 3), *Zu San Li* (St 36), *Pi Shu* (Bl 20), *Shen Shu* (Bl 23)

If there is dry mouth and polydipsia, add supplementing *Cheng Jiang* (CV 24), *Zhao Hai* (Ki 6), and *Lie Que* (Lu 7). If there is liver-kidney yin vacuity, add supplementing *Qu Quan* (Liv 8), *Ge Shu* (Bl 17), and *Gan Shu* (Bl 18). If there is polyphagia and rapid hungering, add draining *Nei Ting* (St 44) and use even supplementing-even draining technique at *Zu San Li*.

Liver-kidney yin vacuity

Main symptoms: Low back and knee soreness and limpness, frequent, numerous, excessive urination which is possibly turbid like rice-washing water, dry mouth and a desire to drink, dizziness or vertigo, a red tongue with scanty fluids, and a deep, fine, slippery pulse

Treatment principles: Enrich and supplement the liver and kidneys

Guiding formula:

Liu Wei Di Huang Wan (Six Flavors Rehmannia Pills)
Shan Yao (Radix Dioscoreae), 9-15g
Shu Di (cooked Radix Rehmanniae), 12-15g
Shan Zhu Yu (Fructus Corni), 9g
Fu Ling (Poria), 9-12g
Ze Xie (Rhizoma Alismatis), 6-9g
Dan Pi (Cortex Moutan), 6-9g

If there is yin vacuity with fire effulgence, add *Zhi Mu* (Rhizoma Anemarrhenae) and *Huang Bai* (Cortex Phellodendri) to enrich yin and downbear fire. If there is yin vacuity and yang hyperactivity with dizziness and vertigo, add *Mai Men Dong* (Tuber Ophiopogonis), *Gui Ban* (Plastrum Testudinis), *Ju Hua* (Flos Chrysanthemi), and *Gou Teng* (Ramulus Uncariae Cum Uncis) to enrich yin and level the liver. If there is bilateral lower leg edema, low back soreness, and turbid urine, add *Xu Duan* (Radix Dipsaci), *Tu Si Zi* (Semen Cuscutae), *Zhu Ling* (Polyporus), and *Sang Bai Pi* (Cortex Mori) to supplement the kidneys and quiet the fetus, disinhibit water and disperse swelling.

Acupuncture & moxibustion: *Tai Xi* (Ki 3), *Qu Quan* (Liv 8), *Ge Shu* (Bl 17), *Gan Shu* (Bl 18), *Shen Shu* (Bl 23)

If there is yin vacuity with yang hyperactivity, add draining *Bai Hui* (GV 20), *Feng Chi* (Bl 20), and *Yin Tang* (M-HN-3) and replace *Qu Quan* with even supplementing-even draining *Tai Chong* (Liv 3). If there is high blood pressure, omit *Qu Quan* and add draining *Qu Chi* (LI 11) and *Feng Chi* (GB 20) and even supplementing-even draining *Tai Chong* and *Zu San Li* (St 36). If there is lower lip edema and turbid urine (meaning obvious proteinemia), add draining *Yin Ling Quan* (Sp 9) and *Zhong Ji* (CV 3).

Remarks:

While the above three patterns may be the main ones in gestational diabetes, these three root patterns may be complicated by a number of other commonly seen disease mechanisms, especially phlegm dampness, depressive or phlegm heat, liver depression qi stagnation, and blood stasis. Therefore, it is likely that the above formulas will have to be modified with additions and subtractions.

Endnotes:

[1] Metzger, B.E., "Proceedings of the Third International Workshop-Conference on Gestational Diabates Mellitus," 1991, p. 201

[2] www.amoc.org/gesdiab.htm

[3] www.diabetes.org/diabetescare/supplement198/s60.htm

[4] wwww.nichd.nih.gov/publications/pubs/gest1.htm

[5] www.diabetes.ca/about_diabetes/gestational.htm

[6] www.nichd.nih.gov/publications/pubs/gest2.htm

[7] www.amoc.org, *op. cit.*

[8] www.nichd.nih.gov/publications/pubs/gest2.htm

29

Placenta Previa

Placenta previa refers to a placenta which has implanted over or too near the cervix. This condition occurs in approximately 0.5% of pregnancies and usually in multiparas, in patients who have had a previous cesarean section, or in patients with such uterine abnormalities as uterine myomas which prevent normal implantation. The placenta may cover the internal os completely (total previa) or partially (partial previa), or it may encroach on the internal os. This latter condition is referred to as low-lying placenta or marginal previa and may be detected during routine prenatal ultrasonography. Happily, in most cases, this condition spontaneously resolves as the uterus enlarges. However, in some cases, it may cause vaginal bleeding in late stage pregnancy or during delivery. This bleeding may be precipitated by vaginal examination or vaginal intercourse. This bleeding is painless, may be recurrent, and may be massive. It is typically bright red in color. If bleeding is profuse, there may be low blood pressure, pallor, spontaneous perspiration, and a rapid pulse. There is no treatment in Western medicine for placenta previa other than cesarean section which is commonly done during the 39th week. If hemorrhage is massive, emergency cesarean-section may have to be performed.

Chinese medical disease categorization

Placenta previa corresponds to fetal leakage, *tai lou*, in Chinese medicine.

Disease causes & disease mechanisms

There are very few discussions in the Chinese medical literature of placenta previa of which I am aware. As previously stated under spontaneous abortion, there are only four possible causes of bleeding in Chinese medicine: 1) heat forcing the blood to move frenetically outside its channels, 2) qi vacuity failing to contain the blood within its vessels, 3) stasis forcing the blood to move outside its pathways, and 4) traumatic injury severing the channels and vessels, with the first three of these mechanisms being the primary ones in gynecology. While it is possible that any of these three mechanisms, either alone or in combination, may be associated with placenta previa, in my experience and based on the scanty Chinese literature, central qi vacuity seems to be the main disease mechanism of this condition.

Treatment based on pattern discrimination:

Central qi downward falling

Main symptoms: Potentially massive, painless vaginal bleeding late in pregnancy accompanied by fresh red blood, spontaneous perspiration, dizziness standing up, fatigue, lack of strength, a pale facial complexion, a pale, enlarged tongue with teeth-marks on its edges and thin, white fur, and a short, fine, forceless pulse

Treatment principles: Fortify the spleen and boost the qi, stop leakage and quiet the fetus

Guiding formula:

***Bu Zhong Yi Qi Tang* (Supplement the Center & Boost the Qi Decoction)**
Huang Qi (Radix Astragali), 9-18g
Ren Shen (Radix Ginseng), 3-9g
Bai Zhu (Rhizoma Atractylodis Macrocephalae), 9g
Dang Gui (Radix Angelicae Sinensis), 9g
Chen Pi (Pericarpium Citri Reticulatae), 6g
Sheng Ma (Rhizoma Cimicifugae), 3-6g
Chai Hu (Radix Bupleuri), 3-9g
mix-fried *Gan Cao* (Radix Glycyrrhizae), 6-9g

If bleeding is due to spleen qi vacuity, add *Xian He Cao* (Herba Agrimoniae), *Ai Ye* (Folium Artemisiae Argyii), and *E Jiao* (Gelatinum Corii Asini). If complicated by kidney qi vacuity, add *Du Zhong* (Cortex Eucommiae), *Tu Si Zi* (Semen Cuscutae), and *Xu Duan* (Radix Dipsaci). If there is complicating blood heat, add carbonized *Di Yu* (Radix Sanguisorbae), carbonized *Huai Hua Mi* (Flos Immaturus Sophorae), and carbonized *Sheng Di* (uncooked Radix Rehmanniae).

Acupuncture & moxibustion: Moxa *Bai Hui* (GV 20) indirectly 1-2 times per day

Abstract of representative Chinese research:

From "The Treatment of 30 Cases of Placenta Previa with *Bu Zhong Yi Qi Tang Jia Wei* (Supplement the Center & Boost the Qi Decoction with Added Flavors)" by Hu Cui-fang, *Zhe Jiang Zhong Yi Za Zhi (Zhejiang Journal of Chinese Medicine)*, #4, 1995, p. 159

Cohort description:

Of the 30 cases included in this study, 20 were multiparas and 10 were primiparas. Their ages ranged from 25-35 years old. Among the multiparas, 14 had had artificial abortions, four had had endometritis during their previous pregnancies, and two had had cesarean deliveries. Among the primiparas, all had had artificial abortions. All these women were in their 22-37 weeks of pregnancy. In each case, there was an abnormal discharge of blood from the vaginal tract without any pain. This was accompanied by scanty qi and disinclination to talk, lassitude of the spirit, and weak limbs. Diagnosis was made by ultrasound. All had either borderline or partial placenta previa or low placental position.

Treatment method:

Bu Zhong Yi Qi Tang Jia Wei consisted of: *Huang Qi* (Radix Astragali), *Dang Shen* (Radix Codonopsitis), *Gan Cao* (Radix Glycyrrhizae), *Chen Pi* (Pericarpium Citri Reticulatae), *Sheng Ma* (Rhizoma Cimicifugae), *Chai Hu* (Radix Bupleuri), *Bai Zhu,* (Rhizoma Atractylodis Macrocephalae), *Dang Gui* (Radix Angelicae Sinensis), carbonized *Di Yu* (Radix Sanguisorbae), carbonized *Huai Hua Mi* (Flos Immaturus Sophorae), carbonized *Shu Di* (cooked Radix Rehmanniae), *Tu Si Zi* (Semen Cuscutae), and *Pu Gong Ying* (Herba Taraxaci). If there was low back soreness, stir-fried *Du Zhong* (Cortex Eucommiae) and *Xu Duan* (Radix Dipsaci) were added. If the face was a sallow yellow and there was dizziness, carbonized *E Jiao* (Gelatinum Corii Asini) and *He Shou Wu* (Radix Polygoni Multiflori) were added. If there was torpid intake, scorched *Shen Qu* (Massa Medica Fermentata) was added.

Treatment outcomes:

After 1/2-3 months of taking this formula, 21 cases of placenta previa returned to normal. In five cases, borderline placenta previa had become low positioned placenta, while in three cases, partial placenta previa had become borderline placenta previa. In one case, after taking five packets of the above formula, the bleeding became excessive like a menstrual period and the woman received surgery to terminate the pregnancy. The other 29 cases were followed up and they all had normal deliveries with scanty bleeding and healthy babies.

Remarks:

Although I have yet to find anything in the Chinese medical literature specifically on abruptio placenta, I have treated several cases of abruptio placentae successfully over the years. Abruptio placentae refers to bleeding from a correctly positioned placenta due to premature partial separation of the placenta from the uterine wall. In Chinese medicine, this is also categorized as *tai lou*, fetal leakage, and treated with Chinese medicinals primarily by fortifying the spleen and supplementing the kidneys in order to stop bleeding and quiet the fetus. Heat evils may or may not complicate these two main disease mechanisms.

30

Malposition of the Fetus

Malposition of the fetus, also referred to as malpresentation of the fetus and abnormal fetal position, describes any abnormal position of the fetus in the uterus which may make natural childbirth difficult. The fetus grows in the womb in an upright position. By weeks 32-36, it is supposed to turn downward to enable the head to be directed to the birth canal.[1] The incidence of spontaneous version after 40 weeks is low. Breech presentation refers to a fetus positioned buttocks down toward the birth canal. Breech presentation occurs in 2-4% of all pregnant women. It can lead to stretching and enlargement of the vaginal tract with increased blood loss postpartum and increased susceptibility to postpartum infection. Its contribution to perinatal morbidity and mortality is markedly disproportionate to the actual numbers of nonvertex fetuses.[2] The breech is the presenting part in 25% of deliveries occurring before 30 weeks. Therefore, prematurity is an important factor in the incidence of this condition. Due to changes in medico-legal climate and patient information, cesarean delivery of breech fetuses has become routine in the U.S. Transverse or oblique presentation describes a fetus positioned horizontally in the uterus causing the shoulder to enter the birth canal first.

According to Western medicine, factors leading to malposition of the fetus include maternal anomalies in the uterine shape, such as anthropoid pelvic brim, android pelvic brim, or a flat sacrum, tumors, placenta previa and fundal placentas, fetal prematurity, fetal structural anomalies, such as hydrocephalus, and chromosomal anomalies, such as trisomy-18.[3] Other factors include multiparity (89% of cases) which induces laxity of the supporting tissues[4] and pendulous abdomen.[5] The primary problem with breech presentation is that the presenting part is a poor dilating wedge, making delivery of the head difficult.[6] Complications or problems caused by breech presentation include fetal intracranial bleeding, neck, shoulder, or hip dislocation, clavicle fracture, internal organ disruption, premature placental rupture, umbilical cord prolapse, entrapment of the head, and/or maternal uterine rupture.[7] For instance, the incidence of umbilical cord prolapse is 5-20 times greater in breech presentation.[8]

In terms of Western medical treatment, knee to chest position and external manual version, *i.e.*, the attempt to turn the fetus manually from the outside of the belly, may be tried first as conservative measures during the 32-36 weeks of pregnancy. Because there is the chance of manual version resulting in rupture of the birth membranes, it is typically performed in a hospital setting. If manual version does result in rupture of the membranes, either delivery must be immediately induced or, more likely these days, a cesarean section is performed. Unfortunately, even if manual version is initially successful, the fetus may spontaneously revert to breech position. If such conservative measures fail to achieve their desired result, cesarean section is typically performed.

Chinese medical disease categorization

Traditionally, this condition was referred to as *nan chan*, difficult birth. Today, it is referred to as *tai wei bu zheng*, incorrect fetal position.

Disease causes & disease mechanisms

In Chinese medicine, the turning of the fetus within the uterus is a function of the qi mechanism which governs upbearing and downbearing. Either there is insufficient qi to accomplish this transformation or something is inhibiting the qi mechanism, such as qi stagnation, blood stasis, or phlegm obstruction. Of course, in real life, there can be a combination of these factors. In terms of qi vacuity, the two main viscera whose qi may be vacuous, weak, and insufficient *vis á vis* this condition are the spleen and kidneys.

Patterns common to this condition

Qi mechanism depression & stagnation
Blood stasis & dampness collecting
Qi & blood insufficiency

Treatment based on pattern discrimination:

Qi mechanism depression & stagnation

Main symptoms: Malposition of the fetus accompanied by chest oppression, abdominal distention, emotional depression and/or fear and fright over birthing, possible frequent sighing, a pale tongue with white fur, and a bowstring, slippery pulse

Treatment principles: Course the qi and abduct stagnation

Guiding formula:

Bao Chan Wu You Fang (Protect Birth No Worries Formula)
Hou Po (Cortex Magnoliae Officinalis), 9g
Zhi Ke (Fructus Aurantii), 6-9g
Chuan Bei Mu (Bulbus Fritillariae Cirrhosae), 6-9g
Dang Gui (Radix Angelicae Sinensis), 9g
Chuan Xiong (Radix Ligustici Wallichii), 9-15g
Bai Shao (Radix Albus Paeoniae Lactiflorae), 9g
Huang Qi (Radix Astragali), 9-18g
Tu Si Zi (Semen Cuscutae), 9g
Gan Cao (Radix Glycyrrhizae), 3-9g
Qiang Huo (Radix Et Rhizoma Notopterygii), 9g
Jing Jie (Herba Schizonepetae), 9g
Ai Ye (Folium Artemisiae Argyii), 9g
Sheng Jiang (uncooked Rhizoma Zingiberis), 6g

If there is marked qi vacuity, add *Ren Shen* (Radix Ginseng) or *Dang Shen* (Radix Codonopsitis).

Blood stasis & dampness collecting

Main symptoms: Malposition of the fetus, abdominal distention, insidious pain, possible lower extremity superficial edema, scanty urination, a pale, moist tongue, and a slippery pulse

Treatment principles: Regulate the blood and seep dampness

Guiding formula:

Dang Gui Shao Yao San (Dang Gui & Peony Powder)
Dang Gui (Radix Angelicae Sinensis), 9g
Chuan Xiong (Radix Ligustici Wallichii), 9-15g
Bai Shao (Radix Albus Paeoniae Lactiflorae), 9g
Bai Zhu (Rhizoma Atractylodis Macrocephalae), 9g
Fu Ling (Poria), 9-12g
Ze Xie (Rhizoma Alismatis), 9g

If blood stasis has transformed heat as evidenced by heart vexation and a bitter taste in the mouth, add *Huang Qin* (Radix Scutellariae) to clear heat and quiet the fetus.

Qi & blood insufficiency

Main symptoms: Malposition of the fetus, a sallow yellow facial complexion, lack of strength in the four extremities, fatigue, disinclination to speak and a weak voice, heart palpitations, shortness of breath, a pale tongue with white fur, and a deep, slippery, forceless pulse

Treatment principles: Supplement the qi and nourish the blood

Guiding formulas:

Ba Zhen Tang Jia Jian
(Eight Pearls Decoction with Additions & Subtractions)
Huang Qi (Radix Astragali), 9-18g
Xu Duan (Radix Dipsaci), 9g
Tu Si Zi (Semen Cuscutae), 9g
Dang Gui (Radix Angelicae Sinensis), 9g
Chuan Xiong (Radix Ligustici Wallichii), 9-15g
Bai Shao (Radix Albus Paeoniae Lactiflorae), 9g
Shu Di (cooked Radix Rehmanniae), 12-15g
Dang Shen (Radix Codonopsitis), 9-15g
Bai Zhu (Rhizoma Atractylodis Macrocephalae), 9g
mix-fried *Gan Cao* (Radix Glycyrrhizae), 6-9g

Unnamed formula
Dang Gui (Radix Angelicae Sinensis), 9g
Shu Di (cooked Radix Rehmanniae), 12-15g
Bai Shao (Radix Albus Paeoniae Lactiflorae), 9g
Chuan Xiong (Radix Ligustici Wallichii), 6-9g
Huang Qi (Radix Astragali), 9-18g
Dang Shen (Radix Codonopsitis), 9-15g
Xu Duan (Radix Dipsaci), 9g
Zhi Ke (Fructus Aurantii), 6-9g
mix-fried *Gan Cao* (Radix Glycyrrhizae), 6-9g

Acupuncture & moxibustion: *Zhi Yin* (Bl 67)

Moxa *Zhi Yin* for 15 minutes bilaterally each day for five days or until version has occurred.

Abstracts of representative Chinese research:

From "A Report on the Treatment of 32 Cases of Breech Birth with *Ba Zhen Tang Jia Jian* (Eight Pearls Decoction with Additions & Subtractions)" by Xue Li-mei, *Bei Jing Zhong Yi (Beijing Chinese Medicine)*, #5, 1994, p. 20

Cohort description:

Of the 32 women treated in this study, all were primiparas between 20-28 years old. Eleven cases were between 30-32 weeks, 14 cases were between 32-34 weeks, five cases were between 34-36 weeks, and two cases were between 36-38 weeks. Fifteen cases had been treated with knee-chest position for one week with no result. Another four cases had been treated with knee-chest position plus moxibustion at *Zhi Yin* (Bl 67) for one week also with no result. All these pregnant women had received ultrasonography at about 30 weeks after their last menstruation and thus the breech presentation was discovered. The fetal membranes had not broken and the amount of amniotic fluid was appropriate. There was no abnormality in uterine form, and fetal heartbeat was good.

Treatment method:

The formula consisted of: *Dang Shen* (Radix Codonopsitis), 10g, *Huang Qi* (Radix Astragali), 10g, *Bai Zhu* (Rhizoma Atractylodis Macrocephalae), *Dang Gui* (Radix Angelicae Sinensis), *Shu Di* (cooked Radix Rehmanniae), *Bai Shao* (Radix Albus Paeoniae Lactiflorae), and *Xu Duan* (Radix Dipsaci), 9g each, *Chuan Xiong* (Radix Ligustici Wallichii), 6g, *Zhi Ke* (Fructus Aurantii), 8g, and *Gan Cao* (Radix Glycyrrhizae), 3g. One packet of the above medicinals were given each day in two divided doses on an empty stomach after having been decocted in water. Three packets equaled one course of treatment. If one course did not get any result, patients were given a second and third course. There was a one day rest between courses.

Treatment outcomes:

Cure meant that the breech presentation turned to become a normal head down presentation. No result meant that, after three courses of treatment, there had been no change in fetal position. Based on these criteria, 29 women (90.6%) were cured. Sixteen (50%) of these were cured in one course, 12 cases (37.5%) were cured in two courses, and one case (3.125%) was cured in three courses. Three cases (9.4%) got no result. One of these cases was between 32-34 weeks, another case was between 34-36 weeks, and the third case was more than 36 weeks pregnant.

From "The Correction of 56 Cases of Malposition of the Fetus with *Da Sheng Yin Jia Jian* (Extend Life Drink with Additions & Subtractions)" by Chen Rui-jun, *Fu Jian Zhong Yi Yao (Fujian Chinese Medicine & Medicinals)*, # 1, 1995, p. 46

Cohort description:

The author has treated 56 cases of malposition of the fetus with *Da Sheng Yin Jia Jian* with excellent results. Of those 56 cases, 34 were primiparas and 22 were multiparas. In 18 cases, the fetus was in arm position, in 22 cases in transverse position, and in 16 cases in foot position. Thirty cases were treated between 29-30 weeks of pregnancy, while 26 cases were more than 30 weeks pregnant. The ages of the pregnant women were between 20-30 years old.

Treatment method:

The formula consisted of: *Su Gen* (Caulis Perillae Frutescentis), 9g, *Ren Shen* (Radix Ginseng), 9g, *Bai Zhu* (Rhizoma Atractylodis Macrocephalae), 10g, *Chen Pi* (Pericarpium Citri Reticulatae), 6g, *Bai Shao* (Radix Albus Paeoniae Lactiflorae), 9g, mix-fried *Gan Cao* (Radix Glycyrrhizae), 3g, *Shu Di* (cooked Radix Rehmanniae), 10g, *Chuan Xiong* (Radix Ligustici Wallichii), 6g, *Xu Duan* (Radix Dipsaci), 9g, *Du Zhong* (Cortex Eucommiae), 9g, *Huang Qi* (Radix Astragali), 15g, *Tu Si Zi* (Semen Cuscutae), 9g, *Cong Bai* (Herba Allii Fistulosi), 5 stalks. Typically, four packets equaled one course of treatment.

Treatment outcomes:

Of the 56 women given the above medicinals, 27 of their fetuses turned to normal position with one course of treatment, while another 28 received two courses of treatment combined with moxibustion at *Zhi Yin* (Bl 67) and, thereafter, their fetuses' position was corrected. Five cases later returned to an abnormal position. However, after administering *Da Sheng Yin* and moxaing *Zhi Yin*, the position of the fetus again returned to normal. Only one case failed to return to a normal position. Therefore, the total amelioration rate was 98.80%.

From "The Artemisia Pole Fumigation of Points in 136 Cases of Rotated Fetus" by Zhou Mei-mei & Xu Qiang-hua, *Zhe Jiang Zhong Yi Za Zhi (Zhejiang Journal of Chinese Medicine)*, #7, 1995, p. 301

Cohort description:

Of the 136 women in this study, 104 were 23-30 years old and 32 were 31-33. Eight cases had been pregnant for six months, 50 for seven months, 70 for eight months, and eight had been pregnant for nine months. Ninety-nine were primiparas and 37 were multigravidas. One hundred two cases were breech and 32 were transverse. There were two cases of twins. The above was ascertained by clinical symptoms and ultrasound.

Treatment method:

The main point chosen for treatment was *Zhi Yin* (Bl 67). This was combined with either *Zu San Li* (St 36) or *Tai Xi* (Ki 3). If the pregnant woman exhibited qi stagnation and spleen vacuity, then *Zhi Yin* was combined with *Zu San Li*. If the pregnant woman exhibited kidney vacuity, *Zhi Yin* was combined with *Tai Xi*. A mugwort moxa pole was used to fumigate each point bilaterally for 5-10 minutes apiece, once each day. Five times equaled one course of treatment.

Treatment outcomes:

Of the 136 cases, 129 cases or 94.8% turned head downward. There was no turn to correct in seven cases. One hundred four turned correct in one course of treatment, and 25 turned correct in two courses. If there was no turn correct after two whole coursse, this was considered as no result.

Representative case histories:

Case 1: The patient was a 30 year-old female whose initial examination was on April 26, 1978. She was seven months pregnant. Her pelvic bone opening was somewhat small. She had already been moxaed at *Zhi Yin* (Bl 67) for half a month while lying in the knee to chest position with no effect. Examination revealed dizziness, a bitter taste in the mouth, chest and epigastric glomus and oppression, vexation and agitation, disquietude, difficult stools, a low back which felt as if it were about to break, a somewhat red tongue with a thin, white coating, and a fine, slippery, rapid pulse. Gynecological examination revealed foot first position. The formula used was: *Dang Gui* (Radix Angelicae Sinensis), 15g, *Chuan Xiong* (Radix Ligustici Wallichii), 10g, *Sang Ji Sheng* (Herba Taxilli), 15g, stir-fried *Zhi Ke* (Fructus Aurantii), 6g, *Zi Su Gen* (Caulis Perillae

Frutescentis), 10g, *Jie Geng* (Radix Platycodi), 3g, stir-fried *Huang Qin* (Radix Scutellariae), 3g, *Mai Men Dong* (Tuber Ophiopogonis), 10g, *Gua Lou Pi* (Pericarpium Trichosanthis), 10g, *Zhu Ru* (Caulis Bambusae In Taeniis), 6g, and *Tu Si Zi* (Semen Cuscutae), 12g.

Three packets were administered and all the symptoms improved. Gynecological examination revealed that the uterus was two finger-widths above the navel and that the head was first but not entering the pelvis. Therefore, the patient was prescribed: *Sheng Di* (uncooked Radix Rehmanniae), 12g, *Mai Men Dong* (Tuber Ophiopogonis), 10g, *Gan Cao* (Radix Glycyrrhizae), 3g, *Dang Gui* (Radix Angelicae Sinensis), 6g, stir-fried *Bai Shao* (Radix Albus Paeoniae Lactiflorae), 10g, stir-fried *Huang Qin* (Radix Scutellariae), 6g, scorched *Bai Zhu* (Rhizoma Atractylodis Macrocephalae), 10g, *Sang Ji Sheng* (Herba Taxilli), 10g, *Su Gen* (Caulis Perillae Frutescentis), 6g, and uncooked *Mu Li*, (Concha Ostreae), 18g, decocted first. Five packets were administered in order to consolidate the treatment effect.

Case 2: The patient was a 35 year-old female cadre who was first examined on March 14, 1970. This woman had stopped menstruating eight months before, and this was her second pregnancy. At a prenatal examination, it was determined that the fetus's position was not correct. The fetus was average size and the amniotic fluid was also average in volume. Therefore, the woman was prescribed the following Chinese medicinals: mix-fried *Huang Qi* (Radix Astragali), 4.5g, *Dang Gui* (Radix Angelicae Sinensis), 4.5g, stir-fried *Bai Shao* (Radix Albus Paeoniae Lactiflorae), 3g, *Zhi Ke* (Fructus Aurantii), 1.8g, *Tu Si Zi* (Semen Cuscutae), 4.5g, *Chuan Xiong* (Radix Ligustici Wallichii), 4.5g, *Qiang Huo* (Radix Et Rhizoma Notopterygii), 1.5g, *Jing Jie* (Herba Schizonepetae), 2.1g, *Zi Su Ye* (Folium Perillae Frutescentis), 2.1g, stir-fried *Hou Po* (Cortex Magnoliae Officinalis), 2.1g, *Ai Ye* (Folium Artemisiae Argyii), 2.1g, mix-fried *Gan Cao* (Radix Glycyrrhizae), 1.5g, and *Chuan Bei Mu* (Bulbus Fritillariae Cirrhosae), 2.1g. The patient was prescribed three packets of the above formula and was re-examined three days later. The patient reported that, after taking the first packet of herbs, the baby's head had turned downward and, therefore, she did not take the two remaining packets of medicinals.

Remarks:

1. Although moxibustion of *Zhi Yin* is widely touted in the People's Republic of China as effective for the correction of malposition of the fetus, my clinical preceptors at the Long Hua Chinese Medical Hospital in China were of the opinion that it does not work as well as many people would like to believe. They felt it was moderately effective for transverse presentation but not very effective for frank breech.

2. Many Western women with malposition of the fetus seek out acupuncture treatment after it is already too late. For moxibustion of *Zhi Yin* to have a good chance of success, it must be carried out between weeks 32-36. By week 40 or beyond, it is probably too late.

3. Moxibustion of *Zhi Yin* combined with external version may give better results than either technique alone. Likewise, moxibustion combined with internally administered Chinese medicinals based on the woman's individual pattern discrimination may also achieve better results than either of those two modalities alone.

Endnotes:

[1] www.kfir.net/fetus.html

[2] Moore, Thomas R., "Abnormal Fetal Presentation," *Gynecology & Obstetrics: A Longitudinal Approach, op. cit.*, p. 589

[3] *Ibid.*, p. 589

[4] www.kfir.net, *op. cit.*

[5] Garrey, Matthew *et al., Obstetrics Illustrated, op. cit.*, p. 232

[6] Beers, Mark H. & Berkow, Robert. *The Merck Manual, op. cit.*, p. 2064

[7] www.dcdoctor.com/pages/rightpages_wellnesscenter/pregnancy/complications.html

[8] Moore, Thomas R., *op. cit.*, p. 590

31
Dystocia

Dystocia literally means difficult labor. Practically speaking, it means the abnormally slow progress of labor. According to Western medicine, there are four potential risk factors for dystocia:

1. Uterine contractions which are too weak or too uncoordinated to ripen the cervix and/or inadequate pushing with the voluntary muscles during the second stage of labor.

2. Malposition of the fetus (see the preceding chapter) or other factors which retard the passage of the fetus through the birth canal.

3. Too narrow maternal pelvis to allow passage of the fetus through the birth canal.

4. Abnormalities of the birth canal other than those of the bony pelvis which obstruct fetal descent.

Of these four, small bony pelvis and/or insufficiently strong and uncoordinated uterine contractions are the two most common causes of dystocia.[1]

Dystocia is more common in primigravidas and also among women undergoing induction as opposed to those who have entered spontaneous labor.[2] Strictly speaking, dystocia should not be diagnosed in a primigravida if her cervix has not yet reached 3-4cm and is near 100% effacement. In a multiparous woman, dystocia should not be diagnosed unless her cervix has reached 5cm and is 70-80% effaced. The Western medical treatment of dystocia consists of active monitoring of the mother and fetus, possible amniotomy (rupturing of the amniotic sac), the manual correction (if possible) of abnormal fetal position, the administration of oxytocin, and/or delivery by cesarean section. Commonly, if a woman has not delivered within 12 hours of entering active labor, she will be delivered via cesarean section. In the U.S., 20-25% of all deliveries are by cesarean section, and dystocia accounts for 30% of all cesarean deliveries.[3] Dystocia is associated with increased mortality and morbidity of both the mother and fetus. Although there is no increased fetal mortality or morbidity due to delivery by cesaraen section, increased maternal mortality and morbidity are associated with cesarean-sections. Many women who had a cesarean-section for dystocia are automatically scheduled for a repeat operation if they become pregnant again.

Chinese medical disease categorization

If the pregnant mother has reached full term and goes into labor but the labor is prolonged and the baby is not delivered expediously, this is called *nan chan* or difficult birth. It is sometimes also referred to as *zhi chan* or stagnant birth in the Chinese medical literature. In Chinese medicine, this disease may also cover prolonged gestation and being post-term.

Disease causes & disease mechanisms

There are two basic mechanisms associated with difficult delivery according to Chinese medicine. Either there is insufficient qi and blood to move the fetus down and out the birth canal or stagnant qi and blood stasis are obstructing its movement. Wan Mi-zhai describes this more colorfully when he says that, if a birth goes on for more than a day, the woman is preoccupied by family and personal affairs, and still has an appetite, this is due to astringing of the uterus, but, if the birth goes on for more than a day, all the woman's affairs are settled, and her appetite is diminished, this is central qi insufficiency not able to transport and move the fetus.

Patterns common to this condition

Qi & blood vacuity weakness
Qi stagnation & blood stasis

Treatment based on pattern discrimination:

Qi & blood vacuity weakness

Main symptoms: Prolonged labor with not too much pain but more obvious fatigue and exhaustion, a somber white facial complexion, lassitude of the spirit, lack of strength in the four extremities, heart palpitations, shortness of breath, a pale tongue with thin fur, and a large, vacuous or deep, fine, weak pulse

Treatment principles: Greatly supplement the qi and blood

Guiding formulas:

Cai Song Ting Nan Chan Fang (Cai Song-ting's Difficult Birth Formula)
mix-fried *Huang Qi* (Radix Astragali), 9-18g
Dang Gui (Radix Angelicae Sinensis), 9g
Fu Shen (Sclerotium Pararadicis Poriae Cocos), 9-15g
Dang Shen (Radix Codonopsitis), 9-15g

vinegar mix-fried *Gui Ban* (Plastrum Testudinis), 9-12g
Chuan Xiong (Radix Ligustici Wallichii), 9g
wine stir-fried *Bai Shao* (Radix Albus Paeoniae Lactiflorae), 9g
Gou Qi Zi (Fructus Lycii), 9g

Jia Wei Si Jun Zi Tang (Added Flavors Four Gentlemen Decoction)
Ren Shen (Radix Ginseng), 3-9g
Bai Zhu (Rhizoma Atractylodis Macrocephalae), 9g
Fu Ling (Poria), 9-12g
mix-fried *Gan Cao* (Radix Glycyrrhizae), 6-9g
Dang Gui (Radix Angelicae Sinensis), 9g
Chuan Xiong (Radix Ligustici Wallichii), 6-9g
Zhi Ke (Fructus Aurantii), 6-9g
Xiang Fu (Rhizoma Cyperi), 6-9g
Rou Gui (Cortex Cinnamomi), 3-9g

Kai Gu San (Open the Bones Powder)
Dang Gui (Radix Angelicae Sinensis), 9g
Chuan Xiong (Radix Ligustici Wallichii), 6-9g
Gui Ban (Plastrum Testudinis), 9-12g

If the birthing woman's pubic bones do not open due to qi and blood insufficiency or due to it being the woman's first delivery, one can use the above formula. If qi and blood insufficiency is pronounced, add *Ren Shen* (Radix Ginseng).

Qi stagnation & blood stasis

Main symptoms: Difficult birth with low back and abdominal aching and pain, a purplish, dark facial complexion, a tense, nervous essence spirit, chest and stomach duct distention and oppression, possible vomiting and nausea, a dark red tongue with either normal or slimy fur, and a bowstring, large, extremely rapid, choppy pulse

Treatment principles: Rectify the qi and quicken the blood, transform stasis and hasten delivery

Guiding formulas:

Cui Sheng Yin Jia Yi Mu Cao (Hasten Birth Drink Plus Leonurus)
Dang Gui (Radix Angelicae Sinensis), 9g
Chuan Xiong (Radix Ligustici Wallichii), 9-15g
Da Fu Pi (Pericarpium Arecae), 6-9g
Zhi Ke (Fructus Aurantii), 6-9g
Bai Zhi (Radix Angelicae Dahuricae), 9g
Yi Mu Cao (Herba Leonuri), 9-18g

Jia Wei Si Wu Tang (Added Flavors Four Materials Decoction)
Dang Gui (Radix Angelicae Sinensis), 9g
Chuan Xiong (Radix Ligustici Wallichii), 9-15g
Chi Shao (Radix Rubrus Paeoniae Lactiflorae), 9-15g

Sheng Di (uncooked Radix Rehmanniae), 12-15g
Rou Gui (Cortex Cinnamomi), 3-9g
Yan Hu Suo (Rhizoma Corydalis), 9-18g
Zhi Ke (Fructus Aurantii), 6-9g
Xiang Fu (Rhizoma Cyperi), 6-9g
Bing Lang (Semen Arecae), 6-9g
Mu Xiang (Radix Auklandiae), 6-9g

Acupuncture & moxibustion: For qi stagnation, blood stasis difficult or stagnant labor, use *He Gu* (LI 4), *San Yin Jiao* (Sp 6), *Zhi Gou* (TH 6), *Tai Chong* (Liv 3), etc. Do not retain the needles.

Or, one may use *He Gu* (LI 4), *San Yin Jiao* (Sp 6), *Zhi Yin* (Bl 67), and *Du Yin* (extra point located on the plantar surface of the center of the proximal phalangeal joint of the second toe). In this case, needle the first two points and moxa the second two.

Yet another commonly used formula in China today is to needle *He Gu* (LI 4), *San Yin Jiao* (Sp 6), and *Huan Tiao* (Bl 30).

Gao Yu-chun also suggests using *He Gu* (LI 4), *San Yin Jiao* (Sp 6), and an extra or non-channel point called *Cuo Chan Xue*, Hastening Birth Point. This is located 3 *cun* lateral to *Guan Yuan* (CV 4) and is needled five *fen* in depth.

If there is pronounced back labor and pain in the sacrum, needle transversely the *Ba Liao* (Bl 31-34). Tape the needles in place flush with the skin and use electrical stimulation.

For qi and blood vacuity weakness, one can needle *Zu San Li* (St 36), *San Yin Jiao* (Sp 6), *Fu Liu* (Ki 7), and *Zhi Yin* (Bl 67)

Abstracts of representative Chinese research:

From "The Treatment of 12 Cases of Difficult Delivery with *Tuo Hua Jian Jia Wei* (Out-thrusting & Transforming Decoction with Added Flavors)" by Chen Ren-yue, *Xin Zhong Yi (New Chinese Medicine)*, #10, 1995, p. 54-55

Cohort description:

There were 12 women in this study, all were between 21-32 years of age. Ten were primiparas and two had had previous children. All were overdue by 12-50 days but had no other symptoms.

Treatment method:

Tuo Hua Jian consists of: *Chuan Xiong* (Radix Ligustici Wallichii), *Chuan Niu Xi* (Radix Cyathulae), 6g each, *Dang Gui* (Radix Angelicae Sinensis), 30g, *Rou Gui* (Cortex Cinnamomi), 3g, *Che Qian Zi* (Semen Plantaginis), 5g. To this was added *Dang Shen* (Radix Codonopsitis) and *Shu Di* (cooked Radix Rehmanniae), 12g each, *Shan Yao* (Radix Dioscoreae), 10g, and *Zhi Ke* (Fructus Aurantii), 2g.

These were decocted in water and administered warm. This was followed by the administration of a suitable amount of rice wine. When this formula is administered before delivery, it can hasten birth as well as treat difficult delivery. If there is a dead fetus which is not precipitated, one should add *Mang Xiao* (Mirabilitum), 10-15g.

Treatment outcomes:

All the women in this study eventually gave birth successfully vaginally to live children, one boy and 11 girls. The median number of packets administered before the birth flowed freely and was disinhibited, thus precipitating the fetus was 3-5.

From "A Short Clinical Discussion of Hastening Birth in 50 Cases by a Combination of Ear and Body Points" by Wang Hua-ju, *Jiang Xi Zhong Yi Yao (Jiangxi Chinese Medicine & Medicinals)*, #5, 1994, p. 46

Cohort description:

Among the 50 women in this study, the youngest was 18 and the oldest was 42 years old. For most, this was a first pregnancy. A small number had given birth before. All the women were suffering from difficult, stagnant deliveries.

Treatment method:

Ear point Uterus was the main point. This was combined with *He Gu* (LI 4), *San Yin Jiao* (Sp 6), and *Zhi Yin* (Bl 67). These points were needled bilaterally, with additions and subtractions depending on the birthing woman's personal condition. Five *fen* and 1-2 inch needles were inserted perpendicularly 0.5-1 inch deep. After insertion, the needles were manipulated using twisting draining technique to induce a sore, electric, or distended sensation. Such stimulation was carried out 2-3 times and then the needles were withdrawn. They were not retained.

Treatment outcomes:

Twenty-five women gave birth after being needled a single time. Another 24 gave birth after being needled 2-5 times. One case developed needle shock and was not able to be needled. Therefore, the total effectiveness rate was 98%.

Representative case histories:

Case 1: The patient was a 32 year-old female who was first examined on April 13, 1965. This was the woman's second pregnancy and she was overdue. Two days prior, the woman had felt a downward sagging feeling in her lower abdomen. The next day, there was severe abdominal pain. That evening, her water broke and she entered labor. When examined in the delivery room, her cervix had not yet dilated. However, she was already lying on her back in preparation for delivery. After nine hours, her cervix had only dilated slightly. At this point, the woman's facial complexion was somber and white and there was shortness of breath with hasty breathing, slightly chilled limbs, and abdominal pain with weak contractions which occurred every 3-5 minutes. The patient's pulse was fine, rapid, and forceless.

In order to hasten delivery, the woman was prescribed the following Chinese medicinals: uncooked *Huang Qi* (Radix Astragali), 30g, *Dang Gui* (Radix Angelicae Sinensis), 15g, uncooked *Gui Ban* (Plastrum Testudinis), 30g. These were decocted quickly and administered to the patient. Thirty minutes later, the woman's facial complexion gradually became red and moist-looking and her limbs regained their warmth. Her breathing became harmonious and normal, her abdominal pain increased, and her cervix completely dilated. At 12 hours, the woman gave birth normally to a healthy boy.

Case 2: The patient was an elementary school teacher of undisclosed age who was first examined on Aug. 23, 1976. When the woman had been pregnant for eight months, she had been diagnosed with chronic cholecystitis with chest and rib-side distention and pain and a bowstring, slippery pulse. She had, therefore, been treated with coursing the liver and harmonizing the stomach assisted by quieting the fetus. However, after taking these medicinals, she felt uncomfortable and stopped taking them. When she stopped these medicinals, she went into labor which was accompanied by severe low back and abdominal distention and pain. In addition, there was chest and rib-side distention and oppression. Labor continued for a long time without delivery.

To hasten delivery, the woman was prescribed the following medicinals based on the principles of rectifying the qi and quickening the blood, abducting the fetus and moving it downward: *Dang Gui* (Radix Angelicae Sinensis), *Chuan Xiong* (Radix Ligustici Wallichii), *Niu Xi* (Radix Achyranthis Bidentatae), processed *Xiang Fu* (Rhizoma Cyperi), *Yu Jin* (Tuber Curcumae), *Che Qian Zi* (Semen Plantaginis), *Qing Pi* (Pericarpium Citri Reticulatae Viride), and *Yi Mu Cao* (Herba Leonuri), 9g each, and *Hong Hua* (Flos Carthami), 4.5g. These were decocted in water and administered to the patient, after which she felt stronger contractions. Each hour, the patient was administered another dose of these medicinals. Two hours later, the woman delivered a healthy boy.

Case 3: The woman was 32 years old and was first seen on May 1, 1983. Her last menstruation had occurred June 7, 1982. Her due date was March 14, 1983. Therefore, she was 50 days overdue. There was no low back ache, abdominal pain, or other such symptoms. She already had a daughter who was eight years old and she had had one artificial abortion. When examined at a hospital, the fetal heartbeat was normal. X-rays showed that the fetus's body was large. It was decided to induce labor and, if that was not successful, to do a cesarean section. On May 1, 1983, she was administered one packet of the following formula: *Chuan Xiong* (Radix Ligustici Wallichii) and *Chuan Niu Xi* (Radix Cyathulae), 6g each, *Dang Gui* (Radix Angelicae Sinensis), 30g, *Rou Gui* (Cortex Cinnamomi), 3g, *Che Qian Zi* (Semen Plantaginis), 5g, *Dang Shen* (Radix Codonopsitis) and *Shu Di* (cooked Radix Rehmanniae), 12g each, *Shan Yao* (Radix Dioscoreae),

10g, and *Zhi Ke* (Fructus Aurantii), 2g. This made her feel comfortable. The next day she was given another packet. The following morning, she felt some low back ache and slight abdominal pain. Her lower abdomen had a numb sensation. She went to the hospital delivery room. At 10 AM that same day she had a normal delivery. The mother and daughter were safe and sound and the baby's weight was 4950g.

Remarks:

1. Since at least the writing of the *Nei Jing Su Wen (Inner Classic: Simple Questions)*, Chinese medicine has traditionally emphasized the importance of preventive care. As much as possible, the practitioner should try to supplement vacuity and drain repletion before the woman goes into labor. According to Zhu Dan-xi, "[If] qi and blood are harmonious, birthing will be normally flowing." Unfortunately, in real life, this is not always possible. Acupuncture is quicker acting than internal medicine for dealing with qi stagnation and, to some extent, blood stasis. However, internally administered decoctions administered during labor can boost the qi in an immediate way. In such cases, one should not skimp on the amounts of *Huang Qi* (Radix Astragali) or substitute *Dang Shen* (Radix Codonopsitis) for *Ren Shen* (Radix Ginseng) if *Ren Shen* is not available.

2. During the first stage of labor, women should be encouraged to remain upright so that the weight of the baby may aid in the dilation and effacement of the cervix.

Endnotes:

[1] www.babyzone.com/drnathan/D/Dystocia.htm

[2] http://sogc.medical.org/SOGCnet/sogc_docs/common/guide/pdfs/ps40.pdf

[3] www.emedicine.com/med/topic3280.htm

32
Retained Placenta

According to modern Western medicine, retained placenta may be due to the placenta's being partially or wholly still attached to the uterus or because of absence of uterine contractions. It is normal to wait up to 30 minutes without attempting to provoke delivery of the placenta. In the West, after 30 minutes, one may attempt to manually separate and express the placenta. However, this may provoke hemorrhage and subsequent shock. Should simple manual expression fail, one may resort to manual removal. However, this procedure is carried out under general anesthesia, and there are risks of infection and damage to the uterus. Risk factors for retained placenta include placental implantation onto a uterine scar (for instance, due to a prior cesarean-section or myomectomy), an unusually shaped uterus, and after midtrimester deliveries. In these cases, failure of placental separation is due to absence of an adequate decidual layer.

Chinese medical disease categorization

Retained placenta is referred to in Chinese as *bao yi bu xia*, birth covering not precipitated.

Disease causes & disease mechanisms

In Chinese medicine, retained placenta is usually due to one of two mechanisms. Either blood stasis prevents the placenta from being precipitated normally or there is vacuity cold affecting the uterus. In this latter case, yang qi is insufficient to promote the movement of the placenta down and out. This is attended by signs and symptoms of qi and blood vacuity weakness.

Patterns common to this condition

Blood stasis

Vacuity cold

Treatment based on pattern discrimination

Blood stasis

Main symptoms: Retention of the placenta with piercing pain in the lower abdomen, lower abdominal distention, refusal of pressure, a scanty, astringent, purplish, dark colored lochia in a patient with robust physique, dizziness and vertigo, a dark, greenish facial color, purplish spots or patches on the tongue, and a wiry, choppy, forceful pulse

Treatment principles: Regulate the qi and activate the blood, transform stasis and descend the placenta

Guiding formulas:

Tao He Cheng Qi Tang (Persica Order the Qi Decoction)
Tao Ren (Semen Persicae), 9g
Gui Zhi (Ramulus Cinnamomi), 6-9g
Da Huang (Radix Et Rhizoma Rhei), 3-9g
Mang Xiao (Mirabilitum), 3-6g
mix-fried *Gan Cao* (Radix Glycyrrhizae), 6-9g

Duo Ming Wan Jia Wei (Rescue Destiny Pills with Added Flavors)
Dan Pi (Cortex Moutan), 9g
Tao Ren (Semen Persicae), 9g
Fu Ling (Poria), 9-12g
Chi Shao (Radix Rubrus Paeoniae Lactiflorae), 9-15g
Rou Gui (Cortex Cinnamomi), 3-9g
Jiang Huang (Rhizoma Curcumae Longae), 9g
Su Mu (Lignum Sappan), 9g

Vacuity cold

Main symptoms: Retained placenta with insidious lower abdominal pain, a heavy, dragging feeling in the lower abdomen, lack of distention or serious pain, scanty lochia, a weak body, dizziness, heart palpitations, spontaneous perspiration, lassitude of the spirit, a pale, moist tongue, and a faint, fine; faint, weak; or vacuous, large pulse

Treatment principles: Supplement the qi and nourish the blood, warm the uterus and precipitate the placenta

Guiding formulas:

Jia Wei Si Jun Zi Tang (Added Flavors Four Gentlemen Decoction)
Ren Shen (Radix Ginseng), 3-9g
Bai Zhu (Rhizoma Atractylodis Macrocephalae), 9g
Fu Ling (Poria), 9-12g
Zhi Ke (Fructus Aurantii), 6-9g
Dang Gui (Radix Angelicae Sinensis), 9g

Chuan Xiong (Radix Ligustici Wallichii), 9g
mix-fried *Gan Cao* (Radix Glycyrrhizae), 6-9g
Xiang Fu (Rhizoma Cyperi), 6-9g
Rou Gui (Cortex Cinnamomi), 3-9g
Bing Lang (Semen Arecae), 6-9g
Mu Xiang (Radix Auklandiae), 6-9g

Bao Sheng Wu You San (Protect Life No Worries Powder)
Dang Gui (Radix Angelicae Sinensis), 9g
Zhi Qiao (Fructus Aurantii), 6-9g
Chuan Xiong (Radix Ligustici Wallichii), 6-9g
Mu Xiang (Radix Auklandiae), 6-9g
Bai Shao (Radix Albus Paeoniae Lactiflorae), 9g
Gan Cao (Radix Glycyrrhizae), 3-9g
Ru Xiang (Resina Olibani), 6g
Xue Yu Tan (Crinis Carbonisatus), 4.5-9g

Sheng Hua Tang Jia Wei
(Engendering & Transforming Decoction with Added Flavors)
Dang Gu (Radix Angelicae Sinensis), 9g
Chuan Xiong (Radix Ligustici Wallichii), 9-15g
mix-fried *Gan Cao* (Radix Glycyrrhizae), 6-9g
Tao Ren (Semen Persicae), 9g
Pao Jiang (blast-fried Rhizoma Zingiberis), 6-9g
Da Zao (Fructus Jujubae), 3 pieces
Ren Shen (Radix Ginseng), 3-9g
Huang Qi (Radix Astragali), 9-18g

Acupuncture & moxibustion: *Jian Jing* (GB 21), *Zhong Ji* (CV 3), *Kun Lun* (Bl 60), *He Gu* (LI 4), *San Yin Jiao* (Sp 6), *Du Yin* (extra point; see above under difficult delivery)

For both blood stasis and vacuity cold retained placenta, needle the first 3 points and moxa the last two. For vacuity cold retained placenta, also moxa *Guan Yuan* (CV 4) and *Qi Hai* (CV 6).

Representative case histories:

Case 1: The patient was a 34 year-old female who was initially examined in Fall, 1954. This woman had a weak body and had had many diseases. This was her third birth that had been quite long and, after which, the placenta was not precipitated. Her lower abdomen was slightly distended, but there was no pain with pressure when palpated. During delivery, the woman had lost a lot of blood. Her facial complexion was somber white and there was dizziness, heart palpitations, shortness of breath, lassitude of the spirit, a predilection for warmth and a fear of cold. Her tongue was pale with thin fur, and her pulse was vacuous (in this case probably meaning forceless) and fine.

Based on these signs and symptoms and on her history of habitual bodily weakness, it was determined that her original qi was insufficient and that this vacuity had been made even worse due to the prolonged labor and blood loss. Therefore, in order to supplement the qi, nourish the blood, and eliminate stasis, she was prescribed one packet of: *Tan Jiang* (carbonized Rhizoma Zingiberis), 8g, *Dang Gui* (Radix Angelicae Sinensis), 10g, *Chuan Xiong* (Radix Ligustici Wallichii), 6g, *Tao Ren* (Semen Persicae), 6g, *Ren Shen* (Radix Ginseng), 6g, and wine stir-fried *Bai Shao* (Radix Albus Paeoniae Lactiflorae), 6g.

At the second examination (the next day), it was learned that, after taking these medicinals, the placenta had been precipitated. However, there was excessive bleeding, heart palpitations, shortness of breath, lassitude of the spirit, and lack of strength, a pale tongue, and a faint, fine, forceless pulse. Now the woman was prescribed two packets of: *Ren Shen* (Radix Ginseng), 10g, *Bai Zhu* (Rhizoma Atractylodis Macrocephalae), 6g, *Sheng Ma* (Rhizoma Cimicifugae), 4g, *Chai Hu* (Radix Bupleuri), 6g, *Hong Hua* (Flos Carthami), 3g, *Tan Jiang* (carbonized Rhizoma Zingiberis), 6g, *Tao Ren* (Semen Persicae), 5g, *Chuan Xiong* (Radix Ligustici Wallichii), 4g, and *Dan Shen* (Radix Salviae Miltiorrhizae), 6g.

At the third examination, all the above symptoms were less. However, there were still heart palpitations, shortness of breath, and dizziness. Therefore, the *Tan Jiang, Tao Ren,* and *Hong Hua* were removed from the above formula and six grams each of *Huang Qi* (Radix Astragali) and *Gao Ben* (Rhizoma Ligustici) were added. After taking four packets of this formula, the woman was considered cured.

Case 2: The patient was a 35 year-old female who was initially examined in Fall, 1957. The patient reported that during the seventh and eighth months of her pregnancy she had developed a predilection for eating chilled things. At her delivery, the placenta had not been precipitated and her lochia was scanty in amount and dark red in color. There was lower abdominal chilly pain that refused pressure. Her facial complexion was greenish white. When the pain was severe, she desired to vomit. Her tongue was pale with no fur, and her pulse was deep, bowstring, and choppy.

Based on the above signs and symptoms as well as the history of eating chilled foods during pregnancy, this patient's pattern was categorized as blood stasis due to cold congelation with cold qi attacking the stomach above. Therefore, she was prescribed one packet of: *Rou Gui* (Cortex Cinnamomi), 6g, *Tan Jiang* (carbonized Rhizoma Zingiberis), 9g, *Dang Gui* (Radix Angelicae Sinensis), 9g, *Shu Di* (cooked Radix Rehmanniae), 10g, *Bai Shao* (Radix Albus Paeoniae Lactiflorae), 6g, *Niu Xi* (Radix Achyranthis Bidentatae), 6g, *Chuan Xiong* (Radix Ligustici Wallichii), 5g, and *Ren Shen* (Radix Ginseng), 4g. These medicinals were decocted in half water and half rice wine. Externally, 30 grams of *Bi Ma Ren* (Semen Ricini Communis) were smashed into a paste and applied to the centers of the woman's feet. This latter is a treatment for nonprecipitation of the placenta.

At the second examination, the patient reported that, after taking the above medicinals, the placenta had been delivered. However, there was still lower abdominal empty pain, lassitude of the spirit, lack of strength, and short, rapid breathing. Therefore, six grams of *Hong Shen* (red Radix Ginseng) were decocted in rice wine and administered, and, two hours later, all the woman's symptoms were decreased. Thus, *Rou Gui* and *Tan Jiang* were removed from the above formula and six grams of *Huang Qi* (Radix Astragali) were added. After three packets of this formula, the patient was switched to *Bu Zhong Yi Qi Wan* (Supplement the Center & Boost the Qi Pills) and the disease was considered cured.

Remarks:

1. I have had occasion to successfully treat retained placenta at a home birth. However, it is not something I would recommend to Western practitioners due to the potential severe legal liabilities.

2. Chinese medicine is most likely to be effective for retained placentas due to lack of uterine contractions and hypotonia. It is less likely to be effective for inadequate decidual layer.

BOOK TWO

Postpartum Diseases

1

Introduction

Western medicine & postpartum care

In Western medicine, the six weeks or so immediately following delivery are referred to as the puerperium. During this time, the body reverses most of the physiological changes that occurred during pregnancy. In addition, there are various psychological adaptions to the outcome of pregnancy which occur during this interval. In healthy women, the clinical manifestations of most of these changes are transient and mild. However, Western medicine recognizes several postpartum complications, including puerperal infection, postpartum hemorrhage, inverted uterus, thrombophlebitis, and pulmonary embolus.

Physiologic changes

Within the first 24 hours after delivery, the mother's pulse rate drops and her temperature may be slightly elevated.[1] The uterus decreases in size to that of 20 weeks gestation. At one week postpartum, the uterus is contained in the true pelvis, at two weeks postpartum, it weighs 100g, and, at the end of six weeks postpartum, it measures 7.5 x 2.5cm and weighs 40-60g.[2] This reduction in size and weight is mostly due to atrophy of the muscular elements of the uterus. Inside the uterus, the endometrium regenerates rapidly, while the cervix thickens. By the end of two weeks postpartum the cervical os is basically closed. The vagina decreases in size. However, it does not return to prepregnant dimensions for several more months when the relaxation of the vagina disappears. Vaginal discharge is red or grossly bloody for the first 3-4 days. This discharge is referred to as the lochia and, while it is red, it is called the *lochia rubra*. After 3-6 days, the lochia become pale brown and more clear. This is referred to as the *lochia serosa*. At 10-12 days postpartum, the lochia becomes yellowish white, at which time it is referred to as the *lochia alba*. The *lochia alba* may persist for several weeks.

Due to the passage of the infant through the pelvis, the bladder wall becomes erythematous and edematous and relatively insensitive to intravesical pressure. This results in a tendency to retention of urine. The abdominal wall remains lax for 6-8 weeks when it has nearly returned to its prepregnant condition. The motility of the gastrointestinal tract quickly returns to normal during the puerperium, and cardiac output resumes its prepregnant values 2-3 weeks after delivery. Varicosities of the lower extremities and hemorrhoids frequently subside after birth, and blood volume returns to its prepregnant levels one week after delivery. In terms of blood analysis, there is leukocytosis for 1-2 weeks postpartum with a relative lymphopenia and an absolute esinopenia. Erythrocyte sedimentation rate is elevated for approximately one week, and elevated triglyceride levels return to normal by the end of six weeks. However, total cholesterol levels take a year to gradually decrease to their prepregnant levels. Approximately 12 pounds of weight is lost immediately after delivery of the infant and placenta and due to blood loss. Another eight pounds are lost via urination during the next seven days. By the end of six weeks, most patients are 110-120 percent of their prepregnant weight.

It takes at least 2-3 months for the mother's endocrine system to return to its prepregnant state. Non-nursing mothers can expect to resume ovulation within two months of delivery, and 90% of non-nursing mothers will have resumed menstruation by three months postpartum. Prolactin levels return to baseline in 1-2 weeks in non-nursing women. Nursing women experience reproductive endocrine adaptations as a result of the baby's suckling, and these adaptations are somewhat dependent on the number of times the woman breast-feeds per day. Oxytocin is released by the pituitary in anticipation of breast-feeding or in response to direct tactile stimulation. Suckling also stimulates the release of prolactin from the pituitary. It also stimulates the release of endogenous opiates. These endogenous opiates may suppress the release of gonadotropicregulating hormone (GnRH), and it is the disruption in the release of GnRH which accounts for anovulation and amenorrhea during the time most women are breast-feeding.

Psychological changes

Becoming a mother and having a baby require a number of psychological adjustments on the part of the mother. The immediate psychological adjustments to becoming a mother are typically divided into three stages each which last from a few days to a week. These three phases are called the taking-in phase, the taking-hold phase, and the letting-go phase. In the taking-in phase, even though the recently delivered mother is physically fatigued, she is typically eager to share her experiences of birth and welcomes assistance from caregivers and family. In the taking-hold phase, the mother becomes anxious over the resumption of her own bodily functions as well as her ability to take care of her new child. During this phase, the mother commonly strives for independence and likes to be the initiator. Finally, during the letting-go phase, the mother establishes her maternal role patterns, and her attention focuses on issues beyond just herself and her infant.

Postpartum blues refer to a transient period of mood changes which occur in 50-80% of mothers beginning three days after delivery. These mood changes may include any or all of the following: weepiness, depression, or anxiety. In addition, there may also be accompanying fatigue, insomnia, headaches, poor concentration, and mental confusion. These mood changes can last anywhere from a few hours to several months postpartum. Primiparas and those women with a history of premenstrual syndrome (PMS) are most at risk for these changes. True postpartum depression affects from 7-30% of postpartum women. It typically begins from 2-6 weeks after delivery and its clinical symptoms are similar to major depression. Postpartum psychosis is an even more serious postpartum psychiatric disorder which one study has found affects 1-2% of postpartum women.[3] Risk factors for postpartum psychosis include a history of nonpostpartum psychosis, being a primipara, being unmarried, giving birth by cesarean section, and perinatal death.

Routine postpartum Western medical care

The mother is observed for one hour after completion of the third stage of labor and given periodic uterine massage to promote uterine contraction and prevent excess bleeding. If the uterus does not remain contracted, oxytocin may be administered by intravenous drip. A regular diet is offered as soon after delivery as the patient requests food, and ambulation is encouraged as soon as possible. Abdominal muscle strengthening exercises may be started after one day. Discomfort from an episiotomy may be relieved by a hot sitz bath several times per day and codeine and/or aspirin may be administered. Postpartum women should be encouraged to urinate and must be monitored to prevent urinary retention. If delivery occurred in a hospital, the woman is encouraged to defecate before being discharged, although this does not always happen, especially if there has been an early discharge. A CBC should be performed before discharge to insure the woman is not anemic. Seronegative women are immunized against rubella on the day of discharge, and women who are Rh negative who have not been previously sensitized and who have given birth to an Rh positive infant are given Rh immune globulin within 72 hours of delivery. These days, discharge from the hospital takes place within 24 hours of delivery, with many family-centered birthing units discharging patients as early as six hours postpartum.

Puerperal sepsis occurs in approximately 5% of postpartum women. It is defined as a temperature of 100.4°F (38° C) or higher occurring on any two of the first 10 days after delivery (excepting the first day). Elevated temperature during the first day postpartum is typically due to dehydration, whereas elevated temperatures occurring after the second or third days indicate infection. Such infection is mainly and most seriously of the uterus and parametria (endomyometritis), although bladder and kidney infections are also common. Mastitis refers to infection of the mammary glands and may also fall under the general category of postpartum infection. Anemia, prolonged rupture of the membranes, prolonged labor, operative or traumatic delivery, repeated examination, retention of placental fragments, and postpartum hemorrhage all predispose a migration of normal vaginal bacteria to the uterine cavity where they may cause disease. The single greatest risk factor for the development of puerperal sepsis is cesarean delivery after which there can be an infection rate as high as 38.5%. The risk of cesarean delivery resulting in puerperal sepsis increases if operative time exceeds 60 minutes or blood loss exceeds 800ml.

In addition to fever, the signs and symptoms of endomyometritis include tenderness of the uterus, chills, headache, malaise, anorexia. Pallor, tachycardia, and leukocytosis ususally occur, and the uterus is typically soft, large, and tender. The lochia may be either scanty or excessive and often smells malodorous. The Western medical treatment of endomyometritis usually consists of administering a broad-spectrum antibiotic, such as ampicillin. This is done intravenously until the woman has been afebrile for 48 hours. In most cases, it is not necessary to continue treatment with oral antibiotics after the IV antibiotics have been discontinued.

Chinese medicine & the puerperium

The treatment of postpartum disorders is one of the four major categories of traditional Chinese gynecology. In Chinese, postpartum disorders or diseases are referred to as *chan hou bing* (Literally, birth after diseases). Chapter 21 of Zhang Zhongjing's *Jin Gui Yao Lue (Essentials from the Golden Cabinet)* is the first chapter in the Chinese medical literature devoted to a discussion of postpartum disorders. It opens with the question:

> After delivery, women [commonly] have three diseases. The first is convulsions, the second is dizziness, and the third is difficulty defecating. Why is this?

The master answers:

> After delivery, the blood is vacuous and there has been profuse perspiration. [This makes postpartum women] susceptible to wind stroke and, hence, convulsions. Loss of blood accompanied by sweating and excessive cold lead to dizziness. Loss of fluids [leads to] stomach dryness and, hence, difficult defecation.

This question and its answer discusses the first and most common cause of postpartum disease, blood vacuity and consumption of water fluids. This then may lead to damage and detriment of the *chong* and *ren*.

The other most common causes of postpartum disease are internal blockage by blood stasis, contraction of the six environmental excesses taking advantage of postpartum vacuity weakness, food stagnation due to overeating in an attempt to recuperate the blood, and sexual taxation due to the premature resumption of sexual relations. These disease causes and the mechanisms they set in train may result in a number of postpartum diseases, the most common of which are: postpartum abdominal pain, fever, retention of the lochia, incessant lochiorrhea, dizziness, fatigue, anxiety and depression, night sweats, insomnia, constipation, low back pain, headache, and scanty lactation.

The three causes

The three main causes of postpartum disease are called the *san yin* or three causes in Chinese. They can be summarized as blood vacuity with stirring of fire, frenetic movement of spoilt, *i.e.*, static, blood, and damage due to excessive food and drink. Chen Liang-fang, in his *Nu Ke Mi Jue Da Quan (The Complete Secrets [of Success] in Gynecology)*, explains these three etiologies thus:

> [If] pospartum, there is profuse loss of blood, blood vacuity leads to stirring of fire which causes vexation, agitation, and fever. Vacuity fire leads to frenetic movement of blood within and dizziness of the head and abdominal pain. [If] postpartum, fire damages the original qi, the spleen and stomach become weak. [If] then food and drink are excessive, this may give rise to [abdominal] fullness and diarrhea. Blood vacuity with fire stirring should be treated by supplementation. Frenetic movement of spoilt blood should be scattered, [and] damage due to excessive eating and drinking should be dispersed.

These basic ideas about postpartum disease causes and mechanisms and their associated treatment then lead to a series of three other key things to remember when dealing with a postpartum patient.

The three examinations

There are three things which should be examined especially carefully in a postpartum woman. These are called the *san zhen* or three examinations. First, the lower abdomen should be examined carefully to see if there is pain or not and if there is a proper lochia or not. These parameters are instrumental in distinguishing between vacuity and repletion. Next, defecation should be examined carefully to see if its is freely flowing or not. This can help tell if fluids are abundant or depleted. Third, one should examine carefully to see whether the breast milk is freely flowing or not and if the intake of food and drink is more or less than normal. These things help tell if the stomach qi is sufficient or insufficient. As Prof.'s Song and Yu of the Zhejiang College of Chinese Medicine in Hangzhou say: "Correct diagnosis can only be made based on assessing these three factors integrated with a consideration of [the patient's other] signs and symptoms, tongue, and pulse."

The three prohibitions

The three prohibitions or *san jin* in terms of postpartum treatment are: 1) It is not all right to cause sweating postpartum, 2) it is not all right to precipitate postpartum, and 3) it is not all right to disinhibit urination postpartum. Since blood and fluids share a common source and are interdependent, unwarranted or excessively forceful sweating, precipitation, and/or disinhibition may further damage and consume yin fluids at a time when such fluids already tend to be depleted. Some Chinese authors say that it is also not all right to use windy natured medicinals which upbear the qi. This is because postpartum one does not want to raise any static blood upward for fear of provoking the *san chong* or three penetrations.

The three penetrations

If the lochia is not discharged completely, this spoilt or static blood may penetrate upward causing various diseases. If such spoilt blood penetrates the heart, it may cause fever, delirium, raving, and madness. If it penetrates the lungs, it may cause rapid dyspneic breathing, chest oppression, vexation, agitation, and a red face. If it penetrates the stomach, it may cause nausea, vomiting, ductal oppression, abdominal distention, and abdominal pain.

Endnotes:

1 Beers & Berkow, *The Merck Manual of Diagnosis and Therapy*, *op. cit.,* p. 2066

2 Gordon, Keith et al., *Gynecology and Obstetrics: A Longitudinal Approach*, *op. cit.*, p. 625

3 Ibid., p. 629

Postpartum Hemorrhage

Postpartum hemorrhage is defined as loss of more than 500ml of blood during or after the third stage of labor. If 2-3 liters of blood are lost, the mother may go into hypovolemic shock. After infection, postpartum hemorrhage is the main cause of maternal mortality in childbirth. The causes of postpartum hemorrhage are uterine atony, lacerations, retained products of conception, and systemic coagulopathies. Uterine atony may be due to overdistention, prolonged or dysfunctional labor, grand multiparity, or anesthesia. Lacerations occurring during delivery may be located on the cervix or vagina, and systemic coagulopathies include idiopathic thrombocytopenia (ITP), preeclampsia, clotting factor deficiency, and the use of anticoagulants, such as warfarin and heparin. Postpartum hemorrhage due to subinvolution of the placental site typically occurs early but may come as late as one month after parturition.

The Western medical treatment of postpartum hemorrhage begins with prevention. This means the correction of anemia before delivery; recognition of uterine myomas, hydramnios, or multiple gestation; and identification of any unusual blood type or history of postpartum hemorrhage. After placental separation, administration of oxytocin usually ensures uterine contraction and reduces blood loss. If, on examination the placenta is found to be incomplete, the uterus is explored manually and missing fragments recovered. Curettage is only seldom required to remove infected placental fragments and decidua. If postpartum hemorrhage does occur, bimanual uterine massage is given and oxytocin is administered intravenously. If a large amount of blood has been lost, this is replaced intravenously. In rare cases, hypogastric artery ligation or hysterectomy may be required.

Chinese medical disease categorization

In Chinese, this condition is referred to as *chan hou xue chu*, postpartum hemorrhage. It also falls under the category of *chan hou lou xia bu jue*, incessant lochiorrhea. If the mother has lost so much blood as to become faint, this is referred to as *chan hou xue yun*, postpartum dizziness. Therefore, please see the separate chapters on these conditions.

Disease causes & disease mechanisms

According to Chinese medicine, postpartum hemorrhaging is mostly due to either qi vacuity or blood stasis. Due to the exertion as well as blood and fluid loss, qi may be so vacuous and insufficient as to be unable to contain the blood within its vessels. However, if static blood remains in the uterus, it may also force the blood to move outside its pathways.

Patterns common to this condition

Qi vacuity not containing
Blood stasis

Treatment based on pattern discrimination

Qi vacuity not containing

Main symptoms: Massive postpartum hemorrhage, spontaneous perspiration, shortness of breath, fatigue, lack of strength, a pale face and lips, a pale tongue, and fine, forceless or possibly vacuous, drumskin, or scallion-stalk pulse depending on the degree of desertion

Note: This pattern mostly describes postpartum hemorrhage due to uterine atony.

Treatment principles: Greatly supplement the qi and stem desertion

Guiding formulas:

Du Shen Tang (Solitary Ginseng Decoction)
Ren Shen (Radix Ginseng), 9-18g

Shen Fu Tang (Ginseng & Aconite Decoction)
Ren Shen (Radix Ginseng), 6-9g
Zhi Fu Zi (Radix Lateralis Praeparatus Aconiti Carmichaeli), 3-9g

This formula is for qi desertion with chilled limbs and cold sweat.

Huang Tu Tang (Yellow Earth Decoction)
Fu Long Gan (Terra Flava Usta), 9g
Bai Zhu (Rhizoma Atractylodis Macrocephalae), 9g
Zhi Fu Zi (Radix Lateralis Praeparatus Aconiti Carmichaeli), 3-9g
Sheng Di (uncooked Radix Rehmanniae), 12-15g
Huang Qin (Radix Scutellariae), 9g
Gan Cao (Radix Glycyrrhizae), 3-9g

If there is pronounced qi vacuity, add *Ren Shen* (Radix Ginseng). If bleeding is profuse, add carbonized *Ai Ye* (Folium Artemisiae Argyii), *Pao Jiang* (blast-fried Rhizoma Zingiberis), and *San Qi* (Radix Notoginseng). In this formula,

Huang Qin is seen as moderating the other warming medicinals. It may be deleted if there is little or no chance of heat transformation and vacuity cold is marked.

Gu Beng Zhi Xue Tang Jia Wei
(Secure the Root & Stop Bleeding Decoction with Added Flavors)
Ren Shen (Radix Ginseng), 3-9g
Huang Qi (Radix Astragali), 9-18g
Shu Di (cooked Radix Rehmanniae), 12-15g
Bai Zhu (Rhizoma Atractylodis Macrocephalae), 9-15g
Dang Gui (Radix Angelicae Sinensis), 9g
Pao Jiang (blast-fried Rhizoma Zingiberis), 6-9g

If dizziness is severe, add *Long Gu* (Os Draconis), *Wu Zei Gu* (Os Sepiae Seu Sepiellae), and *Qian Cao* (Radix Rubiae). If there is abdominal pain, add carbonized *Ai Ye* (Folium Artemesiae Argyii).

Acupuncture & moxibustion: Moxa *Guan Yuan* (CV 4), *Qi Hai* (CV 6), and *Shen Que* (CV 8)

Blood stasis

Main symptoms: Massive or continuous bleeding after delivery with dark, purplish blood mixed with clots, abdominal pain, a dark, purplish face, lips, and tongue, and a choppy pulse

Note: This pattern mostly describes postpartum hemorrhage due to retained remnants of the placenta and fetal membranes.

Treatment principles: Quicken the blood, dispel stasis, and stop bleeding

Guiding formulas:

Sheng Hua Tang (Engendering & Transforming Decoction) plus Duo Ming San (Save Destiny [or Life] Powder)
Dang Gui (Radix Angelicae Sinensis), 9g
Chuan Xiong (Radix Ligustici Wallichii), 9-15g
Tao Ren (Semen Persicae), 9g
Pao Jiang (blast-fried Rhizoma Zingiberis), 6-9g
mix-fried *Gan Cao* (Radix Glycyrrhizae), 6-9g
Mo Yao (Resina Myrrhae), 3-6g
Xue Jie (Sanguis Draconis), 3-6g

If there is a red tongue with yellow fur and rapid pulse, delete *Pao Jiang* and add *Dan Shen* (Radix Salviae Miltiorrhizae), *Huang Qin* (Radix Scutellariae), and *Di Yu* (Radix Sanguisorbae).

Zhu Yu Zhi Beng Tang (Dispel Stasis & Stop Flooding Decoction)
Dang Gui (Radix Angelicae Sinensis), 9g
Chuan Xiong (Radix Ligustici Wallichii), 9-15g
San Qi (Radix Notoginseng), 3g (swallowed with the decocted medicinals)

Mo Yao (Resina Myrrhae), 3-6g
Wu Ling Zhi (Feces Trogopterori Seu Pteromi), 9g
carbonized *Dan Pi* (Cortex Moutan), 9g
stir-fried *Dan Shen* (Radix Salviae Miltiorrhizae), 9-15g
stir-fried *Ai Ye* (Folium Artemesiae Argyii), 9g
E Jiao (Gelatinum Corii Asini), 9g
Wu Zei Gu (Os Sepiae Seu Sepiellae), 9-12g
Long Gu (Os Draconis), 9-12g
Mu Li (Concha Ostreae), 9-12g

Acupuncture & moxibustion: Moxa *Guan Yuan* (CV 4) and *Qi Hai* (CV 6)

Remarks

Except for home and emergency deliveries, most Western practitioners of Chinese medicine have little chance of being called on to treat this condition. It is best handled by Western medical intervention.

3

Postpartum Infection

Postpartum infection or puerperal sepsis occurs in approximately 5% of postpartum women. It is defined as a temperature of 100.4° F (38° C) or higher occurring on any two of the first 10 days after delivery (excepting the first day). Elevated temperature during the first day postpartum is typically due to dehydration, whereas elevated temperatures occurring after the second or third days indicate infection. Such infection is mainly and most seriously of the uterus and parametria (endomyometritis), although bladder and kidney infections are also common. Mastitis refers to infection of the mammary glands and may also fall under the general category of postpartum infection. Anemia, prolonged rupture of the membranes, prolonged labor, operative or traumatic delivery, repeated examination, retention of placental fragments, and postpartum hemorrhage all predispose a migration of normal vaginal bacteria to the uterine cavity where they may cause disease. The single greatest risk factor for the development of puerperal sepsis is cesarean delivery after which there can be an infection rate as high as 38.5%. The risk of cesarean delivery resulting in puerperal sepsis increases if operative time exceeds 60 minutes or blood loss exceeds 800ml.

In addition to fever, the signs and symptoms of endomyometritis include tenderness of the uterus, chills, headache, malaise, anorexia. Pallor, tachycardia, and leukocytosis ususally occur, and the uterus is typically soft, large, and tender. The lochia may be either scanty or ecessive and often smells malodorous. The Western medical treatment of endomyometritis usually consists of administering a broad-spectrum antibiotic, such as ampicillin. This is done intravenously until the woman has been afebrile for 48 hours. In most cases, it is not necessary to continue treatment with oral antibiotics after the IV antibiotics have been discontinued.

Chinese medical disease categorization

Postpartum fever is called *chan hou fa re* in Chinese. Literally, *fa* means to emit and *re* means heat.

Disease causes & disease mechanisms

Postpartum fever is mostly due to excessive blood loss. Yin becomes vacuous and yang thence floats outward. Yin and yang's mutual obedience parts and the constructive and defensive lose their balance. Thus the emission of heat to the exterior or fever occurs.

However, blood stasis may also give rise to postpartum fever. If blood stagnates in the channels and network vessels, the free flow of yang qi is inhibited. This yang qi may then accumulate and float upward and outward as fever.

Postpartum fever may also be due to qi and blood insufficiency. If the constructive and defensive lose their harmony and separate, this may provide an opportunity for external contraction of wind evils. This is described in the Chinese medical literature as external evils taking advantage of vacuity. These wind evils obstruct the flow of the defensive qi in the exterior, and, once again, the accumulation of yang qi manifests as fever. However, if taxation during labor is excessive, it may cause qi and blood insufficiency and this alone may give rise to qi vacuity fever without the presence of external evils.

Another mechanism causing postpartum fever involves the spleen and stomach. Because the spleen and stomach are the latter heaven roots of qi and blood engenderment and transformation, loss of blood during labor and the taxation of labor often result in relative weakness of the spleen postpartum. If the woman eats large quantities of nutritious food high in *wei* or flavor in an effort to replenish and replace her yin blood, this may cause food damage to the spleen and stomach, *i.e.*, food stagnation. If spleen-stomach movement and transformation lose their normalcy, food is not transformed but accumulates in the stomach. This impedes the flow of qi internally and transforms into heat which then is emitted and experienced as fever.

And finally, postpartum infection of the birth canal may result in endometritis which then manifests with fever. This is fever due to invasion of evil toxins according to Chinese medicine.

Patterns common to this condition

Wind cold external contraction

Wind heat external contraction

Evils attacking the shao yang

Infection by evil toxins

Blood vacuity

Yin vacuity with internal heat

Blood stasis

Food damage fever

Treatment based on pattern discrimination

Wind cold external contraction

Main symptoms: Postpartum fever, fear of cold, aches and pains of the head and body, no sweating, a runny nose with clear fluid discharge, cough, a somber white facial complexion, a pale tongue with thin, white, moist fur, and a floating and tight, floating and bowstring, or floating and fine pulse

Treatment principles: Supplement the blood and resolve the exterior

Guiding formulas:

Xing Su Si Wu Tang (Armeniaca & Perilla Four Materials Decoction)
Xing Ren (Semen Armeniacae), 9g
Zi Su Ye (Folium Perillae Frutescentis), 9g
Dang Gui (Radix Angelicae Sinensis), 9g
Shu Di (cooked Radix Rehmanniae), 12g
Bai Shao (Radix Albus Paeoniae Lactiflorae), 9g
Chuan Xiong (Radix Ligustici Wallichii), 9-15g

Zhu Ye Tang (Bamboo Leaf Decoction)
Dan Zhu Ye (Herba Lophatheri), 9g
Fang Feng (Radix Sapshnikoviae), 9g
Ge Gen (Radix Puerariae), 9g
Jie Geng (Radix Platycodi), 6-9g
Gui Zhi (Ramulus Cinnamomi), 6-9g
Ren Shen (Radix Ginseng), 3-9g
mix-fried *Gan Cao* (Radix Glycyrrhizae), 6-9g
Zhi Fu Zi (Radix Lateralis Praeparatus Aconiti Carmichaeli), 3-9g
Sheng Jiang (uncooked Rhizoma Zingiberis), 6g
Da Zao (Fructus Jujubae), 3 pieces

Xiao Chai Hu Tang Jia Jian
(Minor Bupleurum Decoction with Additions & Subtractions)
Chai Hu (Radix Bupleuri), 9g
Ren Shen (Radix Ginseng), 3-9g
Gan Cao (Radix Glycyrrhizae), 3-9g
processed *Ban Xia* (Rhizoma Pinelliae), 9g
Chen Pi (Pericarpium Citri Reticulatae), 6g
Chuan Xiong (Radix Ligustici Wallichii), 9-15g
Bai Shao (Radix Albus Paeoniae Lactiflorae), 9g
Sheng Jiang (uncooked Rhizoma Zingiberis), 6g
Da Zao (Fructus Jujubae), 3 pieces

These last two formulas are for a concomitant righteous qi vacuity.

Acupuncture & moxibustion: *Lie Que* (Lu 7), *He Gu* (LI 4), *Feng Men* (Bl 12), *Feng Chi* (GB 20), *San Yin Jiao* (Sp 6), *Xue Hai* (Sp 10)

Wind heat external contraction

Main symptoms: Fever, aversion to wind, headache, sweating, coughing, dry throat, a desire to drink chilled liquids, a red facial complexion, yellow tongue fur, and a floating, rapid pulse

Treatment principles: Clear heat and resolve the exterior

Guiding Formula:

Yin Qiao San (Lonicera & Forsythia Powder)
Jin Yin Hua (Flos Lonicerae), 9-15g
Lian Qiao (Fructus Forsythiae), 9-15g
Dan Dou Chi (Semen Praeparatus Sojae), 9g
Niu Bang Zi (Fructus Arctii), 9g
Jie Geng (Radix Platycodi), 6-9g
Bo He (Herba Menthae Haplocalycis), 6-9g
Dan Zhu Ye (Herba Lophatheri), 9g
Jing Jie (Herba Schizonepetae), 9g

If there is cough, add *Xing Ren* (Semen Armeniacae) and *Qian Hu* (Radix Peucedani). If heat is more pronounced and accompanied by vexatious thirst and sweating, add *Shi Gao* (Gypsum Fibrosum) and *Mai Men Dong* (Tuber Ophiopogonis). If the lochia does not descend and there is abdominal pain`add *Dan Pi* (Cortex Moutan) and *Tao Ren* (Semen Persicae).

Acupuncture & moxibustion: He Gu (LI 4), *Wai Guan* (TB 5), *Qu Chi* (LI 11), *Da Zhui* (GV 14)

If there is cough, add *Feng Men* (Bl 12) and *Fei Shu* (Bl 13). If there is headache, add *Tai Yang* (M-HN-9) and *Feng Chi* (GB 20).

Evils attacking the shao yang

Main symptoms: Alternating hot and cold, *i.e.*, fever and chills, chest and rib-side fullness, a bitter taste in the mouth, dry throat, possible vomiting, thin, white tongue fur, and a bowstring, possibly rapid pulse

Treatment principles: Harmonize and resolve the shao yang

Guiding formulas:

Xiao Chai Hu Tang (Minor Bupleurum Decoction)
Chai Hu (Radix Bupleuri), 9g
Huang Qin (Radix Scutellariae), 9-12g
processed *Ban Xia* (Rhizoma Pinelliae), 9g
Ren Shen (Radix Ginseng), 3-9g
mix-fried *Gan Cao* (Radix Glycyrrhizae), 6-9g
Sheng Jiang (uncooked Rhizoma Zingiberis), 6g
Da Zao (Fructus Jujubae), 3 pieces

In this formula, the emphasis is on supplementing the middle and supporting the righteous.

San Yuan Tang (Three Origins Decoction)
Chai Hu (Radix Bupleuri), 9g
Sheng Di (uncooked Radix Rehmanniae), 12-15g
Chuan Xiong (Radix Ligustici Wallichii), 9g
Chi Shao (Radix Rubrus Paeoniae Lactiflorae), 9g
Dang Gui (Radix Angelicae Sinensis), 9g
Huang Qin (Radix Scutellariae), 9-12g
Ren Shen (Radix Ginseng), 3-9g
Ban Xia (Rhizoma Pinelliae), 9g
Gan Cao (Radix Glycyrrhizae), 3-9g

In this formula, the emphasis is on nourishing the blood and clearing heat.

Acupuncture & moxibustion: *Wai Guan* (TB 5), *Qu Chi* (LI 11), *He Gu* (LI 4), *Yang Ling Quan* (GB 34)

If there is stomach duct fullness, add *Zhong Wan* (CV 12). If there is chest oppression, add *Dan Zhong* (CV 17). If there is rib-side distention, add *Zhang Men* (Liv 13) and *Qi Men* (Liv 14). If there is vomiting, add *Zhong Wan* (CV 12) and *Zu San Li* (St 36).

Infection by evil toxins

Main symptoms: Postpartum fever, aversion to cold, possible fever and chills, lower abdominal aching and pain which is adverse to pressure, scanty or excessive lochia but purple and dark in color with an offensive odor, vexation and agitation, thirst leading to drinking, scanty, yellow-colored urine, dry, bound stools, a red tongue with yellow fur, and a rapid and forceful, large and rapid, or bowstring, fine, and rapid pulse. In severe cases, there will also be delirium and red skin rashes.

Treatment principles: Clear heat and resolve toxins

Guiding formulas:

Jie Du Huo Xue Tang (Resolve Toxins & Quicken the Blood Decoction)
Lian Qiao (Fructus Forsythiae), 9-15g
Jin Yin Hua (Flos Lonicerae), 9-15g
Chai Hu (Radix Bupleuri), 9g
Zhi Ke (Fructus Aurantii), 6-9g
Dang Gui (Radix Angelicae Sinensis), 9g
Chi Shao (Radix Rubrus Paeoniae Lactiflorae), 9g
Sheng Di (uncooked Radix Rehmanniae), 12-15g
Hong Hua (Flos Carthami), 9g
Tao Ren (Semen Persicae), 9g
Gan Cao (Radix Glycyrrhizae), 3-9g

This formula also cools the blood and transforms stasis.

Zi Ju Jie Du Tang (Viola & Chrysanthemum Resolve Toxins Decoction)
Dan Pi (Cortex Moutan), 9g
Chi Shao (Radix Rubrus Paeoniae Lactiflorae), 9g
uncooked *Pu Huang* (Pollen Typhae), 9g
Wu Ling Zhi (Feces Trogopterori Seu Pteromi), 9g
Ye Ju Hua (Flos Chrysanthemi Indici), 9-15g
Zi Hua Di Ding (Herba Violae), 9-15g
Zi Bei Tian Kui (Radix Semiaquilegiae), 9g
Yu Xing Cao (Herba Houttuyniae), 9-18g

This formula works on the same principles as the preceding formula.

Ren Shen Bai Hu Tang (Ginseng White Tiger Decoction)
Shi Gao (Gypsum Fibrosum), 9-19g
Ren Shen (Radix Ginseng), 3-9g
Jing Mi (Fructus Oryzae), 15g
Zhi Mu (Rhizoma Anemarrhenae), 9-12g
Gan Cao (Radix Glycyrrhizae), 3-9g

This formula is for the treatment of an obstinate high fever with a red face, insatiable thirst, labored breathing, profuse sweating, and a large pulse.

Da Huang Mu Dan Pi Tang (Rhubarb & Moutan Decoction)
Tao Ren (Semen Persicae), 9g
Mang Xiao (Mirabilitum), 3-9g
Dan Pi (Cortex Moutan), 9g
Da Huang (Radix Et Rhizoma Rhei), 3-9g
DongGua Zi (Semen Benincasae), 9-15g

This formula is for use if pain predominates and the lochia is not precipitated accompanied by constipation and an obstinate high fever.

Jie Du Tui Re Fang (Resolve Toxins & Recede Heat Formula)
Jin Yin Hua (Flos Lonicerae), 9-15g
Lian Qiao (Fructus Forsythiae), 9-15g
Niu Bang Zi (Fructus Arctii), 9g
Huang Lian (Rhizoma Coptidis), 3-9g
Huang Qin (Radix Scutellariae), 9-12g
Huang Bai (Cortex Phellodendri), 9g
Dang Gui (Radix Angelicae Sinensis), 9g
Sheng Di (uncooked Radix Rehmanniae), 12-15g
Pu Gong Ying (Herba Taraxaci), 9-19g
Zi Hua Di Ding (Herba Violae), 9-15g

If there is simultaneous external contraction, add *Qian Hu* (Radix Puecedani) and *Jie Geng* (Radix Platycodi). If there is simultaneous yin vacuity with damaged fluids, add uncooked *Shi Gao* (Gypsum Fibrosum), *Xuan Shen* (Radix

Scrophulariae), and *Mai Men Dong* (Tuber Ophiopogonis). If there is blood stasis, add *Dan Shen* (Radix Salviae Miltiorrhizae).

Wu Wei Xiao Du Yin Jia Wei
(Five Flavors Disperse Toxins Drink with Added Flavors)
Jin Yin Hua (Flos Lonicerae), 9-15g
Ye Ju Hua (Flos Chrysanthemi Indici), 9-15g
Pu Gong Ying (Herba Taraxaci), 9-18g
Zi Hua Di Ding (Herba Violae), 9-15g
Zi Bei Tian Kui (purple-backed Herba Semiaquilegiae), 9g
Ru Xiang (Resina Olibani), 3-6g
Mo Yao (Resina Myrrhae), 3-6g
Chi Shao (Radix Rubrus Paeoniae Lactiflorae), 9g
Dan Pi (Cortex Moutan), 9g

This formula is appropriate for an infected episiotomy wound.

Yin Lian Hong Jiang Jie Du Tang
(Lonicera, Forsythia, Sargentodoxa & Patrinia Resolve Toxins Decoction)
Jin Yin Hua (Flos Lonicerae), 9-15g
Lian Qiao (Fructus Forsythiae), 9-15g
Hong Teng (Caulis Sargentodoxae), 9-18g
Bai Jiang Cao (Herba Patriniae), 9-18g
Dan Pi (Cortex Moutan), 9g
uncooked *Zhi Zi* (Fructus Gardeniae), 6-9g
Chi Shao (Radix Rubrus Paeoniae Lactiflorae), 9g
Tao Ren (Semen Persicae), 9g
Yan Hu Suo (Rhizoma Corydalis), 9-18g
Chuan Lian Zi (Fructus Toosendan), 6-9g

This formula is appropriate for an infected cesarean section wound.

Acupuncture & moxibustion: *Guan Yuan* (CV 4), *Zhong Ji* (CV 3), *Wei Bao* (an extra-channel point located in a depression on the medial lower edge of the anterior superior iliac spine at the level of *Guan Yuan* [CV 4]), *Yin Ling Quan* (Sp 9), *Qu Chi* (LI 11), *He Gu* (LI 4)

External therapies for episiotomy and/or cesarean-section wound infection: Mash 120 grams of *Pu Gong Ying* (fresh Herba Taraxaci) into a pulp and wrap in cotton gauze. Apply to the mouth of the wound. After it dries, replace. This is appropriate in the initial stage when there is not transformation of pus.

Make a paste from *Liu Shen Wan* (Six Spirits Pills, a ready-made Chinese medicine) and rice vinegar and apply to the affected area. This may be used with abdominal area wounds which are red and swollen but not ulcerated.

Mix *Jin Huang San* (Golden Yellow Powder) with concentrated tea and make into paste. Apply to the wound on the perineum three times each day. This is suitable for the initial stage when there is no transformation of pus. *Jin Huang San* consists of: *Da Huang* (Radix Et Rhizoma Rhei), *Huang Bai* (Cortex Phellodendri), *Jiang Huang* (Rhizoma Curcumae Longae), and *Bai Zhi* (Radix Angelicae Dahuricae), 500g each, *Cang Zhu* (Rhizoma Atractylodis), *Hou Po* (Cortex Magnoliae Officinalis), and *Gan Cao* (Radix Glycyrrhizae), 200g each, and *Tian Hua Fen* (Radix Trichosanthis), 1000g. These medicinals are ground into fine powder, mixed with boiled water or honey into a paste, and applied to the affected area.

Apply *Huang Lian Gao* (Coptis Ointment) externally to the perineal wound three times each day. This is suitable if there is transformation of pus but no ulceration. *Huang Lian Gao* consists of: powdered *Huang Lian* (Rhizoma Coptidis), 9g, *Dang Gui* (Radix Angelicae Sinensis), 15g, *Huang Bai* (Cortex Phellodendri), 9g, *Sheng Di* (uncooked Radix Rehmanniae) and *Jiang Huang* (Rhizoma Curcumae Longae) in an oil and beeswax base.

Apply *Sheng Ji San* (Engender Flesh Powder) or *Sheng Ji Gao* (Engender Flesh Ointment) to the wound. This is suitable if pus has finished. *Sheng Ji Gao* consists of: powdered *Peng Sha* (Borax), 60g, *Bing Pian* (Borneolum), 60g, *Bo He* (Herba Menthae Haplocalycis), 10g, *Qian Dan* (Minium), 30g, zinc oxide, 120g, powdered *Zhen Zhu* (Margarita), 10g, and phenol, 2g, mixed in an oil and beeswax base.

Blood vacuity

Main symptoms: Postpartum fever after having lost a lot of blood, low-grade fever, no aversion to cold, sweating, a flushed red face, dizziness, tinnitus, heart palpitations, a pale tongue with thin fur, and a large, scallion-stalk pulse

Treatment principles: Supplement the qi and boost the blood

Guiding formulas:

Sheng Yu Tang Jia Wei (Sagely Healing Decoction with Added Flavors)
Di Gu Pi (Cortex Lycii), 9-15g
Mai Men Dong (Tuber Ophiopogonis), 9-12g
Sha Ren (Radix Glehniae), 9g
Wu Wei Zi (Fructus Schisandrae), 9g
Huang Qi (Radix Astragali), 9-18g
Ren Shen (Radix Ginseng), 3-9g
Dang Gui (Radix Angelicae Sinensis), 9g
Chuan Xiong (Radix Ligustici Wallichii), 9-15g
Shu Di (cooked Radix Rehmanniae), 12-15g
Sheng Di (uncooked Radix Rehmanniae), 12-15g

Si Wu Tang Jia Wei (Four Materials Decoction with Added Flavors)
Dang Gui (Radix Angelicae Sinensis), 9g
Shu Di (cooked Radix Rehmanniae), 12-15g
Bai Shao Yao (Radix Albus Paeoniae Lactiflorae), 9g

Chuan Xiong (Radix Ligustici Wallichii), 9-15g
Fu Ling (Poria), 9-12g
Jiao Jiang (scorched Rhizoma Zingiberis), 6g

Acupuncture & moxibustion: *Ge Shu* (Bl 17), *Gan Shu* (Bl 18), *Pi Shu* (Bl 20), *Zu San Li* (St 36), *Qu Chi* (LI 11)

Yin vacuity with internal heat

Main symptoms: Postpartum fever, bilateral malar flushing, oral thirst and a liking for chilled drinks, dry stools, yellow-red urine, a red tongue with scanty fur or thin, dry, yellow fur, and a fine, rapid pulse

Treatment principles: Enrich yin, nourish the blood, and clear heat

Guiding formulas:

Yi Yin Jian (Boost Yin Decoction)
Sheng Di (uncooked Radix Rehmanniae), 12-15g
Bai Shao (Radix Albus Paeoniae Lactiflorae), 9g
Mai Men Dong (Tuber Ophiopogonis), 9-12g
Shu Di (cooked Radix Rehmanniae), 12-15g
Zhi Mu (Rhizoma Anemarrhenae), 9g
Di Gu Pi (Cortex Lycii), 9-15g
Gan Cao (Radix Glycyrrhizae), 3-9g

Han Bai-ling suggests adding *Qing Hao* (Herba Artemisiae Annuae), *Mu Li* (Concha Ostreae), and *Bie Jia* (Carapax Amydae Sinensis) to enrich yin and subdue yang.

Chai Hu Yin Zi (Bupleurum Beverage)
Chai Hu (Radix Bupleuri), 9g
Huang Qin (Radix Scutellariae), 9-12g
Ren She (Radix Ginseng), 3-9g
Gan Cao (Radix Glycyrrhizae), 3-9g
Dang Gui (Radix Angelicae Sinensis), 9g
Di Gu Pi (Cortex Lycii), 9-15g
Da Huang (Radix Et Rhizoma Rhei), 3-9g

This formula addresses a qi and yin dual vacuity with liver depression and constipation due to intestinal dryness. Since the blood and body fluids share a common source, loss of blood during delivery can damage fluids and humors leading to intestinal dryness and constipation. If necessary, one can add *Sheng Di* (uncooked Radix Rehmanniae), *Bai Shao* (Radix Albus Paeoniae Lactiflorae), and *Mai Men Dong* (Tuber Ophiopogonis) to further enrich yin and nourish the blood.

Acupuncture & moxibustion: *Guan Yuan* (CV 4), *Shen Shu* (Bl 23), *San Yin Jiao* (Sp 6), *Tai Xi* (Ki 3)

Blood stasis

Main symptoms: Alternating fever and chills, nondescension of the lochia or a not easily flowing lochia which is dark and purplish in color and contains clots, lower abdominal aching and pain refusing pressure, a dry mouth but no desire to drink, a purplish, dark tongue, and a bowstring, choppy pulse

Treatment principles: Quicken the blood and transform stasis in order to regulate the constructive and defensive

Guiding formula:

Sheng Hua Tang Jia Jian
(Engendering & Transforming Decoction with Additions & Subtractions)
Dang Gui (Radix Angelicae Sinensis), 9g
Chuan Xiong (Radix Ligusticum Wallichii), 9-18g
Tao Ren (Semen Persicae), 9g
mix-fried *Gan Cao* (Radix Glycyrrhizae), 6-9g
Dan Pi (Cortex Moutan), 9g
Yi Mu Cao (Herba Leonuri), 9-18g
Hong Hua (Flos Carthami), 9g

In order to strengthen the clearing of heat transformed from blood stasis, one can add *Chi Shao* (Radix Rubrus Paeoniae Lactiflorae) and *Bo He* (Herba Menthae Haplocalycis).

Acupuncture & moxibustion: San Yin Jiao (Sp 6), *Xue Hai* (Sp 10), *He Gu* (LI 4), *Guan Yuan* (CV 4)

Food damage fever

Main symptoms: Low-grade postpartum fever accompanied by chest and ductal oppression and fullness, stomach and abdominal distention and pain, acid regurgitation, eructation with foul odor, loss of appetite, possible diarrhea and/or vomiting, yellow, slimy tongue fur, and a slippery, rapid pulse

Treatment principles: Fortify the spleen and harmonize the stomach, disperse food and abduct stagnation

Guiding formulas:

Jia Wei Si Jun Zi Tang (Added Flavors Four Gentlemen Decoction)
Ren Shen (Radix Ginseng), 3-9g
stir-fried *Bai Zhu* (Rhizoma Atractylodis Macrocephalae), 9g
Fu Ling (Poria), 12g
mix-fried *Gan Cao* (Radix Glycyrrhizae), 6-9g
processed *Ban Xia* (Rhizoma Praeparata Pinelliae), 9g
Sha Ren (Fructus Amomi), 3-4.5g
Chen Pi (Pericarpium Citri Reticulatae), 6g
Shen Qu (Massa Medica Fermentata), 6-9g
Sheng Jiang (uncooked Rhizoma Zingiberis), 6g

Da Zao (Fructus Jujubae), 2-3 pieces

This formula is for a combination of food stagnation and spleen vacuity. If there is constipation, add a small amount of *Da Huang* (Radix Et Rhizoma Rhei).

Bao He Wan Jia Jian
(Protect Harmony Pills with Additions & Subtractions)
Shan Zha (Fructus Crataegi), 9g
Shen Qu (Massa Medica Fermentata), 9g
ginger-processed *Ban Xia* (Rhizoma Pinelliae), 9g
Chen Pi (Pericarpium Citri Reticulatae), 6g
Lian Qiao (Fructus Forsythiae), 9-15g
Fu Ling (Poria), 9-12g
stir-fried *Zhi Ke* (Fructus Aurantii), 6-9g
Bai Zhu (Rhizoma Atractylodis Macrocephalae)

This formula is for less spleen vacuity but more fever.

Acupuncture & moxibustion: *Zhong Wan* (CV 12), *Liang Men* (St 21), *Nei Ting* (St 44), *He Gu* (LI 4), *Qu Chi* (LI 11)

Abstracts of representative Chinese research

From "The Treatment of 70 Cases of Postpartum Fever with *Xiao Chai Hu Tang Jia Wei* (Minor Bupleurum Decoction with Added Flavors)" by Wang Ya-zhen, *Jiang Su Zhong Yi (Jiangsu Chinese Medicine)*, #10, 1999, p. 24-25

Of the 70 women in this study, 46 had given birth normally and 24 had had cesarean deliveries. The youngest was 23 and the oldest was 34 years old. All developed fever within four days postpartum. The longest duration of fever was seven days, and the shortest was two days. In 48 cases, the temperature was 38.5-39° C, while in the other 22 cases, it was 39.1-39.5° C. Accompanying symptoms included varying degrees of aversion to cold, headache, thirst, and poor appetite.

Treatment method:

The basic formula consisted of: *Chai Hu* (Radix Bupleuri), 20g, *Huang Qin* (Radix Scutellariae), 20g, *Ban Xia* (Rhizoma Pinelliae), 10g, *Dang Shen* (Radix Codonopsitis), 15g, *Dang Gui* (Radix Angelicae Sinensis), 10g, *Tao Ren* (Semen Persicae), 10g, *Chuan Xiong* (Radix Ligustici Wallichii), 10g, *Qing Hao* (Herba Artemisiae Annuae), 30g, *Bai Zhu* (Rhizoma Atractylodis Macrocephalae), 10g, *Gan Cao* (Radix Glycyrrhizae), 6g, *Sheng Jiang* (uncooked Rhizoma Zingiberis), 10g, and *Da Zao* (Fructus Jujubae), 5 pieces. If there was vexatious thirst, *Zhi Mu* (Rhizoma Anemarrhenae) were added. If there was breast swelling and pain, *Jin Yin Hua* (Flos Lonicerae) and *Pu Gong Ying* (Herba Taraxaci) were added, and, if there was poor appetite, *Shen Qu* (Massa Medica Fermentata) and *Shan Zha* (Fructus Crataegi) were added. One packet was administered per day in two divided doses after having been boiled in water. Three packets were given in succession.

Treatment outcomes:

Forty-five patients were judged cured using this protocol. This meant that their temperature lowered to 37° C, their appetite improved, there was no pressure pain in their lower abdomen, and their lochia was normal. Twenty-two patients improved. This meant that their temperature was 38° C or lower but not 37°, their appetite had improved, and their lochia was moderate. Three patients got no effect. Therefore, the cure rate was 64.29% and the total amelioration rate was 95.71%.

From "The Treatment of 100 Cases of Postpartum & Gynecological Surgery Fever with *Bu Zhong Yi Qi Tang Jia Jian* (Supplement the Center & Boost the Qi Decoction with Additions & Subtractions)" by Li Xue-jun, *Jiang Xi Zhong Yi Yao (Jiangxi Chinese Medicine & Medicinals)*, #1, 1993, p. 48

Cohort description:

Among the 100 women in this study, all were between 23-56 years of age, all had been pregnant 1-5 times, and all had a fever of 37.5-39.8° C for 2-13 days. In addition, all had been treated with a combination of Western and Chinese medicine with poor result. Forty-six patients had postpartum fever, 30 had post cesarean-section fever, and 24 had post-gynecological surgery fever.

Treatment method:

The basic formula consisted of: *Huang Qi* (Radix Astragali), 15g, *Dang Shen* (Radix Codonopsitis), 20g, *Bai Zhu* (Rhizoma Atractylodis Macrocephalae), 12g, *Chai Hu* (Radix Bupleuri), 15g, *Chen Pi* (Pericarpium Citri Reticulatae), 12g, *Dang Gui* (Radix Angelicae Sinensis), 12g, *Gan Cao* (Radix Glycyrrhizae), 6g, *Tao Ren* (Semen Persicae), 12g, *E Zhu* (Rhizoma Curcumae), 10g, and *Huang Qin* (Radix Scutellariae), 12g. During the spring, *Jin Yin Hua* (Flos Lonicerae), *Lian Qiao* (Fructus Forsythiae), and *Bo He* (Herba Menthae Haplocalycis) were added. During the summer, *Huo Xiang* (Herba Pogostemonis), *Pei Lan* (Herba Eupatorii), *Xiang Ru* (Herba Elscholtziae), and *Hua Shi* (Talcum) were added. In the fall, *Sang Ye* (Folium Mori), *Xing Ren* (Semen Armeniacae), and *Sha Shen* (Radix Glehniae) were added. During the winter, *Jing Jie* (Herba Schizonepetae), *Fang Feng* (Radix Sapshnikoviae), and *Gui Zhi* (Ramulus Cinnamomi) were added. If evils resided in the exterior, *Bo He* (Herba Menthae Haplocalycis) and *Niu Bang Zi* (Fructus Arctii) were added. If evils resided in the qi aspect and there was a strong fever with perspiration, thirst, and yellow tongue fur, *Shi Gao* (Gypsum Fibrosum) and *Zhi Mu* (Rhizoma Anemarrhenae) were added. If evils resided in the constructive, *Xi Jiao* (Cornu Rhinocerotis), *Xuan Shen* (Radix Scrophulariae), and *Ling Yang Jiao* (Cornu Antelopis Saiga-tatarici) were added. If evils resided in the blood aspect and there was bleeding, *Sheng Di* (uncooked Radix Rehmanniae), *Dan Pi* (Cortex Moutan), *Chi Shao* (Radix Rubrus Paeoniae Lactiflorae), and *E Jiao* (Gelatinum Corii Asini) were added. If there was blood vacuity, *Shu Di* (cooked Radix Rehmanniae) and *E Jiao* (Gelatinum Corii Asini) were added. If there was yin vacuity, *Qing Hao* (Herba Artemisiae Annuae) and *Bie Jia* (Carapax Amydae Sinensis) were added. If there was blood stasis, *Yi Mu Cao* (Herba Leonuri) and *Dan Pi* (Cortex Moutan) or *Pu Huang* (Pollen Typhae) and *Wu Ling Zhi* (Feces Trogopterori Seu Pteromi) were added. If there was infection, *Jin Yin Hua* (Flos Lonicerae) and *Pu Gong Ying* (Herba Taraxaci) were added. If there was constipation, *Da Huang* (Radix Et Rhizoma Rhei) and *Mu Xiang* (Radix Auklandiae) were added, and, if fever was severe, *Shi Gao* (Gypsum Fibrosum) was added. One packet of these medicinals was administered per day unless the fever was serious. In that case, two packets were administered per day, once every six hours.

Treatment outcomes:

Marked effect was defined as normalization of the temperature within two days and disappearance of the clinical symptoms. Some effect was defined as normalization of the temperature within three days and disappearance or reduction in the symptoms. No effect meant that, after four days, the temperature had either not come down at all or only come down slightly. Based on these criteria, 82 cases were judged cured, 14 got some effect, and four cases got no effect. Thus the total amelioration rate was 96%.

Representative case histories

Case 1: The patient was 24 years old. Her initial examination occurred on May 23, 1975. Five days before she had had a cesarean delivery, and, since then, she had had a fever for four days. Chinese medicinals, acupuncture, *Kang Yan Yi Hao* (Anti-inflammatory #1), and gentamicin had been used, but the fever had not receded. The fever got worse as dusk approached and at night was as high as 38.8°C. Sweating was extremely copious and her breasts were distended. Her lower abdomen was aching and painful. The lochia was not copious and she had a cough with phlegm. Her urination was choppy and painful. Her pulse was vacuous, large, and rapid, while her tongue had static macules and slimy fur. Based on these signs and symptoms, it was determined that the patient exhibited a shao yang pattern due to external contraction of evils in turn due to postpartum blood vacuity. Therefore, she was administered one packet of: *Chai Hu* (Radix Bupleuri), 9g, *Huang Qin* (Radix Scutellariae), 9g, processed *Ban Xia* (Rhizoma Pinelliae), 9g, *Dang Shen* (Radix Codonopsitis), 9g, *Pao Jiang* (blast-fried Rhizoma Zingiberis), 3g, *Da Zao* (Fructus Jujubae), 3 pieces, *Dang Gui* (Radix Angelicae Sinensis), 9g, *Chuan Xiong* (Radix Ligustici Wallichii), 9g, *Tao Ren* (Semen Persicae), 9g, and *Yi Mu Cao* (Herba Leonuri), 30g.

The second examination occurred on May 24, 1975. After taking the above medicinals, the fever had gradually receded. That night, her temperature was 37.7°C. The next morning, the fever was gone. The patient's spontaneous perspiration was somewhat diminished and her lochia had increased. The cough still had phlegm. Her pulse had become soggy and rapid, and her tongue fur's sliminess had transformed a little. The previous formula had been effective, but diffusing the lungs needed to be boosted. Therefore, 12 grams of *Xing Ren* (Semen Armeniacae) and nine grams each of *Jie Geng* (Radix Platycodi) and *Zhe Bei Mu (*Bulbus Fritillariae Thunbergii) were added to the above formula and two packets were prescribed.

The third examination took place on May 26, 1975. The patient's fever had continued to gradually recede and clear. On the night of the 24th, it had been 37.5°C. On the night of the 25th, it had been 37.1°C. The cough and spontaneous perspiration had already been cured. The patient's pulse was soggy and fine and the root of her tongue had slimy, white fur. The original treatment methods were continued assisted by harmonizing the stomach: *Chai Hu* (Radix Bupleuri), 4.5g, *Huang Qi* (Radix Scutellariae), 9g, *Ban Xia* (processed Rhizoma Pinelliae), 9g, *Tai Zi Shen* (Radix Pseudostellariae), 9g, *Pao Jiang* (blast-fried Rhizoma Zingiberis), 3g, *Dang Gui* (Radix Angelicae Sinensis), 9g, *Chuan Xiong* (Radix Ligustici Wallichii), 9g, *Yi Mu Cao* (Herba Leonuri), 30g, *Sha Ren* (Fructus Amomi), 4.5g, and *Chen Pi* (Pericarpium Citri Reticulatae) 4.5g. Two packets were administered. On May 28, the patient was discharged from the hospital having been judged cured.

Case 2: The patient was a 28 year-old female who was initially examined on Jan. 9, 1974. The patient was 29 days postpartum and had had a high fever for two days. On Dec. 10, 1973, she had given birth at term normally. Generally, things were good postpartum except that her lochia had not stopped even though its amount was scanty. The previous day, the patient's temperature had risen to 38.9° C. This was accompanied by aversion to cold, headache, dizziness, clear, runny nose, generalized body aching and pain, inability to sleep, heart palpitations, shortness of breath, torpid intake, a dry mouth, thirst, sweating, yellow urine, but ok defecation, a pale tongue with thin, yellow fur, and a deep, slippery, rapid pulse.

Based on the above signs and symptoms, the patient's Western medical diagnosis was common cold, and her Chinese medical pattern discrimination was postpartum blood vacuity with external contraction of wind cold. Therefore, she was prescribed: *Jing Jie* (Herba Schizonepetae), 9g, *Fang Feng* (Radix Sapshnikoviae), 6g, *Chuan Xiong* (Radix Ligustici Wallichii), 6g, *Qiang Huo* (Radix Et Rhizoma Notopterygii), 3g, *Dang Gui* (Radix Angelicae Sinensis), 9g, *Yi Mu Cao* (Herba Leonuri), 9g, *Huang Qin* (Radix Scutellariae), 9g, *Gan Cao* (Radix Glycyrrhizae), 6g, *Jie Geng* (Radix Platycodi), 3g, *Xing Ren* (Semen Armeniacae), 6g, *Sheng Jiang* (uncooked Rhizoma Zingiberis), 3 slices, and *Bo He* (Herba Menthae Haplocalycis), 3g, added later.

The patient was seen again on Jan. 11th after having taken one packet of the above medicinals. However, her fever had not abated and was now 39° C. The headache and runny nose were less, there was a slight cough, and there was sweating, a dry mouth with thrist, but the patient's urination and defecation were both alright. Thus she was prescribed: uncooked *Shi Gao* (Gypsum Fibrosum), 45g, *Zhi Mu* (Rhizoma Anemarrhenae), 9g, *Huang Qin* (Radix Scutellariae), 9g, *Shi Hu* (Herba Dendrobii), 12g, *Lian Qiao* (Fructus Forsythiae), 30g, *Jin Yin Hua* (Flos Lonicerae), 30g, *Chi Shao* (Radix Rubrus Paeoniae Lactiflorae), 6g, *Gan Cao* (Radix Glycyrrhizae), 3g, stir-fried *Lai Fu Zi* (Semen Raphani), 9g, stir-fried *Zhi Ke* (Fructus Aurantii), 9g, *Ji Nei Jin* (Endothelium Corneum Gigeriae Galli), 9g, scorched *Shen Qu* (Massa Medica Fermentata), 9g, *Dan Pi* (Cortex Moutan), 6g, and *Di Gu Pi* (Cortex Lycii), 9g.

The third visit occurred on Jan. 13th when the patient reported that, after taking one packet of the above medicinals, the fever had receded. Her headache and runny nose had already decreased, but there was still a slight cough and her appetite was not great. In addition, there was perspiration, a dark red tongue with whitish yellow fur, and a deep, fine, rapid pulse. She had taken yet another packet and, at that point, still had some headache, dizziness, heart palpitations, insomnia, anxiety, a dry mouth with a desire to drink, and an incessant lochia. The patient's tongue was red with scanty fluids, and her pulse was deep, fine, and forceless. Based on the determination that she had damaged yin, the patient was administered the following medicinals: *Sha Shen* (Radix Glehniae), 15g, *Mai Men Dong* (Tuber Ophiopogonis), 9g, *Shi Hu* (Herba Dendrobii), 12g, *Sheng Di* (uncooked Radix Rehmanniae), 12g, stir-fried *Suan Zao Ren* (Semen Zizyphi Spinosae), 9g, stir-fried *Bai Shao* (Radix Albus Paeoniae Lactiflorae), 9g, *Ye Jiao Teng* (Caulis Polygoni Multiflori), 30g, *E Jiao* (Gelatinum Corii Asini), 15g, *Huang Lian* (Rhizoma Coptidis), 3g, *Gan Cao* (Radix Glycyrrhizae), 6g, and *Wu Wei Zi* (Fructus Schisandrae), 9g. After taking three packets of these medicinals, all the patient's symptoms were eliminated and her condition was judged cured.

Case 3: The patient was a 24 year-old female who was first seen on May 23, 1975 and who was five days post cesarean-section. The patient had developed a fever on the fourth day and had been treated with Chinese medicinals. However, her fever had not abated. In the morning it was not high, but it became high in the evening, reaching 38.8° C. Sweating was profuse, her breasts were distended, and her lower abdomen was achy and painful. The woman's lochia was not much, and she had a cough with phlegm. Her urination was choppy and painful, her tongue had static macules and slimy fur, and her pulse was vacuous, large, and rapid.

Based on these signs and symptoms, the patient's pattern was categorized as postpartum qi and blood depletion with external contraction of evils that had now entered the shao yang aspect. Therefore, she was prescribed one packet of the following version of *Xiao Chai Hu Tang* (Minor Bupleurum Decoction): *Chai Hu* (Radix Bupleuri), 9g, *Huang Qin* (Radix Scutellariae), 9g, processed *Ban Xia* (Rhizoma Pinelliae), 9g, *Dang Shen* (Radix Codonopsitis), 9g, *Pao Jiang* (blast-fried Rhizoma Zingiberis), 3g, *Da Zao* (Fructus Jujubae), 3 pieces, *Dang Gui* (Radix Angelicae Sinensis), 9g, *Chuan Xiong* (Radix Ligustici Wallichii), 9g, *Tao Ren* (Semen Persicae), 9g, and *Yi Mu Cao* (Herba Leonuri), 30g.

The second examination occurred on May 24, 1975. After taking the above medicinals, the patient's fever had gradually receded. The night before, her temperature had been 37.7° C. The patient's spontaneous perspiration was relatively less, her lochia had increased in amount, but she still had a cough with phlegm. At this point, the woman's pulse had turned soggy and rapid and the sliminess of her tongue fur had slightly transformed. Therefore, 12 grams of *Xing Ren* (Semen Armeniacae) and nine grams each of *Jie Geng* (Radix Platycodi) and *Zhe Bei Mu* (Bulbus Fritillariae Thunbergii) were added to the above formula and two more packets were prescribed.

The third examination occurred on May 26, 1975 when the fever had gradually cleared. On the 24th, the patient's temperature had been 37.5°C, and on the 25th, it had been 37.1° C. The cough and spontaneous perspiration were still a problem, however. The pulse was soggy and fine, and the tongue fur was white and slimy at the root. Therefore, she was prescribed two packets of: *Chai Hu* (Radix Bupleuri), 4.5g, *Huang Qin* (Radix Scutellariae), 9g, processed *Ban Xia* (Rhizoma Pinelliae), 9g, *Tai Zi Shen* (Radix Pseudostellariae), 9g, *Pao Jiang* (blast-fried Rhizoma Zingiberis), 3g, *Dang Gui* (Radix Angelicae Sinensis), 9g, *Chuan Xiong* (Radix Ligustici Wallichii), 9g, *Yi Mu Cao* (Herba Leonuri), 30g, *Sha Ren* (Fructus Amomi), 4.5g, *Chen Pi* (Pericarpium Citri Reticulatae), 4.5g. On May 28th, the patient was discharged from the hospital, having been judged cured.

Case 4: The patient was a 28 year-old female who was first seen on March 18, 1999 when she was 15 days postpartum. The patient had had a fever for three days, aversion to cold, and no dry mouth. However, she did have a predilection for hot drinks. The woman had been treated with intravenous antibiotics, but her temperature was still 38° C. Her facial complexion was somber white and there was lassitude of the spirit, a low, weak voice, perspiration, a lochia which had not yet stopped, dizziness, a bland taste in the mouth, poor appetite, a fat tongue with thin, white fur, and a fine, rapid, forceless pulse. Based on these signs and symptoms, the patient's pattern was categorized as constructive and defensive disharmony, and she was prescribed the following medicinals: *Gui Zhi* (Ramulus Cinnamomi), 10g, stir-fried *Bai Shao* (Radix Albus Paeoniae Lactiflorae), 10g, stir-fried *Dang Gui* (Radix Angelicae Sinensis), 15g, *Dang Shen* (Radix Codonopsitis), 15g, *Yi Mu Cao* (Herba Leonuri), 10g, mix-fried *Gan Cao* (Radix Glycyrrhizae), 6g, *Sheng Jiang* (uncooked Rhizoma Zingiberis), 6g, and *Da Zao* (Fructus Jujubae), 7 pieces. After taking three packets of this formula, the fever abated and all her symptoms were cured.

Remarks

Although I have treated a number of patients with postpartum fever with Chinese medicine, all successfully, I would caution great care and close monitoring if there is the possibility of endometritis. Chinese medicine can treat endometritis. However, in a Western setting, there may be legal liabilities incurred if done so without a simultaneous referral to a Western MD.

4

Retention of Lochia

As mentioned above, the lochia is the bloody fluid discharged from the vagina for several days after delivery. It is composed of blood and necrotic decidua and is sterile to begin with. By day 3-4, however, it is colonized by vaginal commensals, such as anaerobic *Streptococcus, E. coli*. In most postpartum women, the lochia begins to taper off after 3-4 days. Its color turns from bright red to a pale red and thence to a pale yellow. The lochia typically stops completely after 7-10 days. Some women, however, do not have a lochia or only a very slight vaginal discharge. In Western gynecology, there is no disease category called retention of the lochia. Since Chinese medicine sees the lochia as the discharge of spoilt blood, if this blood is not completely discharged but is left behind and retained, this turbid stasis may result in fever, abdominal pain, and other immediate postpartum conditions or even such long term complications as abdominal masses. Therefore, retention or nondescension of the lochia is an important disease category in Chinese gynecology.

Chinese disease medical categorization

Postpartum retention of the lochia is called *chan hou e lou bu xia*, postpartum lochia does not descend or is not precipitated. Since this disease category may accompany the signs and symptoms of postpartum infection, the reader is referred to the foregoing chapter as well.

Disease causes & disease mechanisms

This disease is mostly caused by qi and blood movement and transportation not taking place smoothly. Such nonsmooth movement and transportation of the qi and blood is, in turn, due to two causes. First, it may be due to emotional stress, frustration, jealousy, and anger causing the qi mechanism to be inhibited. This leads to qi stagnation. Since qi is the commander of the blood, qi stagnation may lead to binding of the blood. In addition, if stress and frustration, anger and jealousy lead to liver qi depression and binding, since the liver network vessels traverse both rib-sides, the chest and rib-sides may become distended and full.

Secondly, external contraction of wind cold evils may take advantage of the relative vacuity of the postpartum woman. This cold may congeal the blood, causing stasis and stagnation. Hence the lochia does not descend, but stasis accumulates within the uterus. In this case, lack of free flow also leads to pain accompanied by lower abdominal distention.

It is also possible in some women for qi and blood dual vacuity to cause lack of lochia. In this case, there simply is not enough blood to provide for a lochia. If qi and blood vacuity recuperates quickly from any injury experienced during delivery, the blood is able to descend. Otherwise it may not.

Patterns common to this condition

Qi stagnation & blood stasis
Qi & blood vacuity weakness

Treatment based on pattern discrimination

Qi stagnation & blood stasis

Main symptoms: The lochia is choppy in flow, meaning it starts and stops, and is scanty in amount. Its color is dark purple with clots. There is lower abdominal aching and pain which dislikes pressure. There is also heart vexation and lack of tranquility, a dark red facial complexion, thin, yellow tongue fur, and a small, weak pulse.

Treatment principles: Regulate the qi and quicken the blood or quicken the blood and transform stasis depending upon the prominence of either qi stagnation or blood stasis

Guiding formulas:

Xiang Ai Xiong Gui Yin (Cyperus, Mugwort, Ligusticum & Dang Gui Drink)
Xiang Fu (Rhizoma Cyperi), 9g
Ai Ye (Folium Artemesiae Argyii), 9g
Dang Gui (Radix Angelicae Sinensis), 9g
Yuan Hu (Rhizoma Corydalis), 9-15g
Chuan Xiong (Radix Ligustici Wallichii), 9-15g

This formula is for more pronounced qi stagnation. Han Bai-ling suggests adding *Wu Yao* (Radix Linderae), *Qing Pi* (Pericarpium Viridis Citri Reticulatae), and *Chuan Lian Zi* (Fructus Toosendan).

Sheng Hua Tang Jia Wei Yi Hao
(Engendering & Transforming Decoction with Added Flavors #1)
Dang Gui (Radix Angelicae Sinensis), 9g
stir-fried *Chuan Xiong* (Radix Ligustici Wallichii), 9-15g

Pao Jiang (blast-fried Rhizoma Zingiberis), 6-9g
mix-fried *Gan Cao* (Radix Glycyrrhizae), 6-9g
Tao Ren (Semen Persicae), 9g
Yi Mu Cao (Herba Leonuri), 9-18g
Wu Ling Zhi (Feces Trogopterori Seu Pteromi), 9g
Pu Huang (Pollen Typhae), 9g
Yan Hu Suo (Rhizoma Corydalis), 9-15g

If there is qi depression with chest and rib-side distention and fullness, add *Xiang Fu* (Rhizoma Cyperi). If wind chill enters the blood aspect or divison with chilly pain in the lower abdomen and white, slimy tongue fur, add *Rou Gui* (Cortex Cinnamomi) and possibly *Zhi Fu Zi* (Radix Lateralis Praeparatus Aconiti Carmichaeli).

Qi & blood vacuity weakness

Main symptoms: The postpartum lochia is scanty in amount and its color is pale. There is no lower abdominal pain or distention, but there is vertigo and blurred vision. The corners of the eyes are dry and scratchy, the skin is not moist, and movement results in sweating. There is fatigue, lack of strength, a somber white facial complexion, a pale, moist tongue, and a vacuous, fine pulse.

Treatment principles: Boost the qi and supplement the blood, assisted by moving stasis

Guiding formulas:

Ba Zhen Tang (Eight Pearls Decoction)
Ren Shen (Radix Ginseng), 3-9g
Bai Zhu (Rhizoma Atractylodis Macrocephalae), 9g
Fu Ling (Poria), 12g
Gan Cao (Radix Glycyrrhizae), 3-9g
Dang Gui (Radix Angelicae Sinensis), 9g
Chuan Xiong (Radix Ligustici Wallichii), 6-9g
Bai Shao (Radix Albus Paeoniae Lactiflorae), 9-12g
Shu Di (cooked Radix Rehmanniae), 12-15g

Wan Mi-zhai recommends this formula for the treatment of spleen-stomach vacuity weakness and bodily, *i.e.*, constitutional, weakness of the central qi. To these standard ingredients, Han Bai-ling suggests adding *Niu Xi* (Radix Achyranthis Bidentatae) to lead these medicinals downward and simultaneously free the flow of the network vessels.

Jia Jian Ba Zhen Tang (Modified Eight Pearls Decoction)
Ren Shen (Radix Ginseng), 3-9g
Bai Zhu (Rhizoma Atractylodis Macrocephalae), 9g
Fu Ling (Poria), 12g
mix-fried *Gan Cao* (Radix Glycyrrhizae), 6-9g
Dang Gui (Radix Angelicae Sinensis), 9g

Chuan Xiong (Radix Ligustici Wallichii), 6-15g
Chi Shao (Radix Rubrus Paeoniae Lactiflorae), 9g
Shu Di (cooked Radix Rehmanniae), 12-15g
Yan Hu Suo (Rhizoma Corydalis), 9-15g
Xiang Fu (Rhizoma Cyperi), 9g
Sheng Jiang (uncooked Rhizoma Zingiberis), 6g
Da Zao (Fructus Jujubae), 3 pieces

This formula is for qi and blood vacuity complicated by qi stagnation and blood stasis.

Acupuncture & moxibustion: For retention of lochia in general, the main points are: *He Gu* (LI 4), *San Yin Jiao* (Sp 6), and *Zhong Ji* (CV 3).

If there is qi stagnation and blood stasis with lower abdominal distention and pain, add *Qu Quan* (Liv 8), *Tai Chong* (Liv 3), *Da Chang Shu* (Bl 25), and *Ci Liao* (Bl 32). For vacuity non-precipitation of the lochia with an ashen white facial color and no blood moving downward, add moxibustion at *Guan Yuan* (CV 4), *Shen Shu* (Bl 23), *Xiao Chang Shu* (Bl 27), and *Ge Shu* (Bl 17) while needling *Zu San Li* (St 36).

Representative case history

The patient was a 26 year-old female who was 10 days postpartum. Her lochia was choppy in flow and scanty in amount. There was abdominal pain which was most severe in the lower abdomen. This was accompanied by dizziness, chest glomus, torpid stomach and scanty intake, thin, white tongue fur, and a deep, fine pulse. Initially after delivery, this patient's pulse had been empty and vacuous. However, due to the contraction of evils, static blood was obstructing and stagnating within her uterus. Therefore, the treatment principles were to move the blood and dispel stasis, warm and free the flow. The medicinals administered consisted of: stir-fried *Jing Jie* (Herba Schizonepetae), 9g, *Chuan Xiong* (Ligustici Wallichii), 3g, *Dang Gui Wei* (Extremitas Radicis Angelicae Sinensis), 6g, processed *Xiang Fu* (Rhizoma Cyperi), 9g, *Rou Gui* (Cortex Cinnamomi), 3g, *Hong Hua* (Flos Carthami), 3g, *Mu Xiang* (Radix Auklandiae), 3g, *Su Mu* (Lignum Sappan), 4.5g, *Ze Lan* (Herba Lycopi), 9g, scorched *Shan Zha* (Fructus Crataegi), 9g, *Qing Pi* (Pericarpium Citri Reticulatae Viride), 4.5g, and *Gan Cao* (Radix Glycyrrhizae), 3g.

On the second visit, the lochia was now freely flowing and the lower abdominal pain had already stopped. The appetite was gradually increasing and the chest glomus had been soothed. However, there was low back pain, dizziness, and fatigue due to postpartum qi and blood dual vacuity with the spleen not fortifying and moving. Thus, in order to boost the qi and harmonize yin, foster and supplement the liver and kidneys, the patent was prescribed: uncooked *Huang Qi* (Radix Astragali), 9g, stir-fried *Bai Zhu* (Rhizoma Atractylodis Macrocephalae), 9g, *Dan Shen* (Radix Salviae Miltiorrhizae), 9g, *Dang Gui* (Radix Angelicae Sinensis), 4.5g, *Chuan Xiong* (Radix Ligustici Wallichii), 2.4g, *Fu Ling* (Poria), 9g, processed *He Shou Wu* (Radix

Polygoni Multiflori), 9g, *Xu Duan* (Radix Dipsaci), 9g, *Du Zhong* (Cortex Eucommiae), 9g, *Chen Pi* (Pericarpium Citri Reticulatae), 4.5g, stir-fried *Gu Ya* (Fructus Germinatus Oryzae) and *Mai Ya* (Fructus Germinatus Hordei), 9g each, *Gan Cao* (Radix Glycyrrhizae), 3g, and *Ze Lan* (Herba Lycopi), 9g.

On the third visit, the patient reported that the lochia had stopped and that her dizziness had gradually gotten better. Her appetite was good, but there was still some low back and knee soreness and limpness. Therefore, in order to regulate and supplement the qi and blood, support the spleen and nourish yin, she was prescribed: *Dang Shen* (Radix Codonopsitis), 9g, stir-fried *Bai Zhu* (Rhizoma Atractylodis Macrocephalae), 6g, *Fu Ling* (Poria), 9g, *Ju Luo* (Retinervus Citri Reticulatae), 4.5g, *Dang Gui* (Radix Angelicae Sinensis), 4.5g, stir-fried *Bai Shao* (Radix Albus Paeoniae Lactiflorae), 4.5g, *Shu Di* (cooked Radix Rehmanniae), 9g, *Chuan Xiong* (Radix Ligustici Wallichii), 2.4g, processed *Xiang Fu* (Rhizoma Cyperi), 9g, *Du Zhong* (Cortex Eucommiae), 9g, and *Gan Cao* (Radix Glycyrrhizae), 3g.

Remarks

In 25 years of clinical experience, I have yet to see a patient with retention of lochia as her major complaint. Because most Western women are not aware of the Chinese medical interpretations of the lochia, when this condition is not associated with a postpartum infection, most women are happy if their lochia is scanty or ends early.

5

Postpartum Lochiorrhea

Lochiorrhea refers to a lochia which continues for more than three weeks. According to modern Western medicine, this condition may be due to endometritis, in which case there is a bright red lochia with an offensive smell, retained products of conception, hypofibrogenemia, and hemorrhage from the placental site due to atonic uterus, prolonged labor, grand multiparity, and relaxant anesthesia. In Western medicine, this condition is subsumed under postpartum hemorrhage and postpartum infection.

Chinese medical disease categorization

This condition is called *chan hou e lou bu jue* or postpartum lochia not cut off or severed in Chinese. It is also called *e lou bu zhi*, incessant lochia, and *e lou bu jin*, lochia without limit.

Disease causes & disease mechanisms

There are three basic causes of lochiorrhea according to Chinese medical theory. The first is qi vacuity. In this case, the qi is not strong enough to assimilate or absorb the blood. This causes dysfunction in the *chong* and *ren's* ability to astringe and consolidate. This is mostly due to profuse hemorrhaging during the third stage of labor, constitutional vacuity weakness, birthing consuming excessive qi, and postpartum taxation fatigue.

Secondly, if static blood halts and is retained in the uterus, this prevents new blood from returning to the channels due to the presence of this unevacuated blood. Such stasis may be due to postpartum contraction of wind cold, in which case, the cold may congeal the blood causing binding and stasis. It may also be due to accumulation due to internal causes.

Third, blood heat may cause the blood to move frenetically outside its pathways. After giving birth, women commonly experience yin vacuity and yang effulgence. The stirring of this heat results in loss of blood. This type of heat is called vacuity heat. However, evil heat causing the blood to move frenetically may also be due to liver depression transforming heat. This is mostly due to emotional stress and frustration. This kind of heat is called depressive heat. Further, postpartum heat may also be due to toxins. This is called evil toxin heat. In this case, blood and toxins mutually bind and transform into heat that forces the blood to move.

Patterns common to this condition

Qi vacuity not containing the blood
Blood stasis
Vacuity heat
Liver depression, blood heat
Attack by heat toxins

Treatment based on pattern discrimination

Qi vacuity not containing the blood

Main symptoms: Lochiorrhea with dribbling and dripping of a scanty, watery, pale, clear discharge, no abdominal distention or pain, slight pain which is not averse to pressure, or a dragging, heavy feeling in the lower abdomen, dizziness, fatigue, sweating on slight movement, disinclination to talk with a weak voice, lack of strength, shortness of breath, lassitude of the spirit, a yellowish white facial complexion, a pale, red, moist tongue, and a vacuous, moderate (*i.e.,* relaxed/retarded, slightly slow), or weak pulse

Treatment principles: Boost the qi, lift the fallen, and stop bleeding

Guiding formulas:

Bu Zhong Yi Qi Tang Jia Wei **(Supplement the Center & Boost the Qi Decoction with Added Flavors) plus** *Huang Qi* **(Radix Astragali)**
Huang Qi (Radix Astragali), 9-45g
Ren Shen (Radix Ginseng), 3-9g
Bai Zhu (Rhizoma Atractylodis Macrocephalae), 9g
mix-fried *Gan Cao* (Radix Glycyrrhizae), 6-9g
Chen Pi (Pericarpium Citri Reticulatae), 6g
Dang Gui (Radix Angelicae Sinensis), 9g
Sheng Ma (Rhizoma Cimicifugae), 3-4.5g
Chai Hu (Radix Bupleuri), 3-9g
Sheng Jiang (uncooked Rhizoma Zingiberis), 6g
Da Zao (Fructus Jujubae), 3 pieces
E Jiao (Gelatinum Corii Asini), 9g
carbonized *Ai Ye* (Herba Artemesiae Argyii), 9g

Ren Shen Yin (Ginseng Beverage)

Ren Shen (Radix Ginseng), 3-9g
Dang Gui (Radix Angelicae Sinensis), 9g
Sheng Di (uncooked Radix Rehmanniae), 12-15g
Di Yu (Radix Sanguisorbae), 9g

This formula supplements the qi, nourishes the blood, clears heat from the blood, and stops bleeding.

Mu Li San (Oyster Shell Powder)

calcined *Mu Li* (Concha Ostreae), 9-18g
Chuan Xiong (Radix Ligustici Wallichii), 6-9g
Shu Di (cooked Radix Rehmanniae), 9-15g
Fu Ling (Poria), 9-12g
Long Gu (Os Draconis), 9-18g
Xu Duan (Radix Dipsaci), 9g
Dang Gui (Radix Angelicae Sinensis), 9g
carbonized *Ai Ye* (Folium Artemesiae Argyii), 9g
Ren Shen (Radix Ginseng), 3-9g
Wu Wei Zi (Fructus Schisandrae), 9g
carbonized *Di Yu* (Radix Sanguisorbae), 9g
Gan Cao (Radix Glycyrrhizae), 3-9g
Sheng Jiang (uncooked Rhizoma Zingiberis), 6g
Da Zao (Fructus Zizyphi Jujubae), 3 pieces

This formula restores securing and astringing at the same time as supplementing the qi and blood.

Sheng Hua Zhu Yu Zhi Xue Tang
(Engendering & Transforming Dispel Stasis & Stop Bleeding Decoction)

Dang Shen (Radix Codonopsitis), 9-18g
Huang Qi (Radix Astragali), 9-45g
Dang Gui (Radix Angelicae Sinensis), 9g
Chuan Xiong (Radix Ligustici Wallichii), 6-9g
Tao Ren (Semen Persicae), 9g
Pao Jiang (blast-fried Rhizoma Zingiberis), 6-9g
uncooked *Gan Cao* (uncooked Radix Glycyrrhizae), 3-6g
uncooked *Pu Huang* (Pollen Typhae), 9g
Wu Ling Zhi (Feces Trogopterori Seu Pteromi), 9g

This formula is a modification of *Sheng Hua Tang* (Engendering & Transforming Decoction) and *Shi Xiao San* (Loose a Smile Powder). It dispels stasis and engenders new (blood), supplements the qi and contains the blood. It is for the treatment of qi and blood vacuity lochiorrhea complicated by postpartum blood stasis.

Acupuncture & moxibustion: *Yin Bai* (Sp 1), *Zu San Li* (St 36), *Pi Shu* (Bl 20), *Bai Hui* (GV 20)

If there is concomitant kidney qi not securing, add *Shen Shu* (Bl 23) and *Guan Yuan* (CV 4).

Blood stasis

Main symptoms: Lochiorrhea which dribbles and drips incessantly but which is scanty in amount and purplish, dark in color and which contains clots, lower abdominal aching and pain which dislikes pressure, a purplish dark tongue or possible static spots or macules, and a bowstring, choppy or deep, forceful pulse

Treatment principles: Quicken the blood and transform stasis

Guiding formulas:

Sheng Hua Tang (Engendering & Transforming Decoction)
Dang Gui (Radix Angelicae Sinensis), 9g
Chuan Xiong (Radix Ligustici Wallichii), 9-15g
Tao Ren (Semen Persicae), 9g
Pao Jiang (blast-fried Rhizoma Zingiberis), 6-9g
mix-fried *Gan Cao* (Radix Glycyrrhizae), 6-9g

This is Fu Qing-zhu's famous postpartum formula for dispersing spoilt blood while at the same time protecting the righteous. If heat is present, delete *Pao Jiang* and add *Zhi Mu* (Rhizoma Anemarrhenae), *Dan Pi* (Cortex Moutan), and *Huang Qin* (Radix Scutellariae). If there are cold limbs, add *Rou Gui* (Cortex Cinnamomi). If there is abdominal pain, add *Wu Yao* (Radix Linderae), *Chuan Lian Zi* (Fructus Toosendanis), and *Yan Hu Suo* (Rhizoma Corydalis). If there is profuse bleeding, add *Ren Shen* (Radix Ginseng), *Huang Qi* (Radix Astragali), and *Zong Lu* (carbonized Petiolus Trachycarpi). These last additions assume that an element of qi vacuity complicates the case.

Chan Hou E Lou Gong Xin Fang
(Postpartum Lochia Attack the Heart Formula)
Yan Hu Suo (Rhizoma Corydalis), 9-18g
Xue Jie (Sanguis Draconis), 3-6g
Mo Yao (Resina Myrrhae), 3-6g
Gui Shen (Radix Angelicae Sinensis), 9g

Gong xin means to attack the heart. Therefore, this formula is for the treatment of lochiorrhea with fever, delirium, raving, and madness.

Suo Gong Zhu Yu Tang (Shrink the Uterus & Dispel Stasis Decoction)
Dang Gui (Radix Angelicae Sinensis), 9g
Chuan Xiong (Radix Ligustici Wallichii), 9-15g
Tao Ren (Semen Persicae), 9g
Pao Jiang (blast-fried Rhizoma Zingiberis), 6-9g
Yi Mu Cao (Herba Leonuri), 9-18g
Zhi Ke (Fructus Aurantii), 6-9g
Liu Ji Nu (Radix Angelicae Anomalae), 9g

scorched *Shan Zha* (Fructus Crataegi), 6-9g
Zao Xiu (Rhizoma Paridis Polyphyllae), 9g
Gan Cao (Radix Glycyrrhizae), 3-9g

If there is qi vacuity, add *Huang Qi* (Radix Astragali). If there is spleen vacuity, add *Dang Shen* (Radix Codonopsitis) and *Bai Zhu* (Rhizoma Atractylodis Macrocephalae). If there is chilly pain in the lower abdomen, add *Wu Yao* (Radix Linderae) and carbonized *Ai Ye* (Folium Artemesiae Argyii). If the lochia is pale in color and thin in consistency, add *Bu Gu Zhi* (Fructus Psoraleae) and *Chi Shi Zhi* (Hallyositum Rubrum). If heat is marked, delete *Pao Jiang* and *Chuan Xiong*. If there is low back pain, add *Du Zhong* (Cortex Eucommiae) and *Xu Duan* (Radix Dipsaci). If the lochia is mixed with yellow water and has a foul odor, add *Huang Bai* (Cortex Phellodendri) and *Yu Xing Cao* (Herba Houttuyniae).

Acupuncture & moxibustion: *Xue Hai* (Sp 10), *San Yin Jiao* (Sp 6), *He Gu* (LI 4)

Vacuity heat

Main symptoms: Enduring lochiorrhea which is scanty in amount and red in color, no odor, a flushed red facial complexion, a dry mouth and parched throat, however, no desire to drink, a red tongue with scanty fur, and a vacuous, surging, or fine, rapid pulse. There may also be other signs of yin vacuity heat, such as dizziness, heart palpitations, night sweats, heat in the hands, feet, and heart, and tinnitus as well as slight lower abdominal pain but no distention.

Treatment principles: Nourish yin and cool the blood, secure the *chong* and stop bleeding

Guiding formulas:

Bao Yin Jian (Protect Yin Decoction)
Sheng Di (uncooked Radix Rehmanniae), 12-15g
Shu Di (cooked Radix Rehmanniae), 12-15g
Bai Shao (Radix Albus Paeoniae Lactiflorae), 9g
Shan Yao (Radix Dioscoreae), 9g
Xu Duan (Radix Dipsaci), 9g
Huang Qin (Radix Scutellariae), 9-12g
Huang Bai (Cortex Phellodendri), 9g
Gan Cao (Radix Glycyrrhizae), 3-9g

Han Bai-ling suggests adding *E Jiao* (Gelatinum Corii Asini) and *Han Lian Cao* (Herba Ecliptae) to more effectively stop bleeding.

Qing Hua Yin (Clearing & Transforming Drink)
Bai Shao (Radix Albus Paeoniae Lactiflorae), 9g
Mai Men Dong (Tuber Ophiopogonis), 9-12g
Fu Ling (Poria), 9-12g
Huang Qin (Radix Scutellariae), 9-12g
Sheng Di (uncooked Radix Rehmanniae), 12-15g

Shi Hu (Herba Dendrobii), 9g

Acupuncture & moxibustion: *San Yin Jiao* (Sp 6), *Guan Yuan* (CV 4), *Tai Xi* (Ki 3)

If there is concomitant qi vacuity, add *Zu San Li* (St 36) and *Pi Shu* (Bl 20). If there is concomitant blood stasis, add *Xue Hai* (Sp 10) and *He Gu* (LI 4).

Liver depression, blood heat

Main symptoms: Lochiorrhea which is either scanty or profuse in amount and which is deep red in color, chest and abdominal distention and fullness, possible rib-side distention and pain, heart vexation, a red facial complexion, a dry mouth with a bitter taste, dizziness and vertigo, easy anger, a red tongue tip, red tongue sides, or inflated sides and thin, possibly yellow fur, and a bowstring, fine, and rapid pulse

Treatment principles: Regulate the liver and resolve depression, clear heat and stop bleeding

Guiding formulas:

***Dan Zhi Xiao Yao San* (Moutan & Gardenia Rambling Powder)**
Dang Gui (Radix Angelicae Sinensis), 9g
Bai Shao (Radix Albus Paeoniae Lactiflorae), 9g
Chai Hu (Radix Bupleuri), 9g
Fu Ling (Poria), 9-12g
Dan Pi (Cortex Moutan), 9g
Zhi Zi (Fructus Gardeniae), 9g
Bai Zhu (Rhizoma Atractylodis Macrocephalae), 9g
Gan Cao (Radix Glycyrrhizae), 3-9g
Bo He (Herba Menthae Haplocalycis), 3-9g

Han Bai-ling suggests adding stir-fried *Di* Yu (Radix Sanguisorbae) and *Huang Qin* (Radix Scutellariae) to further clear heat and stop bleeding.

Unnamed formula by Zhong Li-mei
Dang Gui (Radix Angelicae Sinensis), 9g
Chuan Xiong (Radix Ligustici Wallichii), 9-15g
Hong Teng (Caulis Sargentodoxae), 9-18g
Tao Ren (Semen Persicae), 9g
Shan Yao (Radix Dioscoreae), 9g
Wu Yao (Radix Linderae), 9g
Chai Hu (Radix Bupleuri), 9g

This formula is recorded by Hu Xi-ming. It is for the treatment of lochiorrhea due to depressive heat when complicated by blood stasis. It quickens the blood and transforms stasis as well as clears heat and rectifies the qi.

Acupuncture & moxibustion: *Xing Jian* (Liv 2), *Yang Ling Quan* (GB 34), *San*

Yin Jiao (Sp 6), *Xue Hai* (Sp 10), *Qu Chi* (LI 11)

If there is concomitant spleen qi vacuity, add *Zu San Li* (St 36) and *Pi Shu* (Bl 20).

Attack by heat toxins

Main symptoms: Lochiorrhea which is excessive in amount and purple and dark in color or muddy and turbid with an offensive odor, fever, lancinating lower abdominal pain, a red facial complexion and tongue, and a bowstring, slippery, rapid pulse

Treatment principles: Clear heat and resolve toxins

Guiding formulas:

**Unnamed formula from *A Barefoot Doctor's Manual*
for Acute Postpartum Endometritis**
Jin Yin Hua (Flos Lonicerae), 9-15g
Lian Qiao (Fructus Forsythiae), 9-15g
Hong Teng (Caulis Sargentodoxae), 9-18g
Bai Jiang Cao (Herba Patriniae), 9-18g
Dan Pi (Cortex Moutan), 9g
Chi Shao (Radix Rubrus Paeoniae Lactiflorae), 9g
Yan Hu Suo (Rhizoma Corydalis), 9-15g
Tao Ren (Semen Persicae), 9g
Yi Mu Cao (Herba Leonuri), 9-18g

**Long Dan Xie Gan Tang Jia Wei
(Gentiana Drain the Liver Decoction with Added Flavors)**
Long Dan Cao (Radix Gentianae), 6-9g
Zhi Zi (Fructus Gardeniae), 9g
Huang Qin (Radix Scutellariae), 9-12g
Ze Xie (Rhizoma Alismatis), 6-9g
Che Qian Zi (Semen Plantaginis), 6-9g
Mu Tong (Caulis Akebiae), 6-9g
Sheng Di (uncooked Radix Rehmanniae), 12-15g
Dang Gui Wei (Extremitas Radicis Angelicae Sinensis), 9g
Chai Hu (Radix Bupleuri), 9g
Gan Cao (Radix Glycyrrhizae), 3-6g
Qian Cao (Radix Rubiae), 9g

Hong Jiang Yin (Sargentodixa & Patrinia Drink)
Hong Teng (Caulis Sargentodoxae), 9-18g
Bai Jiang Cao (Herba Patriniae), 9-18g
Bai Hua She She Cao (Herba Hedyotis Diffusae), 9-18g
Guan Zhong (Rhizoma Cyrtomii), 9-15g
carbonized *Pu Huang* (Pollen Typhae), 9g
Dan Pi (Cortex Moutan), 9g
Zhi Zi (Fructus Gardeniae), 6-9g

Jin Yin Hua (Flos Lonicerae), 9-15g
Gu Ya (Fructus Germinatus Oryzae), 15g

If there is qi vacuity and downward falling, add *Dang Shen* (Radix Codonopsitis), *Huang Qi* (Radix Astragali), and *Sheng Ma* (Rhizoma Cimicifugae). If there is kidney vacuity, add *Gou Ji* (Rhizoma Cibotti), *Xu Duan* (Radix Dipsaci), and *Sang Ji Sheng* (Herba Taxilli). If blood stasis is marked, add *Yi Mu Cao* (Herba Leonuri), *Dang Gui* (Radix Angelicae Sinensis), *Chuan Xiong* (Radix Ligustici Wallichii), etc. And if there is qi stagnation, add *Xiang Fu* (Rhizoma Cyperi) and *Mu Xiang* (Radix Auklandiae).

Acupuncture & moxibustion: *Qu Chi* (LI 11), *He Gu* (LI 4), *San Yin Jiao* (Sp 6), *Zhong Ji* (CV 3), *Gui Lai* (St 29)

Representative case histories

Case 1: The patient was a 30 year-old, married female. Her initial examination occurred on December 15, 1977. It was three months since she had given birth and her lochia was still dribbling and dripping incessantly. Its color was a fresh red, and there was low back soreness and insidious pain in the lower abdomen. The patient's pulse was fine, and her tongue fur was thin and slimy. Therefore, this case was categorized as liver-kidney insufficiency with loss of command over securing and containing. Thus treatment was designed to boost the kidneys and secure and contain: *Sang Ji Sheng* (Herba Taxilli), 12g, *Xu Duan* (Radix Dipsaci), 9g, *Gou Ji* (Rhizoma Cibotii), 9g, *Pao Jiang* (blast-fried Rhizoma Zingiberis), 6g, *Xue Yu Tan* (Crinis Carbonisatus), 9g, carbonized *Pu Huang* (Pollen Typhae), 9g, *Xian He Cao* (Herba Agrimoniae), 15g, *Mu Li* (Concha Ostreae), 30g, *Chi Shi Zhi* (Hallyositum Rubrum), 30g, *Xiang Fu* (Rhizoma Cyperi), 9g, *Huang Bai* (Cortex Phellodendri), 9g, and *Gan Cao* (Radix Glycyrrhizae), 5g.

The patient took five packets of the above formula, and the second examination took place on December 20. The lochia had already diminished, but there was still low back soreness. Therefore, four more packets of the original formula were given. The third examination occurred on December 24. The lochia had already stopped and the abdominal pain was also cured, but there was still low back soreness. The pulse was fine. Treatment, therefore, was in order to nourish the blood and regulate and rectify the liver and kidneys: *Dang Gui* (Radix Angelicae Sinensis), 9g, *Shu Di* (cooked Radix Rehmanniae), 9g, *Sang Ji Sheng* (Herba Taxilli), 12g, *Xu Duan* (Radix Dipsaci), 9g, *Gou Ji* (Rhizoma Cibotii), 9g, *Xian He Cao* (Herba Agrimoniae), 15g, *Xian Tao Cao* (Herba Veronicae Peregrinae), 15g, *Mu Li* (Concha Ostreae), 30g, *Huang Bai* (Cortex Phellodendri), 9g, *Hai Piao Xiao* (Os Sepiae Seu Sepiellae), 15g, and *Gan Cao* (Radix Glycyrrhizae), 6g. After taking five packets of this formula, the patient was judged cured.

Case 2: The patient was a 32 year-old, married female. Her initial examination occurred more than 40 days postpartum. Her lochia lingered and was not cut off.

There was lower abdominal glomus and pain, low back and leg soreness and weakness, and torpid intake. Breast milk was not copious, and the stools were not smoothly and easily flowing. She had previously been treated with ingredients to bank and supplement, secure and astringe, but these had not been effective. On examination, her pulse was fine and also choppy. Her tongue edges deep down appeared purplish and dark. Therefore, it was suggested that, postpartum, her qi and blood were vacuous and had suffered detriment. The *chong* and *ren* were not securing, but stasis and stagnation were being retained. Thus the blood was not returning to its channels. Treatment, therefore, was in order to nourish the blood, dispel stasis, and lead the blood to return to the channels: *Dang Gui* (Radix Angelicae Sinensis), 9g, stir-fried *Chuan Xiong* (Radix Ligustici Wallichii), 4.5g, *Dan Shen* (Radix Salviae Miltiorrhizae), 6g, *Dan Pi* (Cortex Moutan), 6g, *Tao Ren* (Semen Persicae), 9g, *Yi Mu Cao* (Herba Leonuri), 9g, *Gua Lou* (Fructus Trichosanthis), 12g, mix-fried *Gan Cao* (Radix Glycyrrhizae), 3g, *Xu Duan* (Radix Dipsaci), 9g, *Niu Xi* (Radix Achyranthis Bidentatae), 9g, *Mu Tong* (Caulis Akebiae), 3g, and *Shi Xiao San* (Loose a Smile Powder), 9g, wrapped.

The patient was prescribed three packets of the above formula. On the second examination, she reported that, after taking two packets of these medicinals, her lochia had changed to flowing smoothly and easily. Her stomach duct and abdomen felt soothed and comfortable. After three packets, her lochia gradually ceased. Her appetite returned, and her spirit was fine. Her breast milk gradually increased, and her pulse became fine and relatively harmonious. Her tongue appeared clear. Therefore, it was appropriate to bank, nourish, harmonize, and rectify in order to restore the health and tranquility: carbonized *Jing Jie* (Herba Schizonepetae), 3g, *Dang Gui* (Radix Angelicae Sinensis), 9g, *Bai Shao* (Radix Albus Paeoniae Lactiflorae), 6g, carbonized *Shu Di* (cooked Radix Rehmanniae), 9g, *Sha Ren* (Fructus Amomi), 3g, *Bai Zhu* (Rhizoma Atractylodis Macrocephalae), 6g, *Chen Pi* (Pericarpium Citri Reticulatae), 6g, *Gou Ji* (Rhizoma Cibotii), 9g, *Sang Ji Sheng* (Herba Taxilli), 9g, *Dang Shen* (Radix Codonopsitis), 9g, and *Hei Zhi Ma* (black Semen Sesami Indici), 9g. After taking four packets of these medicinals, the patient was judged cured.

Remarks

1. Blood stasis does not typically cause lochiorrhea all by itself. However, because bleeding is, *ipso facto*, blood which is no longer moving within its vessels and it is the vessels which move the blood, bleeding is typically complicated by blood stasis if it has endured for any length of time. Therefore, blood stasis commonly complicates other patterns of lochiorrhea.

2. When lochiorrhea is a symptom of endometritis, see Postpartum Infection above for more treatment options.

6

Postpartum Dizziness

After giving birth, some women experience dizziness of the head and blurred vision. In serious cases, they may be unable to stand up or may feel heart and chest fullness and oppression, nausea and vomiting, phlegm surging and qi anxiety, heart vexation and lack of calm. If even more serious, this may manifest as inability to speak, spirit abstraction, and unconsciousness of human affairs. In Western medicine, postpartum dizziness and syncope are mostly seen as the result of postpartum hemorrhage, in which case, dizziness is not considered a disease category in its own right but rather a symptom of the blood loss. However, dizziness may also be a symptom of postpartum hypertension. In that case, it is commonly complicated by headache.

Chinese medical disease categorization

In Chinese, this condition is called *chan hou xue yun* or postpartum blood dizziness.

Disease causes & disease mechanisms

In Chinese medicine, this condition is divided into vacuity and repletion patterns. Vacuity is due to too much yin blood having been lost during labor. Therefore, the heart spirit loses its construction and nourishment. Women who suffer from this scenario are usually constitutionally qi and blood vacuous and weak to begin with. If the constructive and yin are wrested downward, qi will follow blood desertion. Thus it is important to keep in mind that this vacuity is not just blood vacuity but dual qi and blood vacuity.

Repletion is due to upward attack of blood stasis as discussed in preceding chapters. This spoilt blood harasses and causes chaos to the heart spirit. This is called *bai xue chong xin*, spoilt blood penetrating the heart. Some Chinese medical authors emphasize that it is contraction of external cold during birthing that gives rise to this blood stasis and qi counterflow. However, it may also be due to long-standing emotional causes or iatrogenesis.

Patterns common to this condition

Qi follows blood desertion
Blood stasis & qi counterflow

Treatment based on pattern discrimination:

Qi follows blood desertion

Main symptoms: Dizziness and vertigo following postpartum hemorrhage, a somber white facial complexion, heart palpitations, confusion, oppression, and lack of activity, in serious cases, loss of consciousness of human affairs with the eyes shut but the mouth open and counterflow chilling of the four extremities. In this case, cold sweat dribbles and drips. There is a pale tongue with no or dry fur, and the pulse may be faint as if about to be severed; floating, large, and vacuous; or hollow.

Treatment principles: Boost the qi and stem desertion

Guiding formulas:

***Du Shen Tang* (Solitary Ginseng Decoction)**
Ren Shen (Radix Ginseng), 6-18g

Du Jie-hui says to use this formula for postpartum dizziness and excessive vaginal bleeding or lochiorrhea due to vacuity.

***Qing Hun San* (Clear the Ethereal Soul Powder)**
Ren Shen (Radix Ginseng), 3-9g
stir-fried *Jing Jie* (Herba Schizonepetae), 9g
Ze Lan (Herba Lycopi), 9g
Chuan Xiong (Radix Ligustici Wallichii), 9-15g
Gan Cao (Radix Glycyrrhizae), 3-9g

Han Bai-ling suggests adding *Long Gu* (Os Draconis), *Mu Li* (Concha Ostreae), *E Jiao* (Gelatinum Corii Asini), and stir-fried *Di Yu* (Radix Sanguisorbae) to stop bleeding and stem desertion.

***Shen Fu Tang* (Ginseng & Aconite Decoction)**
Ren Shen (Radix Ginseng), 3-9g
Zhi Fu Zi (Radix Lateralis Praeparatus Aconiti Carmichaeli), 3-9g
Sheng Jiang (uncooked Rhizoma Zingiberis), 6g
Da Zao (Fructus Jujubae), 3-5 pieces

This formula is appropriate if cold complicates vacuity desertion. As Du Jie-hui says, counterflow chilling, unstoppable sweating, and a pulse on the verge of severance are all due to great damage to the original qi due to excessive blood loss. Han Bai-ling also suggests adding *Long Gu* (Os Draconis) and *Mu Li* (Concha Ostreae) to this formula to stem desertion. In addition, to help stop bleeding even more, one can also add *Pao Jiang* (blast-fried Rhizoma Zingiberis), carbonized *Ai Ye* (Folium Artemisiae Argyii), and *E Jiao* (Gelatinum Corii Asini).

Blood stasis & qi counterflow

Main symptoms: Nondescension of the lochia or scanty lochia, pain in the front of the lower abdomen which dislikes pressure, feelings of fullness, anxiety, and tension below the heart, spirit abstraction, lack of speech, if serious, lack of consciousness of human affairs, bilateral clenched hands, tightly closed teeth, a purplish, dark facial complexion, purple lips and tongue, and a bowstring, choppy, forceful pulse. In extremely serious cases, the woman may possibly vomit blood clots, and there may be the sound of phlegm rattling in her throat.

Treatment principles: Move the blood and dispel stasis

Guiding formulas:

Duo Ming San Jia Dang Gui Chuan Xiong
(Rescue Life Powder with Dang Gui & Ligusticum)
Mo Yao (Resina Myrrhae), 3-6g
Xue Jie (Sanguis Draconis), 3-6g
Dang Gui (Radix Angelicae Sinensis), 9g
Chuan Xiong (Radix Ligustici Wallichii), 9-15g

Hei Shen San (Black Spirit Powder)
Dang Gui (Radix Angelicae Sinensis), 9g
Chi Shao (Radix Rubrus Paeoniae Lactiflorae), 9g
Shu Di (cooked Radix Rehmanniae), 9-15g
Niu Xi (Radix Achyranthis Bidentatae), 9-12g
Rou Gui (Cortex Cinnamomi), 6-9g
Pu Huang (Pollen Typhae), 9g
Gan Cao (Radix Glycyrrhizae), 3-9g
Hei Dou (Semen Glycinis), 15g

If there is constipation, add *Da Huang* (Radix Et Rhizoma Rhei) to lead the other medicinals downward and to precipitate.

Jia Wei Sheng Hua Tang
(Added Flavors Engendering & Transforming Decoction)
Chuan Xiong (Radix Ligustici Wallichii), 9-15g
Dang Gui (Radix Angelicae Sinensis), 9g
Pao Jiang (blast-fried Rhizoma Zingiberis), 6-9g
Tao Ren (Semen Persicae), 9g
mix-fried *Gan Cao* (Radix Glycyrrhizae), 6-9g
Jing Jie (Herba Schizonepetae), 9g

Qing Shen Fan Hun Tang (Clear the Spirit & Reverse Clouding Decoction)
Chuan Xiong (Radix Ligustici Wallichii), 9-15g
Dang Gui (Radix Angelicae Sinensis), 9g

Tao Ren (Semen Persicae), 9g
Jiang Tan (carbonized Rhizoma Zingiberis), 6-9g
Jing Jie (Herba Schizonepetae), 9g
Ren Shen (Radix Ginseng), 3-9g
Rou Gui (Cortex Cinnamomi), 3-9g

If there is profuse perspiration, add *Huang Qi* (Radix Astragali). If the pulse on both hands is hidden or deep-lying, add *Mai Men Dong* (Tuber Ophiopogonis) and *Wu Wei Zi* (Fructus Schisandrae). If there are clots and pain, remove *Ren Shen* and do not add *Huang Qi* or simply use *Sheng Hua Tang* (Engendering & Transforming Decoction). If there are no clots or pain, add *Ren Shen* and *Huang Qi* and delete *Tao Ren* and *Rou Gui*. This formula, given by Wang Guo-zhu *et al*. is a version of *Sheng Hua Tang*. However, without *Tao Ren* and *Rou Gui* and with *Ren Shen* and *Huang Qi*, it treats postpartum dizziness due to qi and blood vacuity.

Acupuncture & moxibustion: To arouse the spirit, needle *Mei Xin* (M-HN-3), *Ren Zhong* (GV 26), *Yong Quan* (Ki 1). If there is blood stasis and heat, bleed *Shi Xuan* (M-UE-1). If there is vacuity, moxa *Bai Hui* (GV 20).

Another standard acupuncture protocol uses *Ren Zhong* (GV 26), *Bai Hui* (GV 20), *Nei Guan* (Per 6), *San Yin Jiao* (Sp 6), and *Qi Hai* (CV 6) as the main points. If there is postpartum lochiorrhea, add moxa at *Yin Bai* (Sp 1). If the heart is confused and flustered and the patient has lost control, add *Shen Men* (Ht 7). If there is chilly sweat dribbling and dripping, add *Fu Liu* (Ki 7) and *He Gu* (LI 4). If the limbs are cold and there is dizziness inversion, add moxa at *Guan Yuan* (CV 4) and *Shen Que* (CV 7) and needle *Yin Tang* (M-HN-3).

Representative case histories

Case 1: The patient was a 28 year-old female who was initially examined on April 11, 1960. This patient had given birth normally. However, after delivery, her postpartum lochia was very profuse. The patient's facial complexion was somber white and there was dizziness, heart palpitations, nausea, chest oppression, chilly sweat, and reversal chilling of the four extremities. Gradually, the woman became unconscious with a blood pressure of 60/40mmHg. The woman was given intravenous fluids and oxytoxcin to shrink the uterus and stop the bleeding. However, her condition did not improve. Her pulse was faint and fine and her tongue was pale red. This was a case of postpartum blood flooding. Therefore, she was prescribed *Du Shen Tang* (Solitary Ginseng Decoction): *Ren Shen* (Radix Ginseng), 9g. This succeeded in arousing the patient, and, secondarily, she was administered *Jia Wei Dang Gui Tang* (Added Flavors Dang Gui Decoction): *Dang Gui* (Radix Angelicae Sinensis), 21g, *Huang Qi* (Radix Astragali), 30g, *Lu Rong* (Cornu Parvum Cervi), 1.5g, *Sheng Jiang* (uncooked Rhizoma Zingiberis), 3 slices, and *Da Zao* (Fructus Jujubae), 12g. After this, the patient was judged cured.

Case 2: The patient was a 36 year-old female who had had hypertension during her pregnancy. After delivery, her blood pressure had continued to be 24-26.7kPa/16-18.7kPa for the last five days. In addition, there was headache, dizziness, low back soreness, lack of strength, superficial edema of the face and limbs, a dark tongue with white fur, and a deep, fine, bowstring pulse. Based on these signs and symptoms, the patient's pattern was discriminated as ascendant liver yang hyperactivity with spleen loss of fortification and movement. Therefore, she was prescribed the following medicinals: *Chai Hu Yi Guan Jian* (Bupleurum One Link Decoction) plus *Niu Xi* (Radix Achyranthis Bidentatae) and *Che Qian Zi* (Semen Plantaginis), 15g each, *Mu Li* (Concha Ostreae) and *Shi Jue Ming* (Concha Haliotidis), 30g each, *Gou Teng* (Ramulus Uncariae Cum Uncis), 12g, and *Jiang Can* (Bombyx Batryticatus), 9g. After taking 10 packets of this formula, the headache and dizziness were markedly decreased. However, the patient still felt lack of strength and still had a slight degree of lower extremity superficial edema. Her blood pressure was 21.3/12.3kPa. She stopped taking Western medicines and, after one month of regulating treatment, all her symptoms were leveled.

7

Postpartum Convulsions

Postpartum convulsions and seizures are a progression from the preceding disease categories. Like numerous other Chinese medical postpartum conditions, convulsions and seizures are seen in Western medicine as symptoms of some other disease.

Chinese medical disease categorization

Postpartum spasm and twitching of the four limbs, opisthotonus, and, if severe, lockjaw, are called *chan hou fa jing*, postpartum tetany, *chan hou jing zheng*, postpartum tetanic disorder, or *chan hou zhong feng*, postpartum windstroke.

Disease causes & disease mechanisms

If, during delivery, blood loss is excessive or, due to prolonged and excessive labor, there is excessive sweating, the constructive and blood may become greatly vacuous, and this may lead to liver channel blood vacuity. Since liver blood is responsible for moistening and nourishing the sinews, the sinews and vessels may lose this moistening, causing them to contract. In addition, this blood vacuity may give rise to internal stirring of liver wind.

Likewise, if there is excessive sweating during labor, the muscles and skin may become empty and slack. The interstices are then not dense or tightly packed. This leaves room for wind evils to take advantage of vacuity and enter. Once within the body, these wind evils damage and move within the blood vessels, thus causing twitching and involuntary movement.

Patterns common to this condition

Yin-blood vacuity depletion
Infection by evil toxins

Treatment based on pattern discrimination

Yin-blood vacuity depletion

Main symptoms: Postpartum convulsions, opisthotonus, lockjaw, spasticity of the four limbs, counterflow reversal of the hands and feet, a somber white or sallow yellow facial complexion, closed and/or moving mouth and eyes, a pale red tongue with no fur, and either a fine, forceless, bowstring, fine, or vacuous, scattered pulse

Treatment principles: Enrich yin and nourish the blood, soothe the liver and extinguish wind

Guiding formulas:

San Jia Fu Mai Tang Jia Wei
(Three Shells Restore the Pulse Decoction with Added Flavors)
Bai Shao (Radix Albus Paeoniae Lactiflorae), 9-18g
E Jiao (Gelatinum Corii Asini), 9g
Gui Ban (Plastrum Testudinis), 12-15g
Bie Jia (Carapax Amydae Sinensis), 9g
Mu Li (Concha Ostreae), 9-18g
Mai Men Dong (Tuber Ophiopogonis), 9-12g
Shu Di (cooked Radix Rehmanniae), 12-15g
mix-fried *Gan Cao* (Radix Glycyrrhizae), 6-9g
Shi Chang Pu (Rhizoma Acori Tatarinowii), 6-9g
Tian Ma (Rhizoma Gastrodiae), 9g
Gou Teng (Ramulus Uncariae Cum Uncis), 9-15g
Huo Ma Ren (Semen Cannabis), 9-15g

Shi Quan Da Bu Tang Jia Fu Zi (Ten [Ingredients] Completely & Greatly Supplementing Decoction plus Aconite)
Huang Qi (Radix Astragali), 9-18g
Ren Shen (Radix Ginseng), 3-9g
Bai Zhu (Rhizoma Atractylodis Macrocephalae), 9g
Fu Ling (Poria), 12g
mix-fried *Gan Cao* (Radix Glycyrrhizae), 6-9g
Shu Di (cooked Radix Rehmanniae), 12-15g
Dang Gui (Radix Angelicae Sinensis), 9g
Bai Shao (Radix Albus Paeoniae Lactiflorae), 9g
Chuan Xiong (Radix Ligustici Wallichii), 6-9g
Zhi Fu Zi (Radix Lateralis Praeparatus Aconiti Carmichaeli), 3-9g
Rou Gui (Cortex Cinnamomi), 3-9g
Sheng Jiang (uncooked Rhizoma Zingiberis), 6g
Da Zao (Fructus Jujubae), 3 pieces

This formula is for vacuity convulsions with chilling of the four limbs and a somber white facial complexion. If there is lack of chill, delete *Zhi Fu Zi* and *Rou Gui*.

Zi Rong Huo Xue Tang
(Enrich the Constructive & Quicken the Blood Decoction)
Chuan Xiong (Radix Ligustici Wallichii), 9-15g
Dang Gui (Radix Angelicae Sinensis), 9g
Shu Di (cooked Radix Rehmanniae), 12-15g
Ren Shen (Radix Ginseng), 3-9g
Huang Qi (Radix Astragali), 9-18g
Fu Ling (Poria), 9-12g
Tian Ma (Rhizoma Gastrodiae), 9g
mix-fried *Gan Cao* (Radix Glycyrrhizae), 6-9g
Chen Pi (Pericarpium Citri Reticulatae), 6g
Jing Jie (Herba Schizonepetae), 9g
Fang Feng (Radix Sapshnikoviae), 9g
Qiang Huo (Radix Et Rhizoma Notopterygii), 9g
Huang Lian (Rhizoma Coptidis), 3-6g

This formula is for qi and blood vacuity complicated by qi stagnation and blood stasis as well as an element of depressive heat.

Acupuncture & moxibustion: *Bai Hui* (GV 20), *Feng Fu* (GV 16), *Da Zhui* (GV 14), *Qu Chi* (LI 11), *Tai Chong* (Liv 3), *Yong Quan* (Ki 1), *San Yin Jiao* (Sp 6)

If there is lockjaw, add *Jia Che* (St 6) and *Zhi Gou* (TB 6). If there are tremors of the upper limbs, add *Da Dun* (Liv 1) and *He Gu* (LI 4). If there are tremors of the lower limbs, add *Yang Ling Quan* (GB 34) and *Cheng Shan* (Bl 57).

Infection by evil toxins

Main symptoms: Immediately after giving birth, headache, soreness and pain in the joints, fear of cold, tightly shut teeth, twitching of the corners of the mouth, upward staring, tetany, opisthotonus, a normally colored tongue with thin, white fur, and a floating, bowstring pulse

Treatment principles: Resolve toxins and soothe convulsions, regulate the blood and expel wind

Guiding formulas:

Dang Gui San Jia Jian (Dang Gui Powder with Additions & Subtractions)
Dang Gui (Radix Angelicae Sinensis), 9g
Jing Jie (Herba Schizonepetae), 9g
Chan Tui (Periostracum Cicadae), 9g
Jiang Can (Bombyx Batryticatus), 9g
Gan Cao (Radix Glycyrrhizae), 3-9g
Sheng Jiang (uncooked Rhizoma Zingiberis), 6g
Da Zao (Fructus Jujubae), 3 pieces

If there is wind mixed with evil toxins, add *Quan Xie* (Scorpio) and *Wu Gong* (Scolopendra). If wind evils have transformed heat, add *Da Huang* (Radix Et

Rhizoma Rhei) and *Bai Jiang Cao* (Herba Patriniae). If there is profuse phlegm due to wind evils mixed with phlegm, add *Ban Xia* (Rhizoma Pinelliae), *Tian Ma* (Rhizoma Gastrodiae), and *Nan Xing* (Rhizoma Arisaematis). If phlegm depression has transformed heat, add *Shi Chang Pu* (Rhizoma Acori Tatarinowii), bile-processed *Dan Nan Xing* (Rhizoma Arisaematis), and *Zhu Li* (Succus Bambusae).

Acupuncture & moxibustion: *Ren Zhong* (GV 26), *Shen Ting* (GV 24), *Qu Ze* (Per 3), *Lao Gong* (Per 8), *Wei Zhong* (Bl 40), *Xing Jian* (Liv 2), *Shi Xuan* (M-UE-1-5)

If heat is exuberant, add *Da Zhui* (GV 14). If the spirit is clouded [*i.e.*, if there is dizziness and fainting], add *Shen Men* (Ht 7).

Representative case histories

Case 1: The patient was a 38 year-old female who had developed fever, spirit clouding, tugging and slackening of the four limbs (*i.e.*, spasms or tremors), spontaneous perspiration, oral thirst, a red tongue, and a fine, rapid pulse. This condition was diagnosed as being due to a wind heat external contraction. Therefore, the patient was prescribed two packets of the following formula: *Sang Ye* (Folium Mori), 9g, *Shi Chang Pu* (Rhizoma Acori Tatarinowii), 6g, *Lian Qiao* (Fructus Forsythiae), 12g, *Huang Qin* (Radix Scutellariae), 15g, *Ju Hua* (Flos Chrysanthemi), 9g, *Gou Teng* (Ramulus Uncariae Cum Uncis), 12g, *Mai Men Dong* (Tuber Ophiopogonis), 12g, *Fu Ling* (Poria), 15g, *Bai Zhu* (Rhizoma Atractylodis Macrocephalae), 12g, and uncooked *Long Chi* (Dens Draconis), 15g.

After taking these two packets, the patient's fever had resolved and her perspiration had lessend. There was still slight tugging and slackening of the four limbs, but the mind had turned clear. The tongue was now pale red, and the pulse was fine. This was diagnosed as blood vacuity not nourishing the sinews with stirring of internal wind. Thus the patient was prescribed five packets of the following medicinals: *Dang Gui* (Radix Angelicae Sinensis), 12g, *Gan Cao* (Radix Glycyrrhizae), 6g, *Gou Teng* (Ramulus Uncariae Cum Uncis), 15g, *Chuan Xiong* (Radix Ligustici Wallichii), 9g, *Bai Shao* (Radix Albus Paeoniae Lactiflorae), 12g, and uncooked *Long Chi* (Dens Draconis), 15g.

At the third examination, the slight tugging and slackening had still not stopped. There was profuse phlegm, a red facial complexion, and dry lips. The patient's tongue fur was yellow and slimy, and her pulse was fine and slippery. This was diagnosed as lung-stomach phlegm heat, and the patient was prescribed two packets of: *Huang Qin* (Radix Scutellariae), 15g, *Bai Shao* (Radix Albus Paeoniae Lactiflorae), 12g, *Dan Nan Xing* (bile-processed Rhizoma Arisaematis), 12g, *Ju Hua* (Flos Chrysanthemi), 9g, *Zhu Ru* (Caulis Bambusae In Taeniis), 12g, *Shi Hu* (Herba Dendrobii), 12g, *Yuan Zhi* (Radix Polygalae), 9g, *Sang Ye* (Folium Mori), 12g, *Gou Teng* (Ramulus Uncariae Cum Uncis), 15g, uncooked *Mu Li* (Concha Ostreae), 15g.

On the fourth visit, the patient reported that the tugging and slackening had stopped and her perspiration was less. Her mouth was dry and she desired to drink. There were heart palpitations and restless sleep, a crimson red tongue, and a fine, rapid pulse. Now the patient was deemed to be presenting yin-blood insufficiency with heart spirit loss of nourishment. Therefore, she was prescribed three packets of medicinals to nourish the heart and clear heat: *Huang Qin* (Radix Scutellariae), 15g, *Wu Wei Zi* (Fructus Schisandrae), 4.5g, *Bai Zi Ren* (Semen Platycladi), 9g, lime-processed *Ban Xia* (Rhizoma Pinelliae), 12g, *Mai Men Dong* (Tuber Ophiopogonis), 15g, *Suan Zao Ren* (Semen Zizyphi Spinosae), 12g, *Gan Cao* (Radix Glycyrrhizae), 6g, *Zhu Ru* (Caulis Bambusae In Taeniis), 9g, *Sheng Di* (uncooked Radix Rehmanniae), 15g, *Long Gu* (Os Draconis), 15g, and *Mu Li* (Concha Ostreae), 9g. After this, the patient was judged cured.

Case 2: The patient was a 24 year-old female who was three days postpartum. The patient had a fever of 40° C, and there was aversion to cold, a stuffed nose, heat in her hands, feet, and heart, vexation and agitation, restlessness, and perspiration. She had been treated with antibiotics, but these had not improved her situation. Her skin was burning hot to the touch, her mind was confused, and her limbs were stiff. The woman's abdomen was distended and her breathing was rapid. Her facial complexion was flushed red, her tongue was red and dry with yellow fur, and her pulse was floating, bowstring, and rapid.

Based on the above signs and symptoms, the patient's pattern was categorized as postpartum qi and blood vacuity with insecurity of defensive yang which had allowed for attack by wind cold evils. Evil heat had become blocked internally which had consumed and damaged yin fluids, with extreme heat engendering wind and heat harassing the spirit brilliance. Therefore, the patient was prescribed: wine stir-fried *Bai Shao* (Radix Albus Paeoniae Lactiflorae), 20g, *Dang Gui* (Radix Angelicae Sinensis), *Xiang Fu* (Rhizoma Cyperi), *Gou Teng* (Ramulus Uncariae Cum Uncis), and wine stir-fried *Huang Qin* (Radix Scutellariae), 15g each, *Qiang Huo* (Radix Et Rhizoma Notopterygii), *Du Huo* (Radix Angelicae Pubescentis), *Xuan Shen* (Radix Scrophulariae), *Gui Zhi* (Ramulus Cinnamomi), *Quan Xie* (Scorpio), 10g each, *Hong Hua* (Flos Carthami), 6g. One packet was decocted in water along with the addition of rice wine. During the afternoon at 2 PM, she took the first dose of these medicines and had begun to sweat slightly from her head and body, after which her temperature fell. At 9 PM, the patient took another packet of these medicinals, after which she had had a bowel movement which was profuse. After that, her mind gradually cleared and all her symptoms decreased. The next day she took another packet of this formula in two divided doses, morning and evening, after which her temperature was normal, her limbs were no longer stiff, and all her symptoms were healed.

Case 3: The patient was a 26 year-old female who was initially examined on Aug. 10, 1979 complaining of dizziness, torpor, dimming of consciousness, and tugging and slackening or spasms and contractions. The patient had given birth to twins in December of 1978. At the time of birth, she had lost a lot of blood.

Seventeen days after delivery, she had developed dizziness and blurred vision which eventually evolved into spirit dimming and spasms of the four limbs during which her eyes stared upward and she vomited white foam. It was now 10 days after the first occurrence of these seizures. After arousing from a seizure, the patient's thinking was slow and dulled and she was filled with sorrow. She did not want to see other people. The woman was examined in a psychiatry-neurology department where she had been diagnosed as suffering from epilepsy. She had then be administered antiepileptic medications with only slight improvement. However, if she stopped these drugs, the seizures recurred. At the time of her Chinese medical consultation, her facial complexion was somber white and lusterless, she could not follow a conversation, her tongue was emaciated and pale with thin, white fur, and her pulse was fine, soft, and forceless.

Based on these signs and symptoms, the patient was diagnosed with postpartum epilepsy, and her pattern was categorized as kidney depletion scanty marrow and blood vacuity stirring wind. In order to enrich the kidneys and nourish the liver, extinguish wind and open the orifices, she was prescribed: *Shu Di* (cooked Radix Rehmanniae), *Bai Shao* (Radix Albus Paeoniae Lactiflorae), and *Gou Qi Zi* (Fructus Lycii), 15g each, *Lu Jiao Jiao* (Gelatinum Cornu Cervi), 10g, *Dang Gui* (Radix Angelicae Sinensis), 12g, *Shi Chang Pu* (Rhizoma Acori Tatarinowii) and *Yu Jin* (Tuber Curcumae), 6g each, *Bai Zhu* (Rhizoma Atractylodis Macrocephalae), 9g, *Rou Gui* (Cortex Cinnamomi) and *Ling Yang Jiao* (Cornu Antelopis Saiga-tatarici), 3g each.

After two weeks of taking these medicinals, all the patient's symptoms were markedly improved. However, she had still had two small seizures. Therefore, 10 grams of *Chen Pi* (Pericarpium Citri Reticulatae) were added to the above formula and another 10 packets were prescribed. After taking these medicinals, the patient's epilepsy was eliminated and her mind was again normal. In order to secure and consolidate the treatment results, the patient was advised to alternate *Jin Gui Shen Qi Wan* (*Golden Cabinet* Kidney Qi Pills) with *Liu Wei Di Huang Wan* (Six Flavors Rehmannia Pills). On follow-up after several years, there had been no recurrence.

8

Postpartum
Uterine Prolapse

Postpartum uterine prolapse refers to prolapse and protrusion of the uterus from the vaginal meatus after giving birth. It is a condition which primarily occurs in multiparas. Some Chinese gynecology books discuss this as a miscellaneous disease. However, when it occurs directly after and due to giving birth, it is rightly discussed as a postpartum condition. In Western medicine, it is also called inverted uterus if the corpus of the uterus turns inside out and emerges through the cervix and into the vagina or beyond the introitus. In the West, this condition most commonly occurs when too much pressure is applied to the fundus of the uterus or when too much traction is applied to the cord of a retained placenta. It is typically treated in the West by manually pushing the body of the uterus up into the vaginal canal. In a few cases, a ring may need to be surgically implanted between the uterosacral ligaments in order to hold the uterus in place.

Chinese medical disease categorization

This condition is referred to as *chan hou zi gong tuo chu*, postpartum uterine escaping and exiting, in Chinese.

Disease causes & disease mechanisms

If a woman is chronically vacuous and depleted and, during birthing, she uses greatly excessive force, this may cause the uterus to prolapse out of the vaginal meatus and it may not be able to withdraw itself. Mostly this is due to spleen or central qi failing to hold up the viscera and bowels, the uterus being one of the extraordinary bowels. However, such spleen vacuity may also be complicated by kidney vacuity, in which case there is spleen-kidney dual vacuity.

Treatment based on pattern discrimination

Central qi downward falling

Main symptoms: Chronic vacuity weakness, a history of excessive force being used in labor, fatigue, dizziness on standing up, shortness of breath, disinclination to speak and a feeble voice, lack of appetite, a pale tongue with possible teeth-marks on its edges and thin, white fur, and a weak, small; weak, fine; or weak, short pulse

Treatment principles: Supplement the center, boost the qi, and lift the fallen

Guiding formulas:

Bu Zhong Yi Qi Tang Jia Zhi Ke
(Supplement the Center & Boost the Qi plus Aurantium)
Ren Shen (Radix Ginseng), 3-9g
Huang Qi (Radix Astragali), 9-18g
Bai Zhu (Rhizoma Atractylodis Macrocephalae), 9g
mix-fried *Gan Cao* (Radix Glycyrrhizae), 6-9g
Dang Gui (Radix Angelicae Sinensis), 9g
Chen Pi (Pericarpium Citri Reticulatae), 6g
Sheng Ma (Radix Cimicifugae), 3-4.5g
Chai Hu (Radix Bupleuri), 3-9g
Zhi Ke (Fructus Aurantii), 6g

Bu Zhong Yi Qi Tang Jia Jian (Supplement the Center &
Boost the Qi Decoction with Additions & Subtractions)
Dang Shen (Radix Codonopsitis), 9-18g
Huang Qi (Radix Astragali), 9-18g
Sheng Ma (Rhizoma Cimicifugae), 3-4.5g
Bai Zhu (Rhizoma Atractylodis Macrocephalae), 9g
Huang Jing (Rhizoma Polygonati), 9-12g
Gui Ban (Plastrum Testudinis), 12-15g
Zhi Ke (Fructus Aurantii), 6g
Ba Ji Tian (Radix Morindae), 9g
Dang Gui (Radix Angelicae Sinensis), 9g
Yi Mu Cao (Herba Leonuri), 9-18g

This formula is for the treatment of a spleen-kidney dual vacuity possibly complicated by blood stasis.

External therapy: Wash the protruding section of the uterus with a decoction made from *Zhi Ke* (Fructus Aurantii), *He Zi* (Fructus Terminaliae), *Wu Wei Zi* (Fructus Schisandrae), and *Bai Fan* (Alumen) or take a sit bath in a decoction of *Zhi Ke* (Fructus Aurantii) and *Yi Mu Cao* (Herba Leonuri) daily.

Acupuncture & moxibustion: Moxa *Bai Hui* (GV 20). If that is insufficient, then needle *Guan Yuan* (CV 4), *Qi Hai* (CV 6), *Da He* (Ki 12), *Wei Dao* (GB 28), *Zhao Hai* (Ki 6), and *Tai Chong* (Liv 3).

Remarks

According to Yu Jin, 15 of 20 women with mild to moderate uterine prolapse were cured and the other five experienced improvement when treated with *Bu Zhong Yi Qi Tang Jia Jian* and external therapy as described above.[1]

Endnote:

[1] Yu Jin, *Handbook of Obstetrics & Gynecology in Chinese Medicine: An Integrated Approach*, trans. by Chris Hakim, Eastland Press, Seattle, 1998, p.159

9

Postpartum Aphonia

Postpartum aphonia or lack of voice is related to the previous disease categories of postpartum convulsions and postpartum dizziness. It refers to loss of voice or speech due to mental confusion and loss of consciousness. However, it can also cover postpartum laryngitis and hoarseness.

Chinese medical disease categorization

In Chinese, this condition is referred to as *chan hou bu yu*, postpartum lack of speech.

Disease causes & disease mechanisms

This condition is due to three basic causes. First, if spoilt blood remains in the uterus and stagnates and accumulates, it may penetrate upward to the heart. There, blood stasis may obstruct the orifices of the heart. Because heart qi flows to the tongue, if heart qi is blocked, this may lead to the tongue orifice not being able to utter speech.

Secondly, if excessive blood has been lost during labor, heart blood may be vacuous. Again, since the tongue is the sprout or bud of the heart, heart blood vacuity may fail to nourish the tongue and this may cause withering, shrinkage, rolling up, and shortening of the tongue, with speech being unable exit.

Third, phlegm heat may take advantage of the tendency of qi to counterflow upward after delivery. For the 10 lunar months of pregnancy, the heart has sent down qi and blood to the fetus in the uterus. After delivery, the yin substance of the fetus no longer anchors and attracts this qi. Therefore, if phlegm and heat have been engendered during pregnancy, this can float or counterflow upward, thus also blocking the orifices of the heart and impeding clear speech, not to mention clear consciousness.

Patterns common to this condition

Spoilt blood penetrating the heart
Qi & blood dual vacuity
Phlegm heat obstructing the heart

Treatment based on pattern discrimination

Spoilt blood penetrating the heart

Main symptoms: Postpartum retention of the lochia or scanty lochia, a confused spirit with muddled speech or, in serious cases, delirium and madness with deranged or lack of speech, possible lower abdominal or heart pain, a purple, dark facial complexion, purple lips and tongue or static spots or macules on the tongue, and a bowstring, choppy, forceful pulse

Treatment principles: Quicken the blood and dispel stasis assisted by disinhibiting the tongue

Guiding formula:

***Qi Zhen San* (Seven [Ingredients] Settling Powder)**
Ren Shen (Radix Ginseng), 3-9g
Shi Chang Pu (Rhizoma Acori Tatarinowii), 6-9g
Sheng Di (uncooked Radix Rehmanniae), 12-15g
Chuan Xiong (Radix Ligustici Wallichii), 9g
Xi Xin (Herba Asari), 3-6g
Fang Feng (Radix Sapshnikoviae), 9g
Hu Po (Succinum), 3-6g

Because *Xi Xin* contains aristolochic acid, either it should be omitted from this formula or only prescribed for a day or two. Prior to knowing about aristolochic acid, I prescribed *Xi Xin* to many patients and even took it myself without any apparent damage to the kidneys. However, in the present legal climate, continued use of the medicinal is risky.

Qi & blood dual vacuity

Main symptoms: Weak or faint speech, a hoarse voice due to a pasty, dry mouth and throat, a pale tongue with thin, white, dry fur, and a fine, weak pulse. In serious cases of heart qi and blood vacuity, lack of speech may accompany loss of consciousness or the speech may be confused and muddled. If lung yin is vacuous but heart qi is relatively OK, the tongue will be red with dry or scanty fur and the pulse fine, floating, and possibly rapid.

Treatment principles: Supplement the heart and nourish the blood assisted by disinhibiting the tongue

Guiding formulas:

Ba Zhen Tang (Eight Pearls Decoction)
Ren Shen (Radix Ginseng), 3-9g
mix-fried *Gan Cao* (Radix Glycyrrhizae), 6-9g
Bai Zhu (Rhizoma Atractylodis Macrocephalae), 9g
Fu Ling (Poria), 9-12g
Dang Gui (Radix Angelicae Sinensis), 9g
Bai Shao Yao (Radix Albus Paeoniae Lactiflorae), 9g
Shu Di (cooked Radix Rehmanniae), 12-15g
Chuan Xiong (Radix Ligustici Wallichii), 6-9g

Huang Fu-zhong of the Ming dynasty recommends this formula for postpartum aphonia. He says it is for spoilt blood blocking the heart qi and causing the tongue to be stiff and unable to speak. Although he does not discuss vacuity, this formula is one of the most famous qi and blood supplementing formulas in Chinese medicine. However, it should be noted that both *Dang Gui* and *Chuan Xiong* have blood-quickening and stasis-transforming properties. If, in addition, heart qi is boosted, it can overcome stasis and nourish the tongue, enabling it to speak. Add *Gou Teng* (Ramulus Uncariae Cum Uncis), *Shi Chang Pu* (Rhizoma Acori Tatarinowii), and *Yuan Zhi* (Radix Polygalae) if there is dizziness, convulsions, and syncope.

Jia Wei Sheng Mai San (Added Flavors Engender the Pulse Powder)
Ren Shen (Radix Ginseng), 3-9g
Mai Men Dong (Tuber Ophiopogonis), 9-12g
Wu Wei Zi (Fructus Schisandrae), 9g
Dang Gui (Radix Angelicae Sinensis), 9g
Shu Di (cooked Radix Rehmanniae), 12-15g
mix-fried *Gan Cao* (Radix Glycyrrhizae), 6-9g
Shi Chang Pu (Rhizoma Acori Tatarinowii), 6-9g
Zhu Xin (pig heart), 1 piece

This formula is for chronic postpartum hoarseness and laryngitis due to lung yin-heart qi and blood vacuity. The pig's heart can be omitted. In that case, one can simply make with beef broth.

Phlegm heat obstructing the heart

Main symptoms: Dizziness and unconsciousness with loss of speech and a gurgling sound of phlegm rattling in the throat, a red tongue with yellow, slimy fur, and a slippery, bowstring, rapid pulse

Treatment principles: Clear heat, transform phlegm, and disinhibit the tongue

Guiding formula:

Er Chen Tang Jia Wei
(Two Aged [Ingredients] Decoction with Added Flavors)
Ban Xia (Rhizoma Pinelliae), 9g
Fu Ling (Poria), 12g
Chen Pi (Pericarpium Citri Reticulatae), 6-9g
Gan Cao (Radix Glycyrrhizae), 3-9g
Dan Nan Xing (bile-processed Rhizoma Arisaematis), 6-9g
Huang Lian (Rhizoma Coptidis), 3-9g

10

Postpartum
Rib-Side Pain

Flank or rib-side pain is not considered a common postpartum condition in modern Western medicine. However, rib-side pain is a common symptom associated with stress, and many women are more than usually stressed postpartum. It is also possible for postpartum thrombosis to cause an embolism in the lungs resulting in pluritic pain in the flank. In modern Western medicine, minor pulmonary emboli are treated by heparinisation.

Chinese medical disease categorization

Rib-side pain in postpartum women which causes inability to twist or rotate the trunk is called *chan hou xie tong*, postpartum rib-side pain.

Disease causes & disease mechanisms

Postpartum rib-side pain is mostly caused by emotional agitation, excessive anger, and unresolved depression which cause the liver to lose control over coursing and discharge. Thus the vessels and network vessels lose their free flow and liver qi may counterflow transversely into the intercostal spaces. Qi stagnates and eventually the blood becomes static.

However, some postpartum women's rib-side pain is due to loss of blood and fluids during birthing. The blood and essence share a common source as do the liver and kidneys. Therefore, if there is kidney yin vacuity postpartum, the liver may lose its nourishment. Since the liver governs the rib-side, this may give rise to malnourishment and contraction of the sinews in the intercostal spaces. In this case, it is said that water fails to irrigate wood.

Patterns common to this condition

Liver depression qi stagnation
Liver channel blood stasis
Kidney water insufficiency

Treatment based on pattern discrimination

Liver depression qi stagnation

Main symptoms: Postpartum rib-side distention and pain, burping and belching or hiccup, a tendency towards excessive anger and vertigo, a non-freely flowing or scanty lochia with a deep red color, a purplish, dark facial complexion, yellow, parched tongue fur, and a bowstring, tense, forceful pulse

Treatment principles: Regulate the liver, rectify the qi, and free the flow of the network vessels

Guiding formulas:

Xiao Yao San Jia Wei (Rambling Powder with Added Flavors)
Chai Hu (Radix Bupleuri), 9g
Bai Zhu (Rhizoma Atractylodis Macrocephalae), 9g
Fu Ling (Poria), 9-12g
Gan Cao (Radix Glycyrrhizae), 3-9g
Dang Gui (Radix Angelicae Sinensis), 9g
Bai Shao (Radix Albus Paeoniae Lactiflorae), 9-18g
Bo He (Herba Menthae Haplocalycis), 3-6g
Sheng Jiang (uncooked Rhizoma Zingiberis), 6g
Niu Xi (Radix Achyranthis Bidentatae), 9-12g
Qing Pi (Pericarpium Citri Reticulatae Viride), 6g
Yu Jin (Tuber Curcumae), 9g

Si Wu Tang Jia Shen Zhu Chai Hu
(Four Materials Decoction plus Ginseng, Atractylodes & Bupleurum)
Dang Gui (Radix Angelicae Sinensis), 9g
Bai Shao (Radix Albus Paeoniae Lactiflorae), 9-18g
Shu Di (cooked Radix Rehmanniae), 12g
Chuan Xiong (Rhizoma Ligustici Wallichii), 9g
Ren Shen (Radix Ginseng), 3-9g
Bai Zhu (Rhizoma Atractylodis Macrocephalae), 9g
Chai Hu (Radix Bupleuri), 9g

This formula is for a liver-spleen but with more prominent blood vacuity.

Acupuncture & moxibustion: *Tai Chong* (Liv 3), *He Gu* (LI 4), *Zu Lin Qi* (GB 41) & *Wai Guan* (TB 5) on the unaffected side, *Qi Men* (Liv 14) & *Zhang Men* (Liv 13) on the affected side

Liver channel blood stasis

Main symptoms: Lancinating postpartum abdominal pain with an inability to rotate, a scanty, non-freely flowing lochia which is purple and dark in color, dizziness, heart vexation, a purple, dark facial complexion, a red tongue with parched, yellow fur, and a bowstring, choppy, forceful pulse

Treatment principles: Quicken the blood, regulate the liver, and rectify the qi

Guiding formulas:

Xuan Hu Suo Tang **(Corydalis Decoction)**
Dang Gui (Radix Angelicae Sinensis), 9g
Yan Hu Suo (Rhizoma Corydalis), 9-18g
Chi Shao (Radix Rubrus Paeoniae Lactiflorae), 9g
Pu Huang (Pollen Typhae), 9g
Rou Gui (Cortex Cinnamomi), 3-9g
Ru Xiang (Resina Olibani), 3-6g
Mo Yao (Resina Myrrhae), 3-6g

Xiong Gui Xie Gan Tang
(Ligusticum & Dang Gui Drain the Liver Decoction)
Dang Gui Wei (Extremitas Radicis Angelicae Sinensis), 9g
Chuan Xiong (Radix Ligustici Wallichii), 9g
Qing Pi (Pericarpium Citri Reticulatae Viride), 6-9g
Zhi Ke (Fructus Aurantii), 6-9g
*Xiang Fu (*Rhizoma Cyperi), 9g
Hong Hua (Flos Carthami), 9g
Tao Ren (Semen Persicae), 9g

Acupuncture & moxibustion: *Xue Hai* (Sp 10), *He Gu* (LI 4), *San Yin Jiao* (Sp 6), *Zu Lin Qi* (GB 41) & *Wai Guan* (TB 5) on the unaffected side, *Qi Men* (Liv 14) & *Zhang Men* (Liv 13) on the affected side

Kidney water insufficiency

Main symptoms: Postpartum rib-side and low back pain, foot or heel pain, a scanty, pale red lochia, dizziness, heart palpitations, forgetfulness, heat in the hands, feet, and heart, a red face and flushed cheeks, a red tongue with scanty or no fur, and a bowstring, fine, rapid pulse

Treatment principles: Supplement the kidneys and nourish the liver

Guiding formulas:

Jia Wei Liu Wei Di Huang Tang
(Added Flavors Six Flavors Rehmannia Decoction)
Shu Di (cooked Radix Rehmanniae), 12-15g
Shan Yao (Radix Dioscoreae), 9g
Shan Zhu Yu (Fructus Corni), 9g

Fu Ling (Poria), 9-12g
Ze Xie (Rhizoma Alismatis), 6-9g
Dan Pi (Cortex Moutan), 6-9g
Bai Shao (Radix Albus Paeoniae Lactiflorae), 9-18g
Niu Xi (Radix Achyranthis Bidentatae), 9-12g

Yang Gan Bu Shen Tang
(Nourish the Liver & Supplement the Kidneys Decoction)
Shu Di (cooked Radix Rehmanniae), 12-15g
Bai Shao (Radix Albus Paeoniae Lactiflorae), 9-18g
Niu Xi (Radix Achyranthis Bidentatae), 9-12g
Chuan Lian Zi (Fructus Toosendan), 6-9g
Shan Zhu Yu (Fructus Corni), 9g
Qing Pi (Pericarpium Citri Reticulatae Viride), 6-9g
Dang Gui (Radix Angelicae Sinensis), 9g
Fu Ling (Poria), 9-12g
Dan Pi (Cortex Moutan), 9g

Acupuncture & moxibustion: *San Yin Jiao* (Sp 6), *Tai Xi* (Ki 3), *Shen Shu* (Bl 23), *Zu Lin Qi* (GB 41) & *Wai Guan* (TB 5) on the unaffected side, *Qi Men* (Liv 14) & *Zhang Men* (Liv 13) on the affected side

11

Postpartum Low Back Pain

Women may experience low back pain postpartum for a variety of reasons. While this condition is treated more as a symptom than as a disease in Western medicine, postpartum low back pain is a disease in its own right in Chinese gynecology.

Chinese medical disease categorization

Low back pain which occurs after delivery in women is called *chan hou yao tong*, postpartum low back pain.

Disease causes & disease mechanisms

Postpartum low back pain is mostly due to kidney qi vacuity depletion. Birthing can damage the yin and blood. Thus the *chong* and *ren* may become vacuous and empty. The *dai mai* loses its nourishment and, therefore, low back pain occurs.

Another cause is wind cold entering the channels and network vessels when the interstices have not yet become densely repacked. This wind cold obstructs the flow of qi and blood in the channels and network vessels and, if this obstruction occurs in the area of the low back, low back pain occurs.

A third cause is qi and blood vacuity weakness. Postpartum qi and blood must recover from vacuity. In the meantime, the hundreds of bones of the skeleton lose their nourishment. This can then cause aching and pain in the low back and waist region.

The fourth and final cause of postpartum low back pain is due to constitutional or long-term bodily yang vacuity. External cold and dampness may take this advantage to attack. If the lifegate fire is not sufficient to counteract this attack, cold and dampness settle in the channels and network vessels of this region, obstructing the free flow of qi, and blood and, once again, pain arises in the low back.

Patterns common to this condition

Liver-kidney yin vacuity
Blood stasis in the channels & network vessels
Qi & blood vacuity weakness
Kidney yang insufficiency

Treatment based on pattern discrimination:

Liver-kidney yin vacuity

Main symptoms: Postpartum low back aching and pain extending to both thighs, possible foot and/or heel pain, a scanty lochia which is pale red in color, dizziness, tinnitus, blurred vision, dryness in the corners of the eyes and a rough feeling, heat in the hands, feet, and heart, a red facial complexion with flushed cheeks, a dry, red tongue with no fur, a dry mouth but no particular desire to drink, and a bowstring, fine, rapid pulse

Treatment principles: Enrich and supplement the liver and kidneys

Guiding formulas:

Liu Wei Di Huang Tang Jia Wei
(Six Flavors Rehmannia Decoction with Added Flavors)
Shu Di (cooked Radix Rehmanniae), 12-15g
Shan Yao (Radix Dioscoreae), 9g
Shan Zhu Yu (Fructus Corni), 9g
Dan Pi (Cortex Moutan), 9g
Ze Xie (Rhizoma Alismatis), 6-9g
Fu Ling (Poria), 9-12g
Bie Jia (Carapax Amydae Sinensis), 9-15g
Niu Xi (Radix Achyranthis Bidentatae), 9-12g
Bai Shao (Radix Albus Paeoniae Lactiflorae), 9-18g

Bu Shen Di Huang Tang (Supplement the Kidneys Rehmannia Decoction)
Shu Di (cooked Radix Rehmanniae), 12-15g
Dang Gui (Radix Angelicae Sinensis), 9g
Du Zhong (Cortex Eucommiae), 9-15g
Du Huo (Radix Angelicae Pubescentis), 9g
Rou Gui (Cortex Cinnamomi), 3-9g
Xu Duan (Radix Dipsaci), 9g
Da Zao (Fructus Jujubae), 3 pieces
Sheng Jiang (uncooked Rhizoma Zingiberis), 6g

Acupuncture & moxibustion: Tai Xi (Ki 3), *San Yin Jiao* (Bl 23), *Shen Shu* (Bl 23), *Da Chang Shu* (Bl 25), *a shi* points

Blood stasis in the channels & network vessels

Main symptoms: Postpartum low back pain which is piercing in quality and inability to rotate the torso from the waist, a non-freely flowing lochia which is blackish purple in color, heart vexation and lack of tranquility, a dark, stagnant facial complexion, a dark red tongue, and a bowstring, choppy, forceful pulse

Treatment principles: Free the flow of the channels, quicken the network vessels, and resolve the exterior

Guiding formulas:

Jia Wei Dang Gui Ze Lan Tang
(Added Flavors Dang Gui & Lycopus Decoction)
Dang Gui (Radix Angelicae Sinensis), 9g
Ze Lan (Herba Lycopi), 9g
Chuan Niu Xi (Radix Cyathulae), 9-15g
Hong Hua (Flos Carthami), 9g
Yan Hu Suo (Rhizoma Corydalis), 9-15g
Tao Ren (Semen Persicae), 9g
Du Huo (Radix Angelicae Pubescentis), 9g
Sang Ji Sheng (Herba Taxilli), 9-15g
Fang Feng (Radix Sapshnikoviae), 9g

Tao Ren Tang (Persica Decoction)
Tao Ren (Semen Persicae), 9g
Dang Gui (Radix Angelicae Sinensis), 9g
Niu Xi (Radix Achyranthis Bidentatae), 9-12g
Ze Lan (Herba Lycopi), 9g
Su Mu (Lignum Sappan), 9g

Acupuncture & moxibustion: *Xue Hai* (Sp 10), *San Yin Jiao* (Sp 6), *He Gu* (LI 4), *a shi* points

Qi & blood vacuity weakness

Main symptoms: Postpartum low back and body pain, a scanty, watery, pale lochia, dizziness, impaired memory, heart palpitations, shortness of breath, sweating upon movement, a somber white facial complexion, a pale, moist tongue with thin, white fur, and a faint, fine, weak pulse

Treatment principles: Boost the qi and supplement the blood

Guiding formulas:

Ba Zhen Tang Jia Wei (Eight Pearls Decoction with Added Flavors)
Ren Shen (Radix Ginseng), 3-9g
Bai Zhu (Rhizoma Atractylodis Macrocephalae), 9g
Fu Ling (Poria), 9-12g
mix-fried *Gan Cao* (Radix Glycyrrhizae), 6-9g

Dang Gui (Radix Angelicae Sinensis), 9g
Shu Di (cooked Radix Rehmanniae), 12-15g
Bai Shao (Radix Albus Paeoniae Lactiflorae), 9-18g
Chuan Xiong (Radix Ligustici Wallichii), 9g
Du Zhong (Cortex Eucommiae), 9-15g
Xu Duan (Radix Dipsaci), 9-12g
Sang Ji Sheng (Herba Taxilli), 9-12g
Rou Gui (Cortex Cinnamomi), 3-9g

Shi Quan Da Bu Tang
(Ten [Ingredients] Completely & Greatly Supplementing Decoction)
Huang Qi (Radix Astragali), 9-18g
Rou Gui (Cortex Cinnamomi), 3-9g
Dang Gui (Radix Angelicae Sinensis), 9g
Shu Di (cooked Radix Rehmanniae), 12-15g
Bai Zhu (Rhizoma Atractylodis Macrocephalae), 9g
Bai Shao (Radix Albus Paeoniae Lactiflorae), 9-18g
Chuan Xiong (Radix Ligustici Wallichii), 9g
Fu Ling (Poria), 9-12g
mix-fried *Gan Cao* (Radix Glycyrrhizae), 6-9g
Sheng Jiang (uncooked Rhizoma Zingiberis), 6g
Da Zao (Fructus Jujubae), 3 pieces

Acupuncture & moxibustion: *Zu San Li* (St 36), *San Yin Jiao* (Sp 6), *Ge Shu* (Bl 17), *Pi Shu* (Bl 20), *Wei Shu* (Bl 21), *a shi* points

Kidney yang insufficiency

Main symptoms: Postpartum low back pain and heaviness of the body, inability to rotate or move, a pale lochia, frequent urination, lack of warmth in the four limbs, a dusky, dark facial complexion, possible loose stools, lower leg edema, and a deep, weak, moderate (*i.e.*, relaxed or slightly slow) pulse

Treatment principles: Warm and supplement kidney yang

Guiding formula:

Wen Shen Chu Shi Tang
(Warm the Kidneys & Eliminate Dampness Decoction)
Shan Yao (Radix Dioscoreae), 9g
Cang Zhu (Rhizoma Atractylodis), 9g
Niu Xi (Radix Achyranthis Bidentatae), 9-12g
Fu Ling (Poria), 9-12g
Yi Yi Ren (Semen Coicis), 12-30g
Xu Duan (Radix Dipsaci), 9-12g
Sang Ji Sheng (Herba Taxilli), 9-12g
Dang Gui (Radix Angelicae Sinensis), 9g
Bai Shao (Radix Albus Paeoniae Lactiflorae), 9-18g
Gan Cao (Radix Glycyrrhizae), 3-9g

Acupuncture & moxibustion: Tai Xi (Ki 3), *San Yin Jiao* (Sp 6), *Guan Yuan* (CV 4), *Shen Shu* (Bl 23), *Ming Men* (GV 4), *Yao Yang Guan* (GV 3), *Da Chang Shu* (Bl 25). Moxa *Guan Yuan* and the points on the low back.

Representative case history

The patient was a 27 year-old female outpatient who was first seen on March 26, 1993. On Jan. 27 of that year, the patient had normally delivered a full-term child. Postpartum bleeding was not profuse and her lochia had stopped after one month. That same month, the patient had taken a train to Shanghai, during which time she developed generalized body pain with especially severe chilly pain of her lower and upper back. Bedrest for one month did not result in improvement. In addition, there was lassitude of the spirit, lack of strength, a pale red tongue with thin fur, and a deep, fine, soft pulse.

Based on the above signs and symptoms, the patient's Chinese medical pattern was discriminated as spleen-kidney vacuity weakness, and she was prescribed: *Dang Shen* (Radix Codonopsitis), 15g, mix-fried *Huang Qi* (Radix Astragali), 12g, *Bai Zhu* (Rhizoma Atractylodis Macrocephalae), 9g, *Bai Shao* (Radix Albus Paeoniae Lactiflorae), 9g, *Fu Ling* (Poria), 12g, mix-fried *Gan Cao* (Radix Glycyrrhizae), 6g, *Dang Gui* (Radix Angelicae Sinensis), 12g, *Dan Shen* (Radix Salviae Miltiorrhizae), 12g, *Shu Di* (cooked Radix Rehmanniae) 12g, *Xu Duan* (Radix Dipsaci), 12g, *Sang Ji Sheng* (Herba Taxilli), 12g, *Sang Zhi* (Ramulus Mori), 12g, *Du Zhong* (Cortex Eucommiae), 12g, and processed *Gou Ji* (Rhizoma Cibotii), 12g. After taking these medicinals for one month, the lower and upper back pain gradually ceased, the woman was able to resume her normal life, and her vitality increased.

12
Postpartum Generalized Body Pain

In Chinese medicine, the disease category of postpartum generalized pain refers to pain of the muscles and joints occurring in more than one area of the body. It also includes heaviness and weakness of the muscles as well as numbness. In modern Western medicine, there at least three autoimmune diseases characterized by either muscle-joint pain or muscle weakness and numbness – multiple sclerosis (MS), rheumatoid arthritis (RA), and systemic lupus erythmatosus (SLE) – tend to go into remission during pregnancy but flare postpartum.[1,2] In addition, although fibromyalgia syndrome (FMS) has not been confirmed to be an autoimmune disease, generalized body pain is one of its symptoms, the condition is most common in females, and it too tends to flare postpartum. Therefore, in terms of Chinese medicine, the following protocols are applicable to these Western medical conditions when they occur postpartum.

However, as one of the case histories below evidences, this disease category may also be applied to women experiencing thrombophlebitis. During the puerperium, women are at increased risk for deep venous thrombosis. This increased risk is attributed to venous stasis, increased coaguability, and damage to the vessels. These risks are increased in postpartum women who have had a cesarean delivery. In Western medicine, this condition is treated preventively with heparinisation. Its clinical diagnosis is notoriously poor. Physical examination may or may not reveal cyanosis, erythema, edema, or tenderness in the leg. Suspected thrombophlebitis is confirmed by venography. Heparinisation is also the Western medical remedial treatment of this condition.

Chinese medical disease categorization

Aching and pain of the body and joints in postpartum women is called *chan hou shen tong* or, literally, postpartum body pain in Chinese. Some Chinese gynecology texts also refer to this condition as *chan hou guan jie tong*, postpartum joint pain, and *chan hou tong feng*, postpartum painful wind.

Disease causes & disease mechanisms

This condition is mostly due to postpartum blood vacuity. In this case, the channels and vessels lose their nourishment. If blood loss during labor is excessive, the four limbs and the hundreds of bones of the skeleton become vacuous and empty, while the sinews and vessels lose their moisture and nourishment. Thus there is numbness, and, in serious cases, there may be aching and pain.

If the woman suffers from habitual bodily kidney vacuity *and* loses a great deal of blood during labor, this results in qi and blood vacuity as well. Since the uterine vessel is nourished by the blood and also since the uterine vessel ligates or ties up to the low back, that area of the body may experience pain. In addition, since uterine vessel vacuity due to blood loss leads to additional kidney qi vacuity and the low back is the mansion of the kidneys, this may also aggravate kidney vacuity low back pain.

It is also possible that, after delivery when the qi and blood are completely vacuous, the constructive and defensive lose their harmony and the exterior and interior are not closely connected. Hence wind, cold, and damp evils may take advantage of this vacuity and enter the body. There they accumulate and obstruct the channels and network vessels. Since these vessels narrow around the joints and travel the closest to the exterior at those points, obstruction and blockage by wind, cold and/or damp evils are most prominent at the joints. If wind, cold, and/or damp evils obstruct and hinder the transportation and movement of the qi and blood, stasis and stagnation give rise to pain.

Further, in many women with a pre-existing wind, damp, heat impediment pattern, due to postpartum spleen vacuity, dampness and, therefore, heat, may be worse. Therefore, not only can one see contraction or aggravation of wind, cold, damp evils postpartum, one can also see aggravation of wind, damp, heat.

Patterns common to this condition

Qi & blood insufficiency
Liver-kidney vacuity weakness
Wind cold damp impediment
Wind damp heat impediment

Treatment based on pattern discrimination:

Qi & blood insufficiency

Main symptoms: Postpartum joint pain with low back aching and pain, if serious, inability to rotate the waist, movement leads to aggravation, shortness of breath, spontaneous perspiration, dry skin, dry, scratchy eyes, a pale white facial complexion, a pale, dry tongue with no fur, and a fine, forceless pulse

Treatment principles: Boost the qi and nourish the blood

Guiding formulas:

**Dang Gui Huang Qi Tang Jia Wei
(Dang Gui & Astragalus Decoction with Added Flavors)**
Dang Gui (Radix Angelicae Sinensis), 9g
Huang Qi (Radix Astragali), 9-18g
Bai Shao (Radix Albus Paeoniae Lactiflorae), 9-18g
Ji Xue Ten (Caulis Spatholobi), 9-36g
Qin Jiao (Radix Gentianae Macrophyllae), 9g
Gui Zhi (Ramulus Cinnamomi), 6-9g
Gan Cao (Radix Glycyrrhizae), 3-9g

Si Wu Tang Jia Wei (Four Materials Decoction with Added Flavors)
Dang Gui (Radix Angelicae Sinensis), 9g
Chuan Xiong (Radix Ligustici Wallichii), 9-15g
Bai Shao (Radix Albus Paeoniae Lactiflorae), 9-18g
Shu Di (cooked Radix Rehmanniae), 12-15g
Huang Qi (Radix Astragali), 9-18g
Niu Xi (Radix Achyranthis Bidentatae), 9-15g
Mu Gua (Fructus Chaenomelis), 9g
Xu Duan (Radix Dipsaci), 9-12g
Sang Ji Sheng (Herba Taxilli), 9-12g
Qin Jiao (Radix Gentianae Macrophyllae), 9g

**Huang Qi Gui Zhi Wu Wu Tang Jia Wei Yi Hao (Astragalus & Cinnamon
Twig Five Materials Decoction with Added Flavors #1)**
Huang Qi (Radix Astragali), 9-18g
Gui Zhi (Ramulus Cinnamomi), 6-9g
Dang Gui (Radix Angelicae Sinensis), 9g
Bai Shao (Radix Albus Paeoniae Lactiflorae), 9-18g
Chuan Xiong (Radix Ligustici Wallichii), 9g
Ji Xue Teng (Caulis Spatholobi), 9-36g
Sang Zhi (Ramulus Mori), 9g
Du Huo (Radix Angelicae Pubescentis), 9g
Niu Xi (Radix Achyranthis Bidentatae), 9-12g
Sheng Jiang (uncooked Rhizoma Zingiberis), 6g
Fructus Jujubae (*Da Zao*), 3 pieces

Acupuncture & moxibustion: *Zu San Li* (St 36), *San Yin Jiao* (Sp 6), *Ge Shu*
(Bl 17), *Gan Shu* (Bl 18), *Pi Shu* (Bl 20) plus apropriate local points

Liver-kidney vacuity weakness

Main symptoms: Postpartum lower and upper back aching and pain, lack of
strength in the lower extremities, possible foot or heel pain, dizziness, tinnitus,
and nocturia. If there is mostly kidney yang vacuity, there may also be cold feet,

aversion to cold, decreased sexual desire, a pale tongue with thin fur, and a fine, deep, bowstring pulse. If yin fails to control yang and there is internal heat, there may be malar flushing, night sweats, heat in the hands, feet, and heart, a red or pale but rid-tipped tongue, possible thin, dry, yellow fur, and a fine, bowstring, rapid or surging, rapid pulse

Treatment principles: Nourish the liver and enrich the kidneys, strengthen the sinews and bones and invigorate the low back

Guiding formulas:

Yang Rong Zhuang Shen Tang Jia Shu Di (Nourish the Constructive & Stregnthen the Kidneys Decoction plus Cooked Rehmannia)
Dang Gui (Radix Angelicae Sinensis), 9g
Chuan Xiong (Radix Ligustici Wallichii), 9g
Du Huo (Radix Angelicae Pubescentis), 9g
Rou Gui (Cortex Cinnamomi), 3-9g
Fang Feng (Radix Sapshnikoviae), 9g
Du Zhong (Cortex Eucommiae), 9-15g
Xu Duan (Radix Dipsaci), 9-12g
Sang Ji Sheng (Herba Taxilli), 9-12g
Sheng Jiang (uncooked Rhizoma Zingiberis), 6g

This formula is for a predominantly kidney yang vacuity complicated by liver blood vacuity.

Ba Zhen Tang Jia Jian
(Eight Pearls Decoction with Additions & Subtractions)
Dang Shen (Radix Codonopsitis), 9-18g
Bai Zhu (Rhizoma Atractylodis Macrocephalae), 9g
mix-fried *Gan Cao* (Radix Glycyrrhizae), 6-9g
Dang Gui (Radix Angelicae Sinensis), 9g
Chuan Xiong (Radix Ligustici Wallichii), 6-9g
Bai Shao (Radix Albus Paeoniae Lactiflorae), 9-18g
Shu Di (cooked Radix Rehmanniae), 12-15g
Sang Ji Sheng (Herba Taxilli), 9-12g
Gui Zhi (Ramulus Cinnamomi), 6-9g
Du Zhong (Cortex Eucommiae), 9-15g
Tu Si Zi (Semen Cuscutae), 9g
Suo Yang (Herba Cynomorii), 9g

This formula treats a qi and blood, yin and yang vacuity. If there is only a qi, blood, and yin vacuity, delete *Gui Zhi* and *Suo Yang* and add *Niu Xi* (Radix Achyranthis Bidentatae) and *Nu Zhen Zi* (Fructus Ligustri Lucidi).

Acupuncture & moxibustion: *San Yin Jiao* (Sp 6), *Tai Xi* (Ki 3), *Guan Yuan* (CV 4), *Gan Shu* (Bl 18), *Shen Shu* (Bl 23) plus appropriate local points

If there is yang vacuity, add moxibustion at *Guan Yuan, Shen Shu*, and *Ming Men* (GV 4) as well as at any local points.

Wind cold damp impediment

Main symptoms: Depending on the prevalence of wind cold or blood stasis, there is lancinating pain and the visible veins are purplish in color. Movement makes the condition better, but rest makes it worse. The facial color is dark and stagnant. There is body and joint aching and pain. Bending and stretching are inhibited. There may also be possible limb and body swelling and edema, numbness, and heaviness. Walking is difficult but heat is relaxing. The tongue is pale with thin, white fur, while the pulse is fine and moderate (*i.e.*, relaxed or slightly slow) or bowstring, floating, and moderate.

Treatment principles: Nourish the blood and dispel wind, disperse cold and eliminate dampness

Guiding formulas:

***Du Huo Ji Sheng Tang* (Angelica Pubescens & Loranthus Decoction)**
Du Huo (Radix Angelicae Pubescentis), 9g
Sang Ji Sheng (Herba Taxilli), 9-12g
Qin Jiao (Radix Gentianae Macrophyllae), 9g
Fang Feng (Radix Sapshnikoviae), 9g
Xi Xin (Herba Asari), 1-3g
Dang Gui (Radix Angelicae Sinensis), 9g
Bai Shao (Radix Albus Paeoniae Lactiflorae), 9-18g
Chuan Xiong (Radix Ligustici Wallichii), 6-9g
Sheng Di (uncooked Radix Rehmanniae), 12-15g
Du Zhong (Cortex Eucommiae), 9-15g
Niu Xi (Radix Achyranthis Bidentatae), 9-12g
Ren Shen (Radix Ginseng), 3-9g
Fu Ling (Poria), 9-12g
Gan Cao (Radix Glycyrrhizae), 3-9g
Gui Xin (Cortex Cinnamomi), 3-9g

Ba Zhen Tang Jia Jian
(Eight Pearls Decoction with Additions & Subtractions)
Dang Shen (Radix Codonopsitis), 9-18g
Bai Zhu (Rhizoma Atractylodis Macrocephalae), 9g
mix-fried *Gan Cao* (Radix Glycyrrhizae), 6-9g
Dang Gui (Radix Angelicae Sinensis), 9g
Chuan Xiong (Radix Ligustici Wallichii), 6-9g
Bai Shao (Radix Albus Paeoniae Lactiflorae), 9-18g
Shu Di (cooked Radix Rehmanniae), 12-15g
Sang Ji Sheng (Herba Taxilli), 9-12g
Gui Zhi (Ramulus Cinnamomi), 6-9g
Du Huo (Radix Angelicae Pubescentis), 9g

Qin Jiao (Radix Gentianae Macrophyllae), 9g

Acupuncture & moxibustion: *Feng Chi* (GB 20), *Qu Chi* (LI 11), *Ge Shu* (Bl 17), *Yang Ling Quan* (GB 34)

If generalized body aching and pain is severe and difficult to remit, one should needle *Ren Zhong* (GV 26), *Bai Hui* (GV 20), *Shang Xing* (GV 23), and *Tai Yang* (M-HN-9) in order to arouse the brain and stabilize pain. For severe shoulder area pain, add *Jian Yu* (LI 15), *Jian Liao* (TB 14), and *Pi Shu* (Bl 20). For elbow pain, add *Chi Ze* (Lu 5) and *Zhou Liao* (LI 12). For forearm pain, add *Wai Guan* (TB 5) and *Shou San Li* (LI 10). For wrist pain, add *Wan Gu* (SI 4), *Yang Chi* (TB 4), and *Yang Lao* (SI 6). For upper and lower back pain, add reactive points in the affected area. For sacral and hip pain, add *Huan Tiao* (GB 30), *Zhi Bian* (Bl 54), *Cheng Fu* (Bl 36), *Feng Shi* (GB 31), and *Liang Qiu* (St 34). For knee pain, add *Liang Qiu* (St 34), *Du Bi* (St 35), *He Ding* (St 34) and *Zu San Li* (St 36). For ankle pain, add *Kun Lun* (Bl 60), *Qiu Xu* (GB 40), and *Shen Mai* (Bl 62). If impediment is complicated by blood stasis, add *Xue Hai* (Sp 10), *San Yin Jiao* (Sp 6), and *He Gu* (LI 4). If there is concomitant qi and blood vacuity, add *Gan Shu* (Bl 18), *Pi Shu* (Bl 20), and *Zu San Li* (St 36).

Wind damp heat impediment

Main symptoms: Postpartum joint swelling, redness, pain, heat, heaviness, and restricted movement which occurs more often in the lower half of the body, possible fever, oral thirst but sometimes no desire to drink, a tendency to short, reddish urination, a red tongue with slimy, yellow fur, and a slippery, rapid or soggy, rapid pulse

Note: This pattern may also appear in thrombophlebitis.

Treatment principles: Clear heat, eliminate dampness and alleviate impediment

Guiding formulas:

Si Miao San Jia Wei (Four Wonders Powder with Added Flavors)
Huang Bai (Cortex Phellodendri), 9g
Cang Zhu (Rhizoma Atractylodis), 9g
Yi Yi Ren (Semen Coicis), 15-36g
Mu Gua (Fructus Chaenomelis), 9g

If there is qi vacuity, add *Huang Qi* (Radix Astragali) and *Bai Zhu* (Rhizoma Atractylodis Macrocephalae). If there is concomitant blood vacuity, add *Bai Shao* (Radix Albus Paeoniae Lactiflorae) and *Dang Gui* (Radix Angelicae Sinensis). If there is concomitant yin vacuity, add *Sang Ji Sheng* (Herba Taxilli), *Niu Xi* (Radix Achyranthus Bidentatae), and *Nu Zhen Zi* (Fructus Ligustri Lucidi). If there is simultaneous blood stasis, add *Dan Pi* (Cortex Moutan) and *Chi Shao* (Radix Rubrus Paeoniae Lactiflorae). If there is simultaneous qi stagnation, add *Chuan Lian Zi* (Fructus Toosendan).

Unnamed formula given by Yu Jin for acute thrombophlebitis with fever
Jin Yin Hua (Flos Lonicerae), 9-15g
Ren Dong Teng (Ramulus Lonicerae), 9-15g
Lian Qiao (Fructus Forsythiae), 9-15g
Dang Gui (Radix Angelicae Sinensis), 9g
Sang Ji Sheng (Herba Taxilli), 9-12g
Tian Hua Fen (Radix Trichosanthis), 9g
Chuan Bei Mu (Bulbus Fritillariae Cirrhosae), 9g
Dong Gua Zi (Semen Benincasae), 9-15g

Unnamed formula given by Yu Jin for subacute thrombophlebitis after fever has reduced but pain persists
Shui Zhi (Hirudo), 6-9g
Meng Chong (Tabanus), 6-9g
Tao Ren (Semen Persicae), 9g
Da Huang (Radix Et Rhizoma Rhei), 3-9g
Jin Yin Hua (Flos Lonicerae), 9-15g
Dang Gui (Radix Angelicae Sinensis), 9g
Bai Shao (Radix Rubrus Paeoniae Lactiflorae), 9g
Dong Gua Zi (Semen Benincasae), 9-15g
Mu Tong (Caulis Akebiae), 6-9g
Ze Xie (Rhizoma Alismatis), 6-9g

If qi vacuity symptoms are apparent, after symptoms of redness have disappeared, one can add *Huang Qi* (Radix Astragali) and *Dang Shen* (Radix Codonopsitis). If joint pain is severe, add *Yan Hu Suo* (Rhizoma Corydalis). If the lochia is not smoothly flowing, add *Dan Shen* (Radix Salviae Miltiorrhizae) and *Yi Mu Cao* (Herba Leonuri).

Shi Gao Fang Ji Tang (Gypsum & Stephania Decoction)
Cang Zhu (Rhizoma Atractylodis), 9g
Shi Gao (Gypsum Fibrosum), 30g
Zhi Mu (Rhizoma Anemarrhenae), 9g
Fang Ji (Radix Stephaniae Tetrandrae), 9g
uncooked *Gan Cao* (Radix Glycyrrhizae), 3-9g
Xi He Liu (Herba Tamaricis Chinensis), 15g
Ren Dong Teng (Caulis Lonicerae), 15g
Gui Zhi (Ramulus Cinnamomi), 6g
Yan Hu Suo (Rhizoma Corydalis), 30g

Acupuncture & moxibustion: *San Yin Jiao* (Sp 6), *Yin Ling Quan* (Sp 9), and appropriate local points (see wind, damp, cold impediment above)

Abstract of representative Chinese research:

From "The Treatment of 32 Cases of Postpartum Generalized Pain" by Liu Ai-ying *et al., Ji Lin Zhong Yi Yao (Jilin Chinese Medicine & Medicinals)*, #1, 1999, p. 26

Cohort description:

The youngest of the 32 patients in this study was 24 and the oldest was 38 years old. Sixteen women had given birth at full term normally, three had had spontaneous abortions, five had had cesarean deliveries, and eight had had artificial abortions. The shortest course of disease was seven days and the longest was two months. Twelve cases had generalized soreness and pain with numbness and heaviness and inhibition of the movement of the joints. Nine had lower and upper back pain, and 11 had one-sided upper or lower extremity musculoskeletal pain. Erythrocyte sedimentation rates and anti-O tests were all within normal parameters.

Treatment method:

The basic formula consisted of: mix-fried *Huang Qi* (Radix Astragali) and *Ji Xue Teng* (Caulis Spatholobi), 20g each, *Shu Di* (cooked Radix Rehmanniae), *Bai Shao* (Radix Albus Paeoniae Lactiflorae), and *Dang Shen* (Radix Codonopsitis), 15g each, *Dang Gui* (Radix Angelicae Sinensis), *Qiang Huo* (Radix Et Rhizoma Notopterygii), *Fang Feng* (Radix Sapshnikoviae), *Du Zhong* (Cortex Eucommiae), and *Xu Duan* (Radix Dipsaci), 10g each, and *Chuan Xiong* (Radix Ligustici Wallichii), *Gui Zhi* (Ramulus Cinnamomi), and *Gan Cao* (Radix Glycyrrhizae 6g each. If upper extremity pain was severe, *Jiang Huang* (Rhizoma Curcumae Longae) was added. If lower extremity pain was severe, *Du Huo* (Radix Angelicae Pubescentis) was added. If low back pain was severe, *Gou Ji* (Rhizoma Cibotii) and *Niu Xi* (Radix Achyranthis Bidentatae) were added. If dampness was heavy, *Yi Yi Ren* (Semen Coicis) and *Mu Gua* (Fructus Chaenomelis) were added. One packet was decocted in water per day and administered orally in two divided doses, with seven days equaling one course of treatment. Outcomes were assessed after 1-2 courses.

Treatment outcomes:

Cure was defined as disappearance of aching, pain, soreness, and numbness with resumption of normal joint mobility and normal ambulation. Improvement was defined as decrease in aching, pain, soreness, and numbness and basic normalization of joint mobility. No effect meant that there was no improvement in either subjective symptoms or joint mobility. Based on these criteria, 24 cases were judged cured and eight were judged improved, for a total amelioration rate of 100%.

From "The Treatment of 125 Cases of Generalized Pain with *Jian Yun Tang* (Fortifying & Moving Decoction)" by Guo Shi-wei, *He Nan Zhong Yi (Henan Chinese Medicine)*, #7, 2001, p. 46

Cohort description:

The youngest of the 125 patients in this study was 21 and the oldest was 36 years old. One hundred eight patients were primiparas, and 17 were second-time mothers. One hundred three had normal births, and 22 had c-sections. Fifty-seven had suffered the onset of their pain within one month after delivery, 53 cases experienced the onset of their symptoms 1-6 months after delivery, and 15 cases experienced their onset more than six months after having given birth. Eleven cases presented one-sided upper extremity pain, 33 cases had bilateral upper extremity pain, six cases had one-sided lower extremity pain, 21 cases had bilateral lower extremity pain, 33 cases had lower and upper back pain, and 21 patients had multiple sites of aching and pain. All the patients in this study had been previously treated with wind-dispelling Chinese medicinal formulas, antirheumatics, and corticosteroids but with poor results.

Treatment method:

The basic formula consisted of: *Huang Qi* (Radix Astragali), 30g, *Dang Shen* (Radix Codonopsitis), 15g, *Dang Gui* (Radix Angelicae Sinensis), 15g, *Zhi Mu* (Rhizoma Anemarrhenae), 6g, *Mai Men Dong* (Tuber Ophiopogonis), 15g, *Ru Xiang* (Resina Olibani), 10g, *Mo Yao* (Resina Myrrhae), 10g, *San Leng* (Rhizoma Sparganii), 6g, and *E Zhu* (Rhizoma Curcumae), 6g. One packet was decocted in water and administered orally per day, and one week equaled one course of treatment. Outcomes were assessed after two weeks.

Treatment outcomes:

In 95 cases (76.0%), the aching and pain completely disappeared. Hence the patients were considered cured. In another 22 cases (17.6%), after taking these medicinals, the aching and pain markedly decreased, while in eight cases (6.4%) there was no effect. Thus the total amelioration rate was 93.6%.

Representative case histories

Case 1: The patient was a 27 year-old female who was initially seen on Dec. 12, 1974, at which time the patient had had postpartum generalized pain and fear of chill for three months. This patient had given birth normally seven months previous. The pain was mostly in her upper extremities and wrist joints. There was no redness or swelling in the affected areas. However, after exposure to cold, the pain got worse. Besides aversion to cold and fear of chill, there were heart palpitations and shortness of breath, but the patient's appetite and two excretions were normal. However, her tongue was pale with thin, white fur, and her pulse was fine and moderate (*i.e.*, slightly slow).

Based on the above signs and symptoms, the patient's Western medical diagnosis was postpartum joint pain, while her Chinese medical pattern was categorized as blood vacuity with contraction of cold. Therefore, the patient was prescribed the following medicinals: *Huang Qi* (Radix Astragali), 15g, *Dang Shen* (Radix Codonopsitis), 9g, *Dang Gui* (Radix Angelicae Sinensis), 9g, *Bai Shao* (Radix Albus Paeoniae Lactiflorae), 9g, *Du Huo* (Radix Angelicae Pubescentis), 6g, *Qiang Huo* (Radix Et Rhizoma Notopterygii), 6g, *Qin Jiao* (Radix Gentianae Macrophyllae), 9g, *Ji Xue Teng* (Caulis Spatholobi), 24g, *Fang Feng* (Radix Sapshnikoviae), 4.5g, *Tao Ren* (Semen Persicae), 3g, and *Hong Hua* (Flos Carthami), 3g. The patient was seen a second time on Dec. 20. At that time, the patient reported that, after taking six packets of the above medicinals, her generalized body pain had decreased and her heart palpitations and shortness of breath improved. After another seven packets, all her symptoms had been eliminated.

Case 2: The patient was a 37 year-old female worker. Four years prior, the patient had developed heart palpitations and shortness of breath. Two years after that, these symptoms got worse, and she had had four occasions where she had hacked up blood. Now she was 10 days postpartum and was experiencing right lower extremity chilling, distention, and pain which was better during the day but worse at night. This pain was severe enough so that the woman could not walk or move about. Examination revealed that there was chilling of the right leg below the knee, and no pulse could be palpated in the artery of the affected leg. The patient's pulse was bowstring and fine and sometimes bound. Her lips were slightly purple and the edges of her tongue had purple-colored static macules. Otherwise, the tongue had white fur.

Based on the above, the Western diagnosis was thrombophlebitis, while the patient's Chinese medical pattern was categorized as qi stagnation and blood stasis obstructing and congesting the channels and network vessels. Therefore, based on the treatment principles of supplementing the qi and quickening the blood, dispelling stasis and freeing the flow of the network vessels, the patient was prescribed: *Huang Qi* (Radix Astragali), 60g, *Tao Ren* (Semen Persicae), *Hong Hua* (Flos Carthami), *Di Long* (Pheretima), *Chuan Niu Xi* (Radix Cyathulae), and *Xuan Shen* (Radix Scrophulariae), 15g each, *Dang Gui Wei* (Extremitas Radicis Angelicae Sinensis) and *Chuan Xiong* (Radix Ligustici Wallichii), 12g each, *Pu Huang* (Pollen Typhae), *Wu Ling Zhi* (Feces Trogopterori Seu Pteromi), *Ru Xiang* (Resina Olibani), *Mo Yao* (Resina Myrrhae), and *Shi Chang Pu* (Rhizoma Acori Tatarinowii), 9g each, *Gan Cao* (Radix Glycyrrhizae), 3g, and *Su He Xiang* (Styrax Liquidus), 0.9g swallowed with the decocted medicinals. In addition, acupuncture was performed at *Wei Zhong* (Bl 54), *Cheng Shan* (Bl 57), *Yang Ling Quan* (GB 34), and *Zu San Li* (St 36) which was also moxaed.

After taking five packets of the above medicinals, the patient's symptoms gradually decreased, her right lower leg became warm again, and the pain decreased. However, she was still sometimes short of breath. Therefore, the dose of *Huang Qi* was increased to 90g. After one month of this therapy, all the pain was eliminated and the artery in her lower leg could be felt pulsing again. Five weeks after entering the hospital, the patient was discharged, although she continued taking Chinese medicinals to regulate her condition and nourish her body.

Case 3: The patient was 28 years old and married. Her initial examination was on Jan. 18, 1978. She was 51 days postpartum. Her lochia had already ceased and she was lactating. However, her right shoulder was sore, painful, and lacked strength. Lifting and raising were inhibited. The muscles and flesh in the area were numb and insensitive. Her mouth and eyes were somewhat skewed to the right, and her stools were constipated. She had high blood pressure, her tongue had thin fur, and her pulse was fine and rapid. All this was because, postpartum, the hundreds of vessels are vacuous and empty. Therefore, wind, cold, and damp evils had become mixed with liver wind and phlegm dampness. These then blocked and obstructed the network vessel pathways, and the vessels and network vessels lost their harmony, thus resulting in this condition.

Treatment, therefore, was in order to level the liver and transform dampness, dispel wind and free the flow of the network vessels: *Dang Gui* (Radix Angelicae Sinensis), 9g, *Sang Zhi* (Ramulus Mori), 12g, *Si Gua Luo* (Retinervus Luffae Cylindricae,) 9g, *Jiang Huang* (Rhizoma Curcumae Longae), 9g, *Luo Shi Teng* (Ramus Trachelospermi), 9g, *Lu Dou Yi* (Testa Munginis), 9g, *Xiao Hu Ma* (Semen Lini Usitatissimi), 9g, *Hai Feng Teng* (Caulis Piperis), 9g, *Dan Shen* (Radix Salviae Miltiorrhizae), 9g, *Long Chi* (Dens Draconis), 12g, *Fang Ji* (Radix Stephaniae Tetrandrae), 9g, *Wei Ling Xian* (Radix Clematidis), 9g, *Ci Ji Li* (Fructus Tribuli), 9g, *Qiang Huo* (Radix Et Rhizoma Notopterygii), 9g, *Du Huo* (Radix Angelicae Pubescentis), 9g, *Chuan Xiong* (Radix Ligustici Wallichii), 4.5g, *Shu Jin Huo Luo Wan* (Soothe the Sinews & Quicken the Network Vessels Pills), 1 pill, swallowed with the above decocted medicinals. Separately, the patient was administered nine grams each day of *Sang Ma Wan* (Morus & Sesame Pills).

The second examination took place on Jan. 25. The patient still had postpartum shoulder and upper arm soreness and pain. Her qi and constructive were both vacuous and depleted, and her network vessel pathways had lost their harmony. Her pulse was fine and choppy, and her tongue was fat with thin fur. Treatment, therefore, was in order to quicken the blood and dispel wind, transform phlegm and free the flow of the network vessels. She was given the above formula minus *Lu Dou Yi, Bai Ji Li, Long Chi*, and *Xiao Hu Ma* but plus *Wu Xiao She* (Zaocys Dhumnades), 9g, *Shi Chang Pu* (Rhizoma Acori Tatarinowii), 9g, *Bai Jie Zi* (Semen Sinapis Albae), 9g, and *Qing Qi Hua Tan Wan* (Clear the Qi & Transform Phlegm Pills), 9g, swallowed with the foregoing decoction.

The third examination took place on Feb. 3 after the patient had taken five more packets of the above formula. The shoulder and upper arm soreness and pain were diminished, but the local area muscles and flesh were still numb. There were teeth-marks on the edges of her tongue and its fur was thin. Her pulse was fine and rapid. Instead of the original formula, she was given: *Ju He* (Semen Citri Reticulatae), 9g, *Ju Luo* (Retinervus Citri Reticulatae), 9g, *Gui Zhi* (Ramulus Cinnamomi), 9g, *Si Gua Luo* (Retinervus Luffae Cylindricae), 9g, *Qin Jiao* (Radix Gentianae Macrophyllae), 4.5g, *Qiang Huo* (Radix Et Rhizoma Notopterygii), 9g, *Du Huo* (Radix Angelicae Pubescentis), 9g, *Hai Feng Teng* (Caulis Piperis), 12g, *Wu Jia Pi* (Cortex Acanthopanacis), 9g, *Mu Gua* (Fructus Chaenomelis), 4.5g, *Huang Qi* (Radix Astragali), 9g, *Dang Gui* (Radix Angelicae Sinensis), 9g, *Chuan Xiong* (Radix Ligustici Wallichii), 4.5g, *Sang Zhi* (Ramulus Mori), 12g, *Ci Ji Li* (Fructus Tribuli), 12g, and *Jiang Huang* (Rhizoma Curcumae Longae), 9g.

The fourth examination took place on Feb. 13 after yet another five packets.

After taking these medicinals, the patient's right shoulder's movement and use were uninhibited. However, the aching and pain had increased. Her low back was sore, and there was a white-colored vaginal discharge. At night, the patient's sleep was disturbed by dreams. In the morning when she arose, there was superficial edema of her face. Her tongue edges had the indentations of her teeth and her tongue had thin fur. The woman's pulse was fine and rapid. Based on these signs and symptoms, it was now surmised that this was due to the three qi of wind, cold, and dampness entering and assailing postpartum and the network vessel pathways losing their harmony. Treatment, therefore, was in order to dispel wind and free the flow of the network vessels, and the patient was prescribed five packets of the following medicinals: *Dang Gui* (Radix Angelicae Sinensis), 9g, *Sang Zhi* (Ramulus Mori), 9g, *Si Gua Luo* (Retinervus Luffae Cylindricae), 9g, *Wu Jia Pi* (Cortex Acanthopanacis), 9g, *Fang Ji* (Radix Stephaniae Tetrandrae), 9g, *Wei Ling Xian* (Radix Clematidis), 9g, *Gui Zhi* (Ramulus Cinnamomi), 3g, *Hai Feng Teng* (Caulis Piperis), 12g, *Jiang Huang* (Rhizoma Curcumae Longae), 4.5g, *Dan Shen* (Radix Salviae Miltiorrhizae), 9g, *Chuan Wu* (Radix Aconiti Carmichaeli), 4.5g, *Cao Wu* (Radix Aconiti Kusnezoffi), 4.5g, mix-fried *Gan Cao* (Radix Glycyrrhizae), 9g, *Dang Shen* (Radix Codonopsitis), 12g, *Qiang Huo* (Radix Et Rhizoma Notopterygii), 9g, *Du Huo* (Radix Angelicae Pubescentis), 9g, *Shu Jin Huo Luo Wan* (Soothe the Sinews & Quicken the Network Vessels Pills), 1 pill, swallowed down with the aforementioned decoction.

The fifth examination took place on Feb. 22. There was postpartum shoulder and upper arm soreness and pain. Bending and lifting were difficult. After taking these medicinals, there had been some change for the better. However, the woman could not endure taxation or force. Her pulse was fine and rapid, while her tongue was pale with thin fur. This pattern was discriminated as wind, cold, and dampness brewing internally. Treatment, therefore, was in order to dispel wind, transform dampness, and free the flow of the network vessels assisted by boosting the qi and nourishing the blood so as to attend to the root: *Dang Gui* (Radix Angelicae Sinensis), 9g, *Sang Zhi* (Ramulus Mori), 12g, *Hai Feng Teng* (Caulis Piperis), 12g, *Wei Ling Xian* (Radix Clematidis), 9g, *Wu Jia Pi* (Cortex Acanthopanacis), 9g, *Qiang Huo* (Radix Et Rhizoma Notopterygii), 9g, *Du Huo* (Radix Angelicae Pubescentis), 9g, *Huang Qi* (Radix Astragali), 9g, *Bai Jie Zi* (Semen Sinapis Albae), 9g, *Bu Gu Zhi* (Fructus Psoraleae), 9g, *Qin Jiao* (Radix Gentianae Macrophyllae), 9g, *Ju Ye* (Folium Citri Reticulatae), 9g, *Ju He* (Semen Citri Reticulatae), 9g, *Ban Xia* (Rhizoma Pinelliae), 9g, *Dang Shen* (Radix Codonopsitis), 9g, *Ren Shen Zai Zao Wan* (Ginseng Recreation Pills), 1 pill, swallowed down with the aforementioned decoction. Separately, the patient was administered *Jin Ji Hu Wan* (Golden Cock & Tiger Pills), 1 bottle.

The sixth examination occurred on Feb. 27. The patient was administered five more packets of the above formula, after which she was considered cured.

Case 4: The patient was a 25 year-old female who was first examined on April 5, 1999, at which time she was 30 days postpartum. The woman's lochia had already stopped. However, postpartum, she had perspired relatively profusely and had contracted some wind cold evils. Since then she had had generalized pain, which was most severe in the low back region, for a week. Bending and stretching of the patient's lower limbs were inhibited, her tongue was pale with thin, white fur, and her pulse was floating and moderate (*i.e.*, relaxed or slightly slow). Based on these signs and symptoms, her pattern was categorized as qi and blood vacuity weakness with wind cold blocking and obstructing the channels and vessels. Therefore, she was prescribed the following medicinals: *Gui Zhi* (Ramulus Cinnamomi), 8g, stir-fried *Bai Shao* (Radix Albus Paeoniae Lactiflorae), 10g, mix-fried *Gan Cao* (Radix Glycyrrhizae), 5g, *Da Zao* (Fructus Jujubae), 10g, *Sheng Jiang* (uncooked Rhizoma Zingiberis), 3 slices, mix-fried *Huang Qi* (Radix Astragali), 15g, *Bai Zhu* (Rhizoma Atractylodis Macrocephalae), 12g, *Dang Gui* (Radix Angelicae Sinensis), 12g, *Niu Xi* (Radix Achyranthis Bidentatae), 12g, *Sang Ji Sheng* (Herba Taxilli), 20g, *Du Huo* (Radix Angelicae Pubescentis), 9g, and *Yan Hu Suo* (Rhizoma Corydalis), 10g. After taking four packets of these medicinals, the patient's aching and pain had decreased. However, she had stomach duct distention and discomfort. Therefore, 10 grams of *Chen Pi* (Pericarpium Citri Reticulatae) were added to the formula, four more packets were prescribed, and the patient was cured.

Remarks

1. Rheumatoid arthritis may manifest either wind, cold, damp impediment or wind, damp, heat impediment pain and is commonly complicated by qi and/or blood vacuity as well as by yin and/or yang vacuity. Lupus and FMS tend to manifest more as wind, damp, heat impediment problems combined with qi and yin vacuities. Similarly, MS commonly presents with a qi, blood, and yin vacuity often complicated by damp heat. For more information on the Chinese medical treatment of each of these conditions, see my and Philippe Sionneau's *The Treatment of Modern Western Medical Diseases with Chinese Medicine* also available from Blue Poppy Press.

2. Shortness of breath can be a symptom of pulmonary embolism. Therefore, practitioners should be very careful of patients who manifest this symptom, especially if it is concomitant with localized, unilateral lower extremity pain and swelling. In that case, referral to Western medical services probably makes sense.

Endnotes:

[1] http://my.webmd.com/condition_center_content/rha/article/1680.50442

[2] www.gpfn.sk.ca/health/support/less/lupusbro.html

13

Postpartum Headache

In Western medicine, benign headaches are generally divided into two types—tension and neurovascular headaches. Either of these two types may occur postpartum, although migraines tend to improve with pregnancy and postpartum. Headaches can also be a symptom of hypertension, and, it is possible for hypertension developed during pregnancy to continue postpartum. As with a number of the other Chinese disease categories in this book, there is no category of specifically postpartum headache in modern Western medicine. However, this is a not uncommon complaint in real-life clinical practice.

Chinese medical disease categorization

If there is headache after delivery, this is referred to as *chan hou tou tong*, postpartum headache.

Disease causes & disease mechanisms

There are three main causes of postpartum headache. The first is vacuity of yin-blood with upward ascension of yang qi. After birth, if excessive blood has been lost, yin and blood may be vacuous and insufficient. In that case, yin may be insufficient to control yang qi. Since the head is the reunion of yang, this yang qi may counterflow upward to collect in the head. This results in headache. However, although yang qi counterflows upward, this is only because of a yin and blood vacuity which is the root of this pattern. If yin is supplemented and blood nourished, yang qi will become properly calm and the headache will stop on its own.

It is also possible, according to the theories of Chinese medicine, for spoilt blood to cause headache. If such spoilt blood remains in the uterus, this may counterflow upwards from yin's position in the lower half of the body up the vessels to pierce through to the crown or vertex. This then causes pain at the vertex. This is a species of blood stasis headache.

The third cause of postpartum headache is contraction of wind cold evils in the region of the head due to postpartum blood vacuity. Because the wind evils hinder and obstruct the free flow of the channels and vessels in the region, there is pain.

Patterns common to this condition

Blood vacuity
Blood stasis
Wind cold external contraction

Treatment based on pattern discrimination:

Blood vacuity

Main symptoms: Constant postpartum headache which is worse towards the end of the day or after work and fatigue, a pale facial complexion, pale lips and nails, dry skin, dry, scratchy eyes, a pale tongue with thin, white, possibly dry fur, and a fine, weak pulse

Treatment principles: Supplement and nourish the blood

Guiding formulas:

Ba Zhen Tang Jia Wei (Eight Pearls Decoction with Added Flavors)
Ren Shen (Radix Ginseng), 3-9g
Bai Zhu (Rhizoma Atractylodis Macrocephalae), 9g
Fu Ling (Poria), 9-12g
mix-fried *Gan Cao* (Radix Glycyrrhizae), 6-9g
Dang Gui (Radix Angelicae Sinensis), 9g
Chuan Xiong (Radix Ligustici Wallichii), 9-18g
Bai Shao (Radix Albus Paeoniae Lactiflorae), 9g
Shu Di (cooked Radix Rehmanniae), 12-15g
Man Jing Zi (Fructus Viticis), 9g

Ren Shen Yang Rong Tang Jia Jian (Ginseng Nourish the Constructive Decoction with Additions & Subtractions)
Dang Shen (Radix Codonopsitis), 9g
Gan Cao (Radix Glycyrrhizae), 3-9g
Dang Gui (Radix Angelicae Sinensis), 9g
Bai Shao (Radix Albus Paeoniae Lactiflorae), 9g
Shu Di (cooked Radix Rehmanniae), 12-15g
Rou Gui (Cortex Cinnamomi), 3-9g
Huang Qi (Radix Astragali), 9-18g
Bai Zhu (Rhizoma Atractylodis Macrocephalae), 9g
Fu Ling (Poria), 9-12g
Wu Wei Zi (Fructus Schisandrae), 9g
Yuan Zhi (Radix Polygalae), 6-9g

Chen Pi (Pericarpium Citri Reticulatae), 6g
Chuan Xiong (Radix Ligustici Wallichii), 9-18g
Bai Zhi (Radix Angelicae Dahuricae), 9-15g

If there is occipital pain, add *Ge Gen* (Radix Puerariae) and *Gou Teng* (Ramulus Uncariae Cum Uncis).

Acupuncture & moxibustion: *Zu San Li* (St 36), *He Gu* (LI 4), *Ge Shu* (Bl 17), *Gan Shu* (Bl 18), *Pi Shu* (Bl 20) plus appropriate local points

Blood stasis

Main symptoms: Sharp, vertigeal pain accompanied by a dark-colored, stagnant and astringent lochia, lower abdominal pain, a purplish dark facial complexion or purple lips, a purplish, dark tongue or static spots or macules on the tongue, and a bowstring, choppy pulse

Treatment principles: Quicken the blood and transform stasis

Guiding formulas:

Hei Shen San (Black Spirit Powder)
Gang Gui (Radix Angelicae Sinensis), 9g
Chi Shao (Radix Rubrus Paeoniae Lactiflorae), 9g
Shu Di (cooked Radix Rehmanniae), 12-15g
Niu Xi (Radix Achyranthis Bidentatae), 9-12g
Rou Gui (Cortex Cinnamomi), 3-9g
Pu Huang (Pollen Typhae), 9g
Gan Cao (Radix Glycyrrhizae), 3-9g
Hei Dou (Semen Glycinis), 15g

Tong Qiao Sheng Hua Tang
(Open the Orifices Engendering & Transforming Decoction)
Dang Gui (Radix Angelicae Sinensis), 9g
Chuan Xiong (Radix Ligustici Wallichii), 9-18g
Tao Ren (Semen Persicae), 9g
Pao Jiang (blast-fried Rhizoma Zingiberis), 6-9g
Yi Mu Cao (Herba Leonuri), 9-18g
Di Long (Pheretima), 3-9g
Jiang Can (Bombyx Batryticatus), 9g
Bai Zhi (Radix Angelicae Dahuricae), 9-15g
Gou Teng (Ramulus Uncariae Cum Uncis), 9-15g
San Leng (Rhizoma Sparganii), 9g
Niu Xi (Radix Achyranthis Bidentatae), 9-12g
Shan Yang Jiao (Cornu Caprae), 9-15g

Acupuncture & moxibustion: *Xue Hai* (Sp 10), *San Yin Jiao* (Sp 6), *He Gu* (LI 4) plus appropriate local points

Wind cold external contraction

Main symptoms: Postpartum chilly pain in the forehead with diminishment of the pain if it obtains heat, a scanty lochia which is colored dark and purplish, a thin, white tongue coating, and a wiry, choppy pulse

Treatment principles: Warm the channels, scatter cold, and stop pain

Guiding formula:

Gui Zhi Si Wu Tang (Cinnamon Twig Four Materials Decoction)
Dang Gui (Radix Angelicae Sinensis), 9g
Chuan Xiong (Radix Ligustici Wallichii), 9-18g
Chi Shao (Radix Rubrus Paeoniae Lactiflorae), 9g
Shu Di (cooked Radix Rehmanniae), 12-15g
Gui Zhi (Ramulus Cinnamomi), 6-9g
Bai Zhi (Radix Angelicae Dahuricae), 9-15g
Chang Pu (Rhizoma Acori Tatarinowii), 6-9g
Xi Xin (Herba Asari), 1-3g
Man Jing Zi (Fructus Viticis), 9g
mix-fried *Gan Cao* (Radix Glycyrrhizae), 6-9g
Yi Mu Cao (Herba Leonuri), 9-18g

Acupuncture & moxibustion: *He Gu* (LI 4), *Tai Yang* (M-HN-9), *Feng Chi* (GB 20) plus local points on the head based on the location of the pain

Representative case histories

Case 1: The patient was a 28 year-old female who was first seen on Oct. 5, 1992. During July, the patient had given birth for the first time, during which she had lost a lot of blood. During the puerperium, she had developed empty pain at the vertex of her head. If she wrapped her head in a cotton cloth, this gave her some comfort. When it was very hot and she would go outside to cool off, she dreaded wind on her head. Her tongue was pale but dark with thin, slimy fur, and her pulse was fine and bowstring. Based on the preceding signs and symptoms, her pattern was discriminated as blood vacuity with cold congelation. Therefore, she was prescribed: *Dang Gui* (Radix Angelicae Sinensis), 12g, *Chuan Xiong* (Radix Ligustici Wallichii), 6g, *Bai Shao* (Radix Albus Paeoniae Lactiflorae), 12g, *Bai Zhu* (Rhizoma Atractylodis Macrocephalae), 12g, *Sheng Shu Di* (uncooked and cooked Radix Rehmanniae), 12g each, *Dang Shen* (Radix Codonopsitis), 9g, *Fu Ling* (Poria), 9g, *Huang Qi* (Radix Astragali), 15g, *Xi Xin* (Herba Asari), 3g, stir-fried *Jing Jie* (Herba Schizonepetae), 9g, *Rou Gui* (Cortex Cinnamomi), 3g, *Ye Jiao Teng* (Caulis Polygoni Multiflori), 15g, uncooked *Bai Zhi* (Radix Angelicae Dahuricae), 9g, and *Niu Xi* (Radix Achyranthis Bidentatae), 12g. The patient continued taking this formula for approximately one half year continuously along with getting acupuncture, and her headaches were completely eliminated and her mind and emotions were also vitalized.

Case 2: The patient was a married female of undisclosed age who was initially examined on Jan. 7, 1959 when she was three weeks postpartum. Two weeks postpartum, the patient had caught a cold and had developed a fever and headache. After two days, the fever had healed but the headache had continued. These headaches were worse at night. In addition, there was a dry mouth but no desire to drink, extremely profuse spontaneous perspiration, incessant lochia that was not profuse in amount, thin, yellow tongue fur, and a deep, fine, rapid pulse. Based on these signs and symptoms, the patient's pattern was discriminated as qi and yin dual vacuity with ascendant hyperactivity of liver yang. Therefore, she was prescribed: uncooked *Huang Qi* (Radix Astragali), 15g, *Dang Gui* (Radix Angelicae Sinensis), 9g, *Bai Shao* (Radix Albus Paeoniae Lactiflorae), 9g, uncooked *Long Chi* (Dens Draconis), 15g, uncooked *Mu Li* (Concha Ostreae), 15g, *Sha Yuan Zi* (Semen Astragali Complanati), 9g, *Gou Qi Zi* (Fructus Lycii), 9g, *Fu Xiao Mai* (Fructus Levis Tritici Aestivi), 12g, *Da Zao* (Fructus Jujubae), 4 pieces, and carbonized *Jing Jie* (Herba Schizonepetae), 6g.

After taking five packets of the above medicinals, the headache had disappeared. However, the woman still felt flustered and a bit dizzy. Her perspiration had gradually reduced, but there was still fear of heat, dry mouth, poor appetite, loose stools, thorns or prickles on the tip of the tongue, yellow tongue fur, and a deep, fine pulse. Therefore, she was prescribed another five packets of the following medicinals to foster yin and subdue yang, fortify the spleen and harmonize the stomach: *Dang Shen* (Radix Codonopsitis), 9g, *Bai Zhu* (Rhizoma Atractylodis Macrocephalae), 9g, *Fu Ling* (Poria), 12g, mix-fried *Gan Cao* (Radix Glycyrrhizae), 3g, *Bai Shao* (Radix Albus Paeoniae Lactiflorae), 9g, *Gou Qi Zi* (Fructus Lycii), 9g, uncooked *Long Chi* (Dens Draconis), 15g, uncooked *Mu Li* (Concha Ostreae), 15g, *Chen Pi* (Pericarpium Citri Reticulatae), 3g, *Mu Xiang* (Radix Auklandiae), 3g, *Fu Xiao Mai* (Fructus Levis Tritici Aestivi), 12g, and *Da Zao* (Fructus Jujubae), 4 pieces. These medicinals gradually resulted in a quieting of this patient's mind and the elimination of her dizziness.

14

Postpartum Heart Pain

In Western medicine, there are a number of causes of postpartum pain in the area of the heart, most of which do not involve coronary artery or heart disease. Other possibilities include postpartum panic attacks or other stress reactions[1] and a pulmonary embolism. Postpartum panic attacks occur in approximately 10% of women.[2] A pulmonary embolism is an emergency condition which requires immediate referral to Western medical services. Commonly, a pulmonary embolism is accompanied by sharp chest pain, shortness of breath, and cyanosis.[3]

Chinese medical disease categorization

Postpartum heart pain (*chan hou xin tong*) refers to pain in the precordium or epigastrium just below the ribs. As Fu Qing-zhu says, this is rightly stomach venter or *wei wan* pain.

Disease causes & disease mechanisms

The heart rules the blood. If a woman has long-standing cold hidden or deeply lying internally, after giving birth this may cause vacuity cold. Vacuity cold constricts and contracts, congealing the blood. Stasis does not move and it is axiomatic in Chinese medicine that lack of free flowing causes pain.

The second cause of postpartum heart pain is postpartum yin vacuity leading to fire penetrating the heart wrapper vessels or pericardium. If a woman loses excessive blood during labor, this may result in yin vacuity with stirring of internal fire. Since fire burns upward, it may travel upward to accumulate in the heart. There it scorches and attacks the heart wrapper vessels.

The third cause of postpartum heart pain is due to cold qi attacking above. This refers to external contraction of cold taking advantage of postpartum vacuity and thence causing obstruction to the flow of qi and blood in the region of the heart. According to Fu Qing-zhu, this cold may also be due to eating chilly, cold foods postpartum and, therefore, this condition may be complicated by food stagnation. It is said that if such cold stasis attacks below it causes abdominal pain, but, if it attacks above, it causes heart pain.

The last cause of postpartum heart pain is blood vacuity. In this case, excessive blood loss during labor and a tendency to spleen vacuity result in insufficient blood to nourish the heart. Thus the flow through the heart vessels loses its free flow and pain arises.

Patterns common to this condition

Vacuity cold & blood congelation
Yin vacuity with fire penetrating the wrapper network vessels
Cold qi attacking above
Blood vacuity heart pain

Treatment based on pattern discrimination:

Vacuity cold & blood congelation

Main symptoms: Lancinating precordial pain accompanied by a purplish dark facial complexion, purple lips, a scanty, non-freely flowing, dark, purplish lochia with clots, chilled limbs, lack of strength, fatigue, a pale, purplish tongue or possible static spots or macules, and a slow, tight, choppy; deep and slow; or regularly irregular pulse

Note: This pattern may present in pulmonary thrombosis.

Treatment principles: Warm the channels and transform stasis

Guiding formulas:

Da Yan Mi Tang (Greatly Spreading Honey Decoction)
Shu Di (cooked Radix Rehmanniae), 12-15g
Dang Gui (Radix Angelicae Sinensis), 9g
wine stir-fried *Bai Shao* (Radix Albus Paeoniae Lactiflorae), 9g
Du Huo (Radix Angelicae Pubescentis), 9g
Wu Zhu Yu (Fructus Evodiae), 6-9g
Gan Jiang (dry Rhizoma Zingiberis), 6-9g
Xi Xin (Herba Asari), 1-3g
Gui Xin (Cortex Cinnamomi), 3-9g
Gan Cao (Radix Glycyrrhizae), 3-9g
Yuan Zhi (Radix Polygalae), 6-9g
Bai Mi (honey), a suitable amount

Gua Lou Xie Bai Ban Xia Tang Jia Wei
(Trichosanthes, Allium & Pinellia Decoction with Added Flavors)
Dan Shen (Radix Salviae Miltiorrhizae), 9-15g

Gua Lou (Fructus Trichosanthis), 9g
Xie Bai (Bulbus Allii Macrostemi), 9g
Chuan Xiong (Radix Ligustici Wallichii), 9g
Pu Huang (Pollen Typhae), 9g
Xiang Fu (Rhizoma Cyperi), 9g
Ban Xia (Rhizoma Pinelliae), 9g
Hong Hua (Flos Carthami), 9g
Gui Zhi (Ramulus Cinnamomi), 6-9g
powdered *Xue Jie* (Sanguis Draconis), 3-6g (swallowed in divided
    doses with the liquid decoction)
powdered *San Qi* (Radix Notoginseng), 1-3g (swallowed in
    divided doses with the liquid decoction)

This formula is for more prominent blood stasis. For severe cold impediment, add *Zhi Fu Zi* (Radix Lateralis Praeparatus Aconiti Carmichaeli) and *Yin Yang Huo* (Herba Epimedii). For concomitant heart yang vacuity, add *Huang Qi* (Radix Astragali), *Xi Xin* (Herba Asari), and *Zhi Fu Zi* (Radix Lateralis Praeparatus Aconiti Carmichaeli). For qi vacuity with fatigue, shortness of breath, and weakness of the limbs, add *Huang Qi* (Radix Astragali) and *Dang Shen* (Radix Codonopsitis). For severe chest oppression, add *Hou Po* (Cortex Magnoliae Officinalis) and *Zhi Ke* (Fructus Aurantii). For profuse phlegm, add *Jie Geng* (Radix Platycodi). For severe heart pain, add *Yan Hu Suo* (Rhizoma Corydalis).

Acupuncture & moxibustion: *Xin Shu* (Bl 15), *Ju Que* (CV 14), *Nei Guan* (Per 6), *Ge Shu* (Bl 17)

If there is severe chest oppression, add *Dan Zhong* (CV 17). For cold hands or a cold sensation in the cardiac area, add moxibustion on *Xin Shu*, *Ju Que*, and *Ge Shu*. If there is profuse phlegm or slimy tongue fur, add *Feng Long* (St 40). For concomitant qi vacuity, add *Zu San Li* (St 36). For concomitant asccendant liver yang hyperactivity, add *Tai Chong* (Liv 3) and *Feng Chi* (GB 20).

Yin vacuity with fire penetrating the wrapper network vessels

Main symptoms: Postpartum precordial pain accompanied by vexation and agitation, night sweats, tidal fever, heat in the hands, feet, and heart, malar flushing, a red tongue with scanty fur; a red, cracked, and fissured tongue with thin, dry, yellow coating; or a red tongue with slimy, yellow, somewhat dry, and geographic coating, and a fine, wiry, rapid pulse

Treatment principles: Enrich yin, abduct yang back down to its lower source, and free the flow of the network vessels

Guiding formula:

Tian Wang Bu Xin Dan Jia Jian (Heavenly Emperor Supplement the Heart Elixir with Additions & Subtractions)
Dan Shen (Radix Salviae Miltiorrhizae), 9-15g
Xuan Shen (Radix Scrophulariae), 9-15g

Tian Men Dong (Tuber Asparagi), 9-12g
Fu Ling (Poria), 9-12g
Mai Men Dong (Tuber Ophiopogonis), 9-12g
Yuan Zhi (Radix Polygalae), 6-9g
Ren Shen (Radix Ginseng), 3-9g
Dang Gui (Radix Angelicae Sinensis), 9g
Suan Zao Ren (Semen Zizyphi Spinosae), 9-15g
Bai Zi Ren (Semen Platycladi), 9g
Wu Wei Zi (Fructus Schisandrae), 9g

If there are heart palpitations, add *Long Chi* (Dens Draconis) and *Mu Li* (Concha Ostreae). For severe yin vacuity, add *Sheng Di* (uncooked Radix Rehmanniae) and *Bai Shao* (Radix Albus Paeoniae Lactiflorae). For dizziness and tinnitus, add *Shi Jue Ming* (Concha Haliotidis), *Gou Teng* (Ramulus Uncariae Cum Uncis), and *Ju Hua* (Flos Chrysanthemi). For low back pain and weakness of the lower limbs, add *Sang Ji Sheng* (Herba Taxilli), *Niu Xi* (Radix Achyranthis Bidentatae), and *Du Zhong* (Cortex Eucommiae). For easy anger, severe restlessness, a red facial complexion, and aversion to heat, add *Xia Ku Cao* (Spica Prunellae), *Zhi Zi* (Fructus Gardeniae), and *Dan Pi* (Cortex Moutan). For night sweats and hot flashes in the face, add *Di Gu Pi* (Cortex Lycii), *Dan Pi* (Cortex Moutan), and *Zhi Mu* (Rhizoma Anemarrhenae). For dry mouth with profuse drinking, add *Tian Hua Fen* (Radix Trichosanthis) and *Shan Yao* (Radix Dioscoreae). If there is concomitant phlegm heat, add *Gua Lou Pi* (Pericarpium Trichosanthis), *Ban Xia* (Rhizoma Pinelliae), and *Huang Qin* (Radix Scutellariae).

Acupuncture & moxibustion: *Xin Shu* (Bl 15), *Shen Men* (Ht 7), *Tai Xi* (Ki 3), *San Yin Jiao* (Sp 6), *Nei Guan* (Per 6)

If there are heart palpitations, add *Ju Que* (CV 14) and *Dan Zhong* (CV 17). For dizziness, tinnitus, and high blood pressure, add *Xing Jian* (Liv 2) and *Feng Chi* (GB 20). For low back pain and weakness of the lower limbs, add *Fu Liu* (Ki 7) and *Shen Shu* (Bl 23). For easy anger, severe restlessness, a red facial complexion, and aversion to heat, add *Xing Jian* (Liv 2) and *Xia Xi* (GB 43). For night sweats and hot flashes in the face, add *Da Zhui* (GV 14) and *Yin Xi* (Ht 6). If there is concomitant phlegm heat, add *Feng Long* (St 40), *Nei Ting* (St 44), and *Zhong Wan* (CV 12).

Cold qi attacking above

Main symptoms: Lancinating or tight, gripping precordial pain, a pale, scanty, dark lochia which contains clots, cyanotic facial complexion, possible static spots or macules on the tongue, and a floating, tight pulse

Note: This pattern may present in cases of pulmonary thrombosis.

Treatment principles: Quicken the blood and transform stasis, warm the channels and scatter cold

Guiding formula:

**Sheng Hua Tang Jia Wei
(Engendering & Transforming Decoction with Added Flavors)**
Dang Gui (Radix Angelicae Sinensis), 9g
Chuan Xiong (Radix Ligustici Wallichii), 9-15g
mix-fried *Gan Cao* (Radix Glycyrrhizae), 6-9g
Pao Jiang (blast-fried Rhizoma Zingiberis), 6-9g
Tao Ren (Semen Persicae), 9g
Rou Gui (Cortex Cinnamomi), 6-9g

Chen Liang-fang says that if this does not stop the pain, add *Wu Zhu Yu* (Fructus Evodiae) and *Sheng Jiang* (uncooked Rhizoma Zingiberis). This formula as written above does not address complicating food stagnation. For this, Fu Qing-zhu suggests deleting *Tao Ren* and adding *Sha Ren* (Fructus Amomi) and *Wu Zhu Yu*. If food damage is due to cereal foods, add *Shen Qu* (Massa Medica Fermentata) and *Mai Ya* (Fructus Germinatus Hordei). If food stagnation is due to overeating meat, then add *Shan Zha* (Fructus Crataegi). If there is constipation, add *Rou Cong Rong* (Herba Cistanchis Huo).

Acupuncture & moxibustion: Same as for vacuity cold and blood congelation above.

Blood vacuity heart pain

Main symptoms: Chronic, low-grade precordial aching and pain which is aggravated by fatigue, a pale, watery, scanty lochia, lack of strength and fatigue, a pale facial complexion and lips, a pale, dry tongue with thin, white fur, and a fine, forceless pulse

Treatment principles: Supplement the blood and nourish the network vessels

Guiding formula:

Ba Zhen Tang (Eight Pearls Decoction)
Dang Gui (Radix Angelicae Sinensis), 9g
Bai Shao (Radix Albus Paeoniae Lactiflorae), 9g
Shu Di (cooked Radix Rehmanniae), 12-15g
Chuan Xiong (Radix Ligustici Wallichii), 9g
Ren Shen (Radix Ginseng), 3-9g
Bai Zhu (Rhizoma Atractylodis Macrocephalae), 9g
Fu Ling (Poria), 9-12g
mix-fried *Gan Cao* (Radix Glycyrrhizae), 6-9g

Acupuncture & moxibustion: *Zu San Li* (St 36), *Nei Guan* (Per 6), *Dan Zhong* (CV 17), *Xin Shu* (Bl 15), *Ge Shu* (Bl 17), *Gan Shu* (Bl 18), *Pi Shu* (Bl 20)

Remarks:

Heart or chest pain should never be underestimated. Because, in postpartum women, it may be a sign of pulmonary embolism, careful examination and questioning are required. If there is the possibility of either a pulmonary embolism or true cardiac disease, a timely referral is highly advised.

Endnotes:

[1] www.wellmother.com/postpartum

[2] www.obgyn.net/pb/articles/pp_psychiatric_indman_0299.htm

[3] www.babycenter.com/recap/baby/phyrecovery/12257.htm

15

Postpartum Cough

In Chinese medicine, any cough occurring during the puerperium is called post-partum cough no matter what its origin. As the reader will see, this Chinese disease category includes pulmonary embolism as well as the common cold, and every-thing in between.

Chinese medical disease categorization

Postpartum cough, called *chan hou ke sou* in Chinese, can cover both the cough that accompanies a common cold and also a chronic, lingering cough.

Disease causes & disease mechanisms

If the lochia is not completely discharged and spoilt blood remains behind in the uterus, this may penetrate upward to the lungs. In this case, there may be rapid breathing, dyspnea, chest oppression, vexation, etc. As seen below, if spoilt blood plays a part in this scenario, this can be determined by examining the lochia and the presence of any abdominal pain.

If excessive blood and body fluids are lost during labor and the woman has a ten-dency toward habitual bodily yin vacuity, it is also possible for yin vacuity of the lungs alone to cause postpartum cough. In this case, there is insufficient yin fluids to moisten the lungs. The lungs cannot control their function of depurating and downbearing, and and so their yang qi tends to counterflow upwards.

It is also possible for external evils to take advantage of postpartum vacuity to enter the body. The lungs rule the qi, and the defensive is a species of qi. If the woman is vacuous and insufficient after delivery due to excessive sweating, the interstices of the skin and hair may not be closely or densely packed. Wind cold may thus invade and enter the lungs, thus disturbing their function of depurative downbear-ing. Hence the lung qi counterflow upwards and there is coughing.

Patterns common to this condition

Wind cold external contraction
Blood stasis penetrating upward
Yin vacuity with fire flaring

Treatment based on pattern discrimination

Wind cold external contraction

Main symptoms: Fever, aversion to cold, a stuffed nose, sneezing, clear, watery nasal discharge, and coughing, a pale tongue, and a floating, fine, and tight or bowstring pulse. There may or may not be sweating depending on the state of the defensive qi.

Treatment principles: Resolve the exterior and scatter cold, transform phlegm and stop coughing

Guiding formulas:

Xuan Fu Hua Tang **(Inula Decoction)**
Jing Jie (Herba Schizonepetae), 9g
Qian Hu (Radix Peucedani), 9g
Ma Huang (Herba Ephedrae), 6-9g
Xing Ren (Semen Armeniacae), 9g
Ban Xia (Rhizoma Pinelliae), 9g
Fu Ling (Poria), 9-12g
Chi Shao (Radix Rubrus Paeoniae Lactiflorae), 9g
Wu Wei (Fructus Schisandrae), 9g
Gan Cao (Radix Glycyrrhizae), 3-9g
Xuan Fu (Flos Inulae), 9g
Sheng Jiang (uncooked Rhizoma Zingiberis), 6g
Da Zao (Fructus Jujubae), 3 pieces

If there is sweating, delete *Ma Huang* and add *Gui Zhi* (Ramulus Cinnamomi) instead.

Ding Fei Sheng Hua Tang
(Stabilize the Lungs Engendering & Transforming Decoction)
Chuan Xiong (Radix Ligustici Wallichii), 9g
Dang Gui (Radix Angelicae Sinensis), 9g
Xing Ren (Semen Armeniacae), 9g
Sha Shen (Radix Glehniae), 9-12g
Gan Cao (Radix Glycyrrhizae), 3-9g
Gan Jiang (dry Rhizoma Zingiberis), 3-6g
Jie Gen (Radix Platycodi), 6-9g

If there is phlegm, add *Tian Hua Fen* (Radix Trichosanthis). If there is vacuity with perspiration, add *Ren Shen* (Radix Ginseng). Wang Guo-zhu *et al.* recommend this formula for the treatment of external contraction of wind cold occurring less than a half month after delivery.

Shen Su Yin (Ginseng & Perilla Beverage)
Ren Shen (Radix Ginseng), 3-9g
Zi Su Ye (Folium Perillae Frutescentis), 9g
Chen Pi (Pericarpium Citri Reticulatae), 6g
Ge Gen (Radix Puerariae), 9-15g
Qian Hu (Radix Peucedani), 9g
Ban Xia (Rhizoma Pinelliae), 9g
Fu Ling (Poria), 9-12g
Zhi Ke (Fructus Aurantii), 6g
Jie Gen (Radix Platycodi), 6-9g
Mu Xiang (Radix Auklandiae), 9g
Gan Cao (Radix Glycyrrhizae), 3-9g

Huang Fu-zhong suggests this formula for the treatment of external contraction of wind cold.

Acupuncture & moxibustion: *He Gu* (LI 4), *Lie Que* (Lu 7), *Feng Men* (Bl 12), *Fei Shu* (Bl 13), *Zu San Li* (St 36), *Ge Shu* (Bl 17)

Blood stasis penetrating upward

Main symptoms: Postpartum coughing, distention and oppression in the region of the diaphragm, a scanty, non-freely flowing, dark-colored, possibly clotty lochia, pain in the lower abdomen which is averse to pressure, a purplish, dark facial complexion, static spots or macules on the tongue, and a fine, bowstring, and choppy pulse

Note: This pattern may present in pulmonary embolism.

Treatment principles: Quicken the blood and transform stasis

Guiding formulas:

Fo Shou San Jia Wei (Buddha's Hand Powder with Added Flavors)
Dang Gui (Radix Angelicae Sinensis), 9g
Chuan Xiong (Radix Ligustici Wallichii), 9-15g
Tao Ren (Semen Persicae), 9g
Hong Hua (Flos Carthami), 9g
Xing Ren (Semen Armeniacae), 9g
Sha Shen (Radix Glehniae), 9-12g
Yan Hu Suo (Rhizoma Corydalis), 9-15g

Er Mu Tang (Two Mothers Decoction)[1]
Sha Shen (Radix Glehniae), 9-12g

Chuan Bei Mu (Bulbus Fritillariae Cirrhosae), 9g
Fu Ling (Poria), 9-12g
Ren Shen (Radix Ginseng), 3-9g
Xing Ren (Semen Armeniacae), 9g
Tao Ren (Semen Persicae), 9g

Acupuncture & moxibustion: *Xue Hai* (Sp 10), *San Yin Jiao* (Sp 6), *He Gu* (LI 4), *Fei Shu* (Bl 13), *Dan Zhong* (CV 17)

Yin vacuity with fire flaring

Main symptoms: Chronic, dry, unproductive postpartum cough which is often provoked by speaking and tends to be worse in the afternoon and evening, a dry mouth and throat but no particular desire to drink, night sweats, heat in the hands, feet, and heart, tinnitus, heart palpitations, malar flushing, a red tongue with scanty fur, and a floating, fine, and rapid pulse

Treatment principles: Nourish yin and supplement the lungs

Guiding formulas:

Mai Wei Di Huang Tang (Ophiopogon & Schisandra Rehmannia Decoction)
Shu Di (cooked Radix Rehmanniae), 9-012g
Shan Zhu Yu (Fructus Corni), 9g
Shan Yao (Radix Dioscoreae), 9g
Fu Ling (Poria), 9g
Dan Pi (Cortex Moutan), 6-9g
Ze Xie (Rhizoma Alismatis), 6-9g
Mai Men Dong (Tuber Ophiopogonis), 9-12g
Wu Wei Zi (Fructus Schisandrae), 9g

Jia Wei Si Wu Tang (Added Flavors Four Materials Decoction)
Dang Gui (Radix Angelicae Sinensis), 9g
Sheng Di (uncooked Radix Rehmanniae), 9-12g
Chuan Xiong (Radix Ligustici Wallichii), 9g
Shan Yao (Radix Dioscoreae), 9g
He Zi (Fructus Terminaliae), 9g
Gua Lou Ren (Semen Trichosanthis), 9g
Zhi Mu (Rhizoma Anemarrhenae), 9g
Kuan Dong Hua (Flos Farfarae), 9g
Bai Bu (Radix Stemonae), 9g
Jie Gen (Radix Platycodi), 6-9g
Gan Cao (Radix Glycyrrhizae), 3-9g

Acupuncture & moxibustion: *Fei Shu* (Bl 13), *Lie Que* (Lu 7), *Zhao Hai* (Ki 6), *San Yin Jiao* (Sp 6), *Dan Zhong* (CV 17)

Remarks

If cough is associated with marked signs of blood stasis, there is the possibility of pulmonary embolism, in which case, a timely referral to Western medical services is advised.

Endnote:

[1] An alternate Chinese name of Radix Glehniae *(Sha Shen)* is *Zhi Mu*, Benefit the Mother. Since Bulbus Fritillariae Cirrhosae *(Chuan Bei Mu)* also has the word *mu* or mother in its name and these two are the ruling medicinals in this formula, thus its Chinese and English language names.

16

Postpartum Dyspnea and/or Asthma

In terms of modern Western medicine, this Chinese disease category covers both asthma and dyspnea due to pulmonary embolism. This disease is an extension or worsening of the previous disease category.

Chinese medical disease categorization

Postpartum qi panting is referred to as *chan hou qi chuan* in Chinese.

Disease causes & disease mechanisms

The premodern Chinese gynecological literature identifies basically two mechanisms resulting in postpartum qi panting. The first is spoilt blood penetrating the lungs. We have discussed this above. The second is due to great blood loss during delivery. If the blood deserts and the qi scatters, the constructive and defensive lose their harmony. Because of this, yang counterflows upward from its lower source and the kidneys lose their ability to grasp the qi sent down by the lungs.

Patterns common to this condition

Spoilt blood penetrating the lungs
Kidneys not grasping the qi

Treatment based on pattern discrimination

Spoilt blood penetrating the lungs

Main symptoms: Panting and coughing with distention and oppression in the chest and diaphragmatic region, a scanty, stagnant, non-freely flowing lochia which is dark and purplish in color and may contain clots, lower abdominal pain which is averse to pressure, a dark, purplish tongue or possible static spots or macules, and a bowstring, choppy pulse

Note: This pattern may present in cases of pulmonary embolism.

Treatment principles: Quicken the blood and transform stasis assisted by supporting the righteous

Guiding formula:

Jia Shen Sheng Hua Tang
(Added Ginseng Engendering & Transforming Decoction)
Ren Shen (Radix Ginseng), 3-9g
Chuan Xiong (Radix Ligustici Wallichii), 9-15g
Dang Gui (Radix Angelicae Sinensis), 9g
Tao Ren (Semen Persicae), 9g
Gan Jiang (dry Rhizoma Zingiberis), 3-6g
mix-fried *Gan Cao* (Radix Glycyrrhizae), 6-9g

If there are blood clots in the lochia, do not add *Bai Zhu* (Rhizoma Atractylodis Macrocephalae) or *Huang Qi* (Radix Astragali).

Acupuncture & moxibustion: *Fei Shu* (Bl 13), *Dan Zhong* (CV 17), *Nei Guan* (Per 6), *Xue Hai* (Sp 10), *San Yin Jiao* (Sp 6), *He Gu* (LI 4)

Kidneys not grasping the qi

Main symptoms: Postpartum qi panting in a woman who is constitutionally vacuous and weak, low back and knee soreness and limpness, lack of warmth in the four limbs, fatigue, spontaneous perspiration on slight exertion, lack of strength, disinclination to talk with a feeble voice and speaking makes the panting worse, inability to breathe when lying down, a pale tongue with thin, white fur, and a deep, weak, slow pulse

Treatment principles: Warm and supplement the lower source

Guiding formula:

Bu Qi Yang Rong Tang
(Supplement the Qi & Nourish the Constructive Decoction)
Ren Shen (Radix Ginseng), 3-9g
Dang Gui (Radix Angelicae Sinensis), 9g
Chuan Xiong (Radix Ligustici Wallichii), 9g
Shu Di (cooked Radix Rehmanniae), 9-15g
Huang Qi (Radix Astragali), 9-18g
Bai Zhu (Rhizoma Atractylodis Macrocephalae), 9g
Gan Cao (Radix Glycyrrhizae), 3-9g
Chen Pi (Pericarpium Citri Reticulatae), 6g
Jiang Tan (carbonized Rhizoma Zingiberis), 6-9g

This formula is recommended by Wang Guo-zhu *et al*. Their discrimination is that it is for postpartum panting with blood lumps, *i.e.*, clots, but no pain—in other words, for vacuity panting with only a slight complication of spoilt blood. If there is thirst, add *Mai Men Dong* (Tuber Ophiopogonis) and *Wu Wei* (Fructus Schisandrae). If there is spontaneous perspiration, add *Ma Huang Gen* (Radix Ephedrae) and *Fu Xiao Mai* (Fructus Levis Tritici Aestivi). If there is food damage due to cereals, add *Shen Qu* (Massa Medica Fermentata) and *Mai Ya* (Fructus Germinatus Hordei). If there is food damage due to meat, add *Sha Ren* (Fructus Amomi) and *Shan Zha* (Fructus Crataegi). If the stools are not freely flowing, add *Huo Ma Ren* (Semen Cannabis) and *Rou Cong Rong* (Herba Cistanchis).

Acupuncture & moxibustion: *Fei Shu* (Bl 13), *Dan Zhong* (CV 17), *Shen Shu* (Bl 23), *Ming Men* (GV 4), *Guan Yuan* (CV 4)

If there is some blood stasis, add *Xue Hai* (Sp 10), *San Yin Jiao* (Sp 6), and *He Gu* (LI 4). If there is food stagnation, add *Shang Wan* (CV 13), *Zhong Wan* (CV 12), and *Xia Wan* (CV 10). If there is concomitant constipation, add *Tian Shu* (St 25) and *Da Chang Shu* (Bl 25). If there's thirst, add *Zhao Hai* (Ki 6) and *Nei Ting* (St 44).

17
Postpartum Thirst

If a woman is more than usually thirsty postpartum, this is referred to as postpartum thirst in Chinese medicine. It is mostly due to fluid and blood loss, including the loss of fluids from breast-feeding. It is considered a disease category in its own right in at least some Chinese gynecology texts.

Chinese medical disease categorization

Excessive thirst and desire to drink after delivery is called *chan hou ke* in Chinese.

Disease causes & disease mechanisms

The stomach is the sea of water and grains and the bowels are the sea of fluids and humors. If blood loss is excessive during delivery, fluids and humors within may be consumed. If yin fluids in the stomach are vacuous, this can lead to pronounced stomach qi vacuity as well. Further, this condition may also allow for the engenderment of internal heat. Thus the mouth is parched, the throat is dry, and the mother is thirsty.

Treatment based on pattern discrimination

Stomach yin vacuity

Main symptoms: Postpartum thirst and dryness of the mouth and throat with dry tongue fur. If internal heat has been engendered, there may be a fever and the tongue may be red with dry, yellow fur. If stomach qi is vacuous, the tongue may be pale and have teeth-marks along its edges with dry, white fur.

Treatment principles: Nourish yin and engender fluids, supplement the qi and clear heat as necessary

Guiding formulas:

Shen Mai Yin (Ginseng & Ophiopogon Beverage)
Ren Shen (Radix Ginseng), 3-9g
Mai Men Dong (Tuber Ophiopogonis), 9-12g

This formula is for qi vacuity and fluid insufficiency. This combination can be added to other formulas where there is thirst due to yin vacuity accompanied by qi vacuity.

Si Wu Fen Mai Jian (Four Materials Divide the Vessels Decoction)
Dang Gui (Radix Angelicae Sinensis), 9g
Shu Di (cooked Radix Rehmanniae), 9-15g
Bai Shao (Radix Albus Paeoniae Lactiflorae), 9g
Chuan Xiong (Radix Ligustici Wallichii), 6-9g
Tian Hua Fen (Radix Trichosanthis), 9g
Mai Men Dong (Tuber Ophiopogonis), 9-12g

This formula is for marked blood vacuity complicating fluid insufficiency.

Zhu Ye Gui Qi Tang (Bamboo Leaf, Dang Gui & Astragalus Decoction)
Ren Shen (Radix Ginseng), 3-9g
Bai Zhu (Rhizoma Atractylodis Macrocephalae), 9g
Dang Gui (Radix Angelicae Sinensis), 9g
Huang Qi (Radix Astragali), 9-18g
Dan Zhu Ye (Herba Lophatheri), 9g
Gan Cao (Radix Glycyrrhizae), 3-9g

If the above formulas fail to resolve the thirst, one can use the following acupuncture formula which also clears heat:

Acupuncture & moxibustion: *Cheng Jiang* (CV 24), *Di Cang* (St 4), *Zhao Hai* (Ki 6), *Nei Ting* (St 44)

If there is marked blood vacuity, add *Zu San Li* (St 36), *Ge Shu* (Bl 17), and *Gan Shu* (Bl 18). If there is additional qi vacuity, also add *Pi Shu* (Bl 20). If there is heat damaging fluids, add *Qu Chi* (LI 11) and *He Gu* (LI 4).

Remarks

In my experience, orally administered Chinese medicinals are more effective for treating postpartum thirst than acupuncture. In any case, thirst is typically a complicating symptom in Western postpartum patients, not the major complaint.

18

Postpartum Edema

This Chinese disease category covers any swelling of the body, face, and/or extremities after delivery. In modern Western medicine, this condition is seen as a symptom as opposed to its own disease category. In most cases, postpartum edema is due to the body's not yet eliminating the extra fluid it retained during the last trimester. When this is the case, postpartum edema is rarely serious and typically subsides within one week after delivery. However, sudden edema of a single leg accompanied by fixed pain may be a sign of deep venous thrombosis for which emergency medical care may be indicated. Other emergency conditions associated with postpartum edema include peripartum eclampsia and peripartum cardiomyopathy, both of which often present bilateral lower leg edema. Eclampsia has been dealt with in Book 1, and its Chinese medical pattern discrimination and treatment postpartum are not significantly different than what is discussed in that chapter. Peri- or postpartum cardiomyopathy is a relatively rare disease affecting four in every 10,000 near-term or recently delivered women. The normalization of fluids in the body postpartum causes wide fluctuations in cardiac function that may lead to heart disease. Such postpartum cardiomyopathy occurs most frequently in multiparas, women over 30, those carrying twins, and those with preeclampsia. This condition has 50% mortality rate within five years and a high probability of recurrence. Therefore, women who have experienced this condition are counseled against future pregnancies.

Chinese medical disease categorization

Postpartum edema is called *chan hou fu zhong* in Chinese.

Disease causes & disease mechanisms

Immediately after delivery, spoilt blood which is not yet exhausted or completely discharged may take advantage of vacuity to flow into the channels and network vessels. Because qi and blood flow together, if blood stasis obstructs the channels and network vessels, this causes stagnation of the qi. Because the qi moves fluids in the body and fluids and blood move together, such qi stagnation and blood stasis may result in concomitant water swelling.

It is also possible that, after delivery, the patient is vacuous and weak. Her interstices are not densely packed, and the interior and exterior are not harmonious, *i.e.*, united interdependently. In this case, wind damp evils may take advantage of this vacuity and attack externally. These evil qi cause obstruction to the flow of qi and blood in the channels and network vessels which negatively impacts the circulation of fluids. Thus accumulation of fluids manifests as swelling.

However, not every case of vacuity edema involves external contraction. Since the spleen governs the movement and transformation of water fluids in the body, should qi and blood vacuity affect spleen function, this organ may lose its control over this movement and transformation. In this case, fluids may spill over from the middle to seep into the space beneath the skin causing edema and swelling of the extremities.

Patterns common to this condition

Qi stagnation & blood stasis
External contraction of wind evils
Spleen vacuity not moving & transforming

Treatment based on pattern discrimination

Qi stagnation & blood stasis

Main symptoms: Edematous swelling and chilling of the four extremities, possible swelling of a single leg accompanied by fixed pain of the leg and which may be either hot or cold, a scanty, stagnant, dark lochia which may contain clots, possible lower abdominal pain which is adverse to pressure, and a fine, bowstring, choppy pulse

Treatment principles: Rectify the qi and quicken the blood, transform stasis and move water

Guiding formula:

Tiao Jing Tang **(Regulate the Menses Decoction)**
Dang Gui (Radix Angelicae Sinensis), 9g
Chi Shao (Radix Rubrus Paeoniae Lactiflorae), 9g
Dan Pi (Cortex Moutan), 9g
Rou Gui (Cortex Cinnamomi), 3-9g
Chi Fu Ling (Sclerotium Rubrum Poriae Cocos), 9-15g
mix-fried *Gan Cao* (Radix Glycyrrhizae), 6-9g
Chen Pi (Pericarpium Citri Reticulatae), 6g
Xi Xin (Herba Asari), 1-3g
Gan Jiang (dry Rhizoma Zingiberis), 3-6g
Sheng Jiang (uncooked Rhizoma Zingiberis), 6g

Acupuncture & moxibustion: Xue Hai (Sp 10), Yin Ling Quan (Sp 9), San Yin Jiao (Sp 6), Zhong Ji (CV 3), Guan Yuan (CV 4)

If qi stagnation is marked, add *Tai Chong* (Liv 3) and *He Gu* (LI 4).

External contraction of wind evils

Main symptoms: Edematous face, eyes, and limbs, a slightly fat, swollen tongue with white fur, and a floating, fine pulse. Since external evils are affecting lung function in this case, there may also be chest oppression and/or panting as well as possible inhibition of urination.

Treatment principles: Diffuse the lungs and disinhibit dampness

Guiding formulas:

Jia Wei Wu Pi Tang (Added Flavors Five Skins Decoction)
Sang Bai Pi (Cortex Mori), 9g
Chen Pi (Pericarpium Citri Reticulatae), 6g
Jiang Pi (Cortex Rhizomatis Zingiberis), 6-9g
Fu Ling Pi (Cortex Sclerotii Poriae Cocos), 9-15g
Da Fu Pi (Pericarpium Arecae), 9g
Fang Ji (Radix Stephaniae Tetrandrae), 9g
stir-fried *Zhi Ke* (Fructus Aurantii), 6g
Zhu Ling (Polyporus), 9-15g
mix-fried *Gan Cao* (Radix Glycyrrhizae), 6-9g
Sheng Jiang (uncooked Rhizoma Zingiberis), 6g

Wu Pi San (Five Skins Powder)
Wu Jia Pi (Cortex Acanthopanacis), 9g
Di Gu Pi (Cortex Lycii), 9g
Da Fu Pi (Pericarpium Arecae), 9g
Fu Ling Pi (Cortex Sclerotii Poriae Cocos), 9-15g
Jiang Pi (Cortex Rhizomatis Zingiberis), 6-9g

Wang Guo-zhu *et al.* recommend this formula for postpartum swelling of the face and eyes, swelling and distention of the four limbs, and panting when these are due to wind damp damaging the spleen channel with qi and blood stasis and stagnation.

Acupuncture & moxibustion: He Gu (LI 4), Lie Que (Lu 7), Feng Men (Bl 12), Fei Shu (Bl 13), Yin Ling Quan (Sp 9)

Spleen vacuity not moving & transforming

Main symptoms: Postpartum edema, fatigue, lack of strength, abdominal distention after meals, possible loose stools, reduced appetite, a bland, sticky taste in the mouth, a pale facial complexion, slimy, white tongue fur, and a sodden, moderate (*i.e.*, relaxed or slightly slow) or fine, forceless pulse

Treatment principles: Fortify the spleen and transform dampness

Guiding formulas:

Xiao Tiao Jing Tang (Minor Regulate the Menses Decoction)
Fu Ling (Poria), 9-15g
Dang Gui (Radix Angelicae Sinensis), 9g
Bai Shao (Radix Albus Paeoniae Lactiflorae), 9g
Chen Pi (Pericarpium Citri Reticulatae), 6g
Bai Zhu (Rhizoma Atractylodis Macrocephalae), 9g

This formula treats spleen vacuity complicated by blood vacuity. If one adds *Chai Hu* (Radix Bupleuri), then it treats a liver-spleen disharmony complicated by blood vacuity and water swelling.

Jian Pi Li Shui Bu Zhong Tang
(Fortify the Spleen, Rectify Water & Supplement the Center Decoction)
Ren Shen (Radix Ginseng), 3-9g
Bai Zhi (Rhizoma Atractylodis Macrocephalae), 9g
Fu Ling (Poria), 9-15g
Bai Shao (Radix Albus Paeoniae Lactiflorae), 9g
Chen Pi (Pericarpium Citri Reticulatae), 6g
Mu Gua (Fructus Chaenomelis), 9g
Zi Su Ye (Folium Perillae Frutescentis), 9g
Cang Zhu (Rhizoma Atractylodis), 9g
Hou Po (Cortex Magnoliae Officinalis), 9g
Da Fu Pi (Pericarpium Arecae), 9g

This formula treats a liver-spleen disharmony with more dampness and turbidity than the previous formula. In addition, the edema is specifically located in the lower extremities.

Si Jun Zi Tang Jia Cang Zhu (Four Gentlemen Decoction plus Atractylodes)
Ren Shen (Radix Ginseng), 3-9g
mix-fried *Gan Cao* (Radix Glycyrrhizae), 6-9g
Bai Zhu (Rhizoma Atractylodis Macrocephalae), 9g
Cang Zhu (Rhizoma Atractylodis), 9g
Fu Ling (Poria), 9-15g

Huang Fu-zhong recommends this formula for postpartum superficial edema if there is great vacuity of the qi and blood.

Acupuncture & moxibustion: *San Yin Jiao* (Sp 6), *Yin Ling Quan* (Sp 9), *Zu San Li* (St 36), *Pi Shu* (Bl 20), *Wei Shu* (Bl 21)

Remarks

1. Because postpartum edema may be associated with potentially life-threatening conditions, care should be exercised in its diagnosis and treatment.

2. When edema accompanies hypertension and/or albuminuria, see the chapter on preeclampsia/eclampsia in Book 1 for further treatment options.

19

Postpartum Hematuria

According to modern Western medicine, there are a number of potential causes of postpartum hematuria, some of them relatively common and others relatively rare. First of all, birthing may have caused damage to the bladder. In a very few cases, the bladder may spontaneously rupture (a medical emergency) due to postpartum urinary retention. This condition is primarily found in women with perineal laceration repair and is characterized by abdominal pain, oliguria, and hematuria. It is also possible for stones in the urinary tract to cause bleeding postpartum the same as at other times in a woman's life, and women are three times more likely to develop nephrolithiasis than men (although not necessarily more likely to develop this postpartum). Urinary tract stones are characterized by fever and chills, intense, hard-to-bear, lancinating flank pain, nausea, and cold sweats to name several of this condition's prominent clinical features. In addition, a urinary tract infection may also cause postpartum hematuria, and urinary tract infection is the single most common of all extrapelvic postpartum infections.[1]

Chinese medical disease categorization

Blood in the urine seen with the naked eye in a postpartum woman is called *chan hou nao xue*, postpartum hematuria in Chinese.

Disease causes & disease mechanisms

In Chinese medicine, there are two main causes of postpartum hematuria. First, spoilt blood may enter the bladder. There, this blood stasis forces the blood to flow outside its pathways. Secondly, internal heat due to yin vacuity may cause the blood to boil over and run recklessly outside its vessels. It is also possible for injury during labor to result in blood in the urine. This last mechanism (and its associated pattern) is discussed under postpartum polyuria and incontinence.

Patterns common to this condition

Spoilt blood
Internal heat

Treatment based on pattern discrimination

Spoilt blood

Main symptoms: Postpartum hematuria with darkish colored blood which may even contain small clots, a scanty, dark-colored, nonfreely flowing lochia which may also contain clots, lower abdominal pain which is averse to pressure, a dark, purplish tongue or possible static spots or macules, and a bowstring, choppy pulse

Treatment principles: Quicken the blood and transform stasis, disinhibit dampness and stop bleeding

Guiding formula:

Xiao Ji Tang Jia Wei Yi Hao
(Small Thistle Decoction with Added Flavors #1)
Xiao Ji (Radix Cephalanoploris), 9-12g
Sheng Di (uncooked Radix Rehmanniae), 12-15g
Chi Shao (Radix Rubrus Paeoniae Lactiflorae), 9g
Mu Tong (Caulis Akebiae), 6-9g
Pu Huang (Pollen Typhae), 9g
Gan Cao (Radix Glycyrrhizae), 3-9g
Dan Zhu Ye (Herba Lophatheri), 9g
Hua Shi (Talcum), 9-15g
Deng Xin Cao (Medulla Junci), 1.5-4.5g

Acupuncture & moxibustion: *Xue Hai* (Sp 10), *Yin Ling Quan* (Sp 9), *San Yin Jiao* (Sp 6), *Guan Yuan* (CV 4), *Zhong Ji* (CV 3), *He Gu* (LI 4)

Internal heat

Main symptoms: Postpartum hematuria which is bright red in color, a bright red, possibly voluminous or incessant lochia, a dry mouth and parched throat, a red facial complexion, a red tongue with dry, white or slightly yellow fur, and a fine, rapid pulse

Treatment principles: Nourish yin, clear heat, and stop bleeding

Guiding formula:

Xiao Ji Tang Jia Wei Er Hao
(Small Thistle Decoction with Added Flavors #2)
Xiao Ji (Radix Cephalanoploris), 9-12g
Sheng Di (uncooked Radix Rehmanniae), 12-15g
Chi Shao (Radix Rubrus Paeoniae Lactiflorae), 9g

Mu Tong (Caulis Akebiae), 6-9g
Pu Huang (Pollen Typhae), 9g
Gan Cao (Radix Glycyrrhizae), 3-9g
Dan Zhu Ye (Herba Lophatheri), 9g
Hua Shi (Talcum), 9-15g
Deng Xin Cao (Medulla Junci), 1.5-4.5g
Huang Qin (Radix Scutellariae), 9-12g
Mai Men Dong (Tuber Ophiopogonis), 9-12g

Acupuncture & moxibustion: *San Yin Jiao* (Sp 6), *Tai Xi* (Ki 3), *Yin Ling Quan* (Sp 9), *Xue Hai* (Sp 10), *Shen Shu* (Bl 23), *Zhong Ji* (CV 3), *Guan Yuan* (CV 4)

Remarks

As the reader can see, the Chinese medicinal treatment of these two patterns is extremely similar, and, in real life, it is possible to have some combination of these two pattern–blood stasis and internal heat.

Endnote:

[1] O'Brien, William, "Puerperal Complications," *Gynecology & Obstetrics: A Longitudinal Approach, op. cit.,* p. 652

20

Postpartum Hemafecia

Postpartum hemafecia manifests as fresh red blood streaking the outside of the stools or fresh red blood dribbling and dripping from the anus after defecation. According to modern Western medicine, this condition is mostly associated with internal hemorrhoids. It is not considered a disease diagnosis in modern Western medicine.

Chinese medical disease categorization

Postpartum hemafecia is called *chan hou da bian chu xue* or *chan hou bian xue* for short.

Disease causes & disease mechanisms

During the last trimester of pregnancy, great weight is exerted by the growing fetus on the bottom of the lower burner. This tends to obstruct the free flow of the bowels and can cause the accumulation of stagnant heat in the bowels. After delivery, blood loss may cause an element of fluid dryness in the bowels which then allows for the engenderment of more obvious internal heat. This mechanism may be aggravated by overeating greasy, highly nutritious food postpartum in an attempt to recuperate from pregnancy and delivery. In this case, it is heat which causes the blood to move frenetically outside its pathways.

It is also possible for a postpartum woman to experience hemafecia due to spleen qi vacuity not containing the blood. This may be associated with qi and blood vacuity from excessive blood loss further weakening the spleen. It may also be associated with enduring spleen vacuity aggravated by the weight of the fetus during the last trimester and excessive use of force during delivery. Whether there is qi and blood vacuity affecting the spleen or downward falling of central qi, it is the spleen's inability to contain the blood within its vessels that causes the bleeding.

Patterns common to this condition

Large intestine heat accumulation
Spleen vacuity not containing

Treatment based on pattern discrimination

Large intestine heat accumulation

Main symptoms: Bright red blood accompanying the stools, often smeared along the outside of the feces, possible pain on defecation, a tendency to dry, bound stools, a red tongue with dry, yellow fur, and a fine, bowstring, rapid pulse

Treatment principles: Nourish and cool the blood, clear the large intestine and stop bleeding

Guiding formula:

**Jia Wei Qin Lian Si Wu Tang
(Added Flavors Scutellaria & Coptis Four Materials Decoction)**
Dang Gui (Radix Angelicae Sinensis), 9g
Sheng Di (uncooked Radix Rehmanniae), 12-15g
Chi Shao (Radix Rubrus Paeoniae Lactiflorae), 9g
Chuan Xiong (Radix Ligustici Wallichii), 6-9g
Huang Qin (Radix Scutellariae), 9-12g
Huang Lian (Rhizoma Coptidis), 3-9g
Di Yu (Radix Sanguisorbae), 6-9g
E Jiao (Gelatinum Corii Asini), 9g
carbonized *Jing Jie* (Herba Schizonepetae), 9g
mix-fried *Sheng Ma* (Rhizoma Cimicifugae), 3-6g

Acupuncture & moxibustion: *Tian Shu* (St 25), *Da Chang Shu* (Bl 25), *Shang Ju Xu* (St 37), *Chang Jiang* (GV 1), *Cheng Shan* (Bl 57)

If there is concomitant dampness, add *Yin Ling Quan* (Sp 9) and *Xing Jian* (Liv 2). If there is fever, add *He Gu* (LI 4) and *Qu Chi* (LI 11).

Spleen vacuity not containing

Main symptoms: Bleeding after defecation with no pain but pale, thin blood, a pale facial complexion, shortness of breath, fatigue, lack of strength in the four extremities, dizziness when standing up, a swollen, fat tongue with teeth-marks on its edges and thin fur, and a fine, forceless or vacuous pulse. If there is qi and blood dual vacuity, a pale facial complexion, pale lips, and a pale tongue are even more marked. If there is central qi falling downward, there is a heavy, dragging feeling in the anus after defecation or at the bottom of the pelvis upon standing and a deep or short pulse in the inch position.

Treatment principles: Fortify the spleen and supplement the qi. If there is qi and blood dual vacuity, supplement the qi and nourish the blood. If there is downward falling of the central qi, fortify the spleen and boost the qi, lift the fallen and stop bleeding.

Guiding formulas:

Gui Pi Tang (Restore the Spleen Decoction)
Ren Shen (Radix Ginseng), 3-9g
Huang Qi (Radix Astragali), 9-18g
Dang Gui (Radix Angelicae Sinensis), 9g
Long Yan Rou (Arillus Euphoriae Longanae), 9g
Bai Zhu (Rhizoma Atractylodis Macrocephalae), 9g
Mu Xiang (Radix Auklandiae), 6-9g
Fu Ling (Poria), 9-12g
Yuan Zhi (Radix Polygalae), 6-9g
Suan Zao Ren (Semen Zizyphi Spinosae), 9-12g
mix-fried *Gan Cao* (Radix Glycyrrhizae), 6-9g
Sheng Jiang (uncooked Rhizoma Zingiberis), 6g
Da Zao (Fructus Jujubae), 3 pieces

This formula is for a heart qi & blood-spleen qi vacuity possibly and commonly complicated by liver depression. To increase its bleeding-stopping effect, one can add *E Jiao* (Gelatinum Corii Asini).

Bu Zhong Yi Qi Tang (Supplement the Center & Boost the Qi Decoction)
Huang Qi (Radix Astragali), 9-18g
Ren Shen (Radix Ginseng), 3-9g
Bai Zhu (Rhizoma Atractylodis Macrocephalae), 9g
mix-fried *Gan Cao* (Radix Glycyrrhizae), 6-9g
Dang Gui (Radix Angelicae Sinensis), 9g
Chen Pi (Pericarpium Citri Reticulatae), 6g
Chai Hu (Radix Bupleuri), 3-9g
Sheng Ma (Rhizoma Cimicifugae), 3-4.5g

This formula is for qi vacuity falling downward. To increase its bleeding-stopping effect, one can add *Xian He Cao* (Herba Agrimoniae).

Acupuncture & moxibustion: *Pi Shu* (Bl 20), *Xiao Chang Shu* (Bl 22), *Tai Bai* (Sp 1), *Zu San Li* (St 36), *Guan Yuan* (CV 4), *San Yin Jiao* (Sp 6)

If there is accompanying indigestion, add *Zhang Men* (Liv 13) and *Gong Sun* (Sp 4). If qi vacuity not containing the blood is unstoppable, add moxibustion at *Ming Men* (GV 4).

Remarks

1. If large intestine heat is associated with overeating fatty, greasy, fried and/or hot, spicy food or drinking alcohol, of course, the patient should be switched to a clear, bland diet.

2. In case of central qi downward falling, bed rest should be encouraged and fatigue definitely avoided.

21

Postpartum Spontaneous Perspiration & Night Sweats

In Chinese medicine, there are two main abnormalities of perspiration—spontaneous perspiration and night sweats—and each may be considered a disease category or major complaint in its own right. In modern Western medicine, abnormalities in perspiration are considered symptoms, not diseases. In the case of postpartum night sweats, these are mostly due to hormonal changes experienced during the puerperium and breast-feeding. As the reader will remember, abnormal sweating is considered one of the three postpartum emergencies in Chinese medicine. This is because, postpartum women are typically vacuous to begin with and sweating is both a loss of yang qi and yin fluids.

Chinese medical disease categorization

Postpartum women may suffer from sweating while awake during the day which occurs spontaneously or by only slight exertion. In Chinese medicine, this is called spontaneous perspiration, *zi han*. It is also common for postpartum women to experience outbreaks of sweating which wake them from sleep in the middle of the night. This is called thief sweating or *dao han* in Chinese.

Disease causes & disease mechanisms

If the woman is habitually vacuous and weak, birthing may further damage her qi and blood. Thus the qi vacuity becomes more severe and defensive yang may fail to secure. In that case, the interstices are not densely packed and the qi or ghost gates (*i.e.*, the pores) are left wide open. This results in spontaneous perspiration. If both qi and blood are vacuous and weak, it may also result in night sweats.

On the other hand, if the birthing woman is habitually yin and constructive vacuous and, during birth, she loses a lot of blood, yin and blood may become even more vacuous and depleted. In this case, insufficient yin fails to control yang, thus giv-

349

ing rise to the engenderment of internal heat. Since yin rules the night, if yin is vacuous, yang may counterflow upward and outward at night. Since defensive yang rules the pores, the pores are thrown open. Then, since qi moves water, this results in night sweats. In addition, yin vacuity with yang jumping upward may also cause sweating specifically from the head since the head is the reunion of yang.

Patterns common to this condition

Qi vacuity spontaneous perspiration
Yin vacuity night sweats

Treatment based on pattern discrimination

Qi vacuity spontaneous perspiration

Main symptoms: Excessive postpartum perspiration which does not stop on its own and is exacerbated by slight movement or exertion, aversion to wind, a lusterless, white facial complexion, shortness of breath, disinclination to speak and a feeble voice, fatigue, lack of strength, dizziness standing up, a pale tongue with thin fur, and a fine, forceless or weak pulse

Treatment principles: Supplement the qi and secure the exterior, harmonize the constructive and stop sweating

Guiding formulas:

Huang Qi Tang (Astragalus Decoction)
Huang Qi (Radix Astragali), 9-45g
Bai Zhu (Rhizoma Atractylodis Macrocephalae), 9g
Fang Feng (Radix Sapshnikoviae), 9g
Shu Di (cooked Radix Rehmanniae), 9-15g
calcined *Mu Li* (Concha Ostreae), 9-18g
Fu Ling (Poria), 9-12g
Mai Men Dong (Tuber Ophiopogonis), 9-12g
Gan Cao (Radix Glycyrrhizae), 3-9g
Da Zao (Fructus Jujubae), 3 pieces

Gui Zhi Jia Long Gu Mu Li Tang
(Cinnamon Twigs plus Dragon Bone & Oyster Shell Decoction)
Gui Zhi (Ramulus Cinnamomi), 6-9g
Bai Shao (Radix Albus Paeoniae Lactiflorae), 9-18g
mix-fried *Gan Cao* (Radix Glycyrrhizae), 6-9g
Pao Jiang (blast-fried Rhizoma Zingiberis), 6-9g
Hong Hua (Flos Carthami), 9g
calcined *Mu Li* (Concha Ostreae), 9-18g
calcined *Long Gu* (Os Draconis), 9-18g

If there is fear of cold and lack of strength, this is due to lung qi vacuity. In this case, add *Huang Qi* (Radix Astragali).

Ma Huang Gen Tang (Ephedra Root Decoction)
Dang Gui (Radix Angelicae Sinensis), 9g
Huang Qi (Radix Astragali), 9-45g
Ma Huang Gen (Radix Ephedrae), 9g
Ren Shen (Radix Ginseng), 3-9g
mix-fried *Gan Cao* (Radix Glycyrrhizae), 6-9g
calcined *Mu Li* (Concha Ostreae), 9-18g

Wang Guo-zhu *et al.* include *Bai Zhu* (Rhizoma Atractylodis Macrocephalae), *Gui Zhi* (Ramulus Cinnamomi), and *Fu Xiao Mai* (Fructus Levis Tritici Aestivi) in their version of this formula. They then go on to recommend the following modifications: If there is vacuity desertion and the feet and hands are chilly, add *Zhi Fu Zi* (Radix Lateralis Praeparatus Aconiti Carmichaeli) and *Gan Jiang* (dry Rhizoma Zingiberis). If there is thirst, add *Mai Men Dong* (Tuber Ophiopogonis), *Wu Wei Zi* (Fructus Schisandrae), and *Shu Di* (cooked Radix Rehmanniae). If there is phlegm, add *Zhu Li* (Succus Bambusae) and *Jiang Ye* (Succus Rhizomatis Zingiberis). If urination is not free-flowing, add medicinals to disinhibit water. If there is alternating hot and cold, it is *not* alright to add *Chai Hu* (Radix Bupleuri). If there is headache and fever, it is *not* alright to use *Ma Huang* (Herba Ephedrae), *Huang Qin* (Radix Scutellariae), *Huang Bai* (Cortex Phellodendri), or excessive windy herbs. If there is fever and great thirst, *Ban Xia* (Rhizoma Pinelliae) and *Sheng Jiang* (uncooked Rhizoma Zingiberis) are forbidden.

Acupuncture & moxibustion: He Gu (LI 4), *Fu Liu* (Ki 7), *Zu San Li* (St 36), *Pi Shu* (Bl 20)

If there is blood vacuity, add *Ge Shu* (Bl 17) and *Gan Shu* (Bl 18).

Yin vacuity night sweats

Main symptoms: Postpartum night sweats, a flushed red facial complexion, dizziness, tinnitus, a dry mouth and parched throat, thirst but no particular desire to drink, possible heat in the hands, feet, and heart, low back and knee soreness and limpness, a red tongue with scanty or no fur, and a fine, rapid, possibly forceless; a vacuous; or a surging pulse

Treatment principles: Nourish yin and boost the qi, engender fluids and stop sweating

Guiding formulas:

Dang Gui Liu Huang Tang (Dang Gui Six Yellows Decoction)
Huang Lian (Rhizoma Coptidis), 3-9g
Huang Qin (Radix Scutellariae), 9-12g
Huang Bai (Cortex Phellodendri), 9g
Dang Gui (Radix Angelicae Sinensis), 9g

Huang Qi (Radix Astragali), 9-18g
Sheng Di (uncooked Radix Rehmanniae), 12-15g
Shu Di (cooked Radix Rehmanniae), 12-15g

This formula clears internal heat as well as nourishes yin and blood.

Unnamed formula for night sweating given by Wang Guo-zhu *et al.*
Ren Shen (Radix Ginseng), 3-9g
Dang Gui (Radix Angelicae Sinensis), 9g
Ma Huang Gen (Radix Ephedrae), 9g
Shu Di (cooked Radix Rehmanniae), 12-15g
Huang Qin (Radix Scutellariae), 9-12g
Fu Xiao Mai (Fructus Levis Tritici Aestivi), 25-45g

This formula treats qi and yin vacuity night sweats.

Acupuncture & moxibustion: *He Gu* (LI 4), *Fu Liu* (Ki 7), *San Yin Jiao* (Sp 6), *Gan Shu* (Bl 18), *Shen Shu* (Bl 23)

Representative case history

The patient was a 36 year-old female who was initially examined on Aug. 3, 1993. This woman had had a cesarean delivery. During her pregnancy, she had developed hypertension and diabetes. At the time of delivery, it was the height of summer heat. After delivery, the patient sweated extremely profusely. During the daytime, her perspiration was normal, but, at night, she drenched her bedclothes. The patient was anxious and worried and there was lassitude of the spirit, limpness of the limbs, poor appetite, noncrisp bowel movements, a dry mouth and parched throat, lower and upper back soreness, joint pain, a tendency to catch cold, a somewhat red tongue with slimy, thin fur, and a fine, bowstring pulse.

Based on the above signs and symptoms, the patient's pattern was discriminated as yin fluid depletion and detriment. Therefore, in order to boost the qi and nourish yin, stop sweating and secure the exterior, she was prescribed *Sheng Mai San* (Engender the Pulse Powder) plus *Dang Gui Liu Huang Tang* (Dang Gui Six Yellows Decoction) with additions and subtractions: *Dang Shen* (Radix Codonopsitis), 12g, *Sha Shen* (Radix Glehniae), 12g, *Mai Men Dong* (Tuber Ophiopogonis), 6g, *Wu Wei Zi* (Fructus Schisandrae), 6g, *Dang Gui* (Radix Angelicae Sinensis), 12g, *Huang Qi* (Radix Astragali), 15g, *Sheng Di* (uncooked Radix Rehmanniae), 12g, *Huang Qin* (Radix Scutellariae), 9g, *Huang Lian* (Rhizoma Coptidis), 9g, *Huang Bai* (Cortex Phellodendri), 9g, *Jin Ying Zi* (Fructus Rosae Laevigatae), 12g, *Gou Qi Zi* (Fructus Lycii), 9g, *Xu Duan* (Radix Dipsaci), 12g, and *Da Zao* (Fructus Jujubae), 10g.

At the second examination, the prescribing physician removed *Jin Ying Zi* and *Huang Bai* and added three grams each of *Sha Ren* (Fructus Amomi) and *Fo Shou* (Fructus Citri Sacrodactylis) in order to fortify the spleen and harmonize the stomach. After two weeks of taking these medicinals, the patient's perspiration decreased, however, if she discontinued the treatment, the condition recurred. Therefore, she continued this treatment for three months, after which her sweating was basically cured. However, her joint pain was not cured, and, for this, the woman received acupuncture combined with Chinese medicinals in order to nourish the blood and free the flow of the network vessels.

Remarks

1. Basically, Chinese medicine posits only one main disease mechanism each for spontaneous perspiration and night sweats. For spontaneous perspiration, that is qi vacuity, while for night sweats, it is yin vacuity. Therefore, these should be the first hypotheses explored for either of these two complaints. In a few cases, damp heat may also cause night sweats. However, this is not so likely postpartum.

2. Whenever dealing with abnormal sweating, it is usually a good idea and often absolutely necessary to include one or more medicinals with an empirically known ability to stop sweating. In Chinese medicine, such medicinals tend to fall under one of three categories: qi supplementing, securing and astringing medicinals, or heavy, settling, spirit-quieting medicinals. For instance, *Huang Qi* (Radix Astragali) is a qi-supplementing medicinal with a pronounced effect on stopping sweating. Among the securing and astringing, *Fu Xiao Mai* (Fructus Levis Tritici Aestivi), *Wu Wei Zi* (Fructus Schisandrae), and *Ma Huang Gen* (Radix Ephedrae) are the medicinals of choice. Among the heavy, settling, spirit-quieting medicinals, it is *Mu Li* (Concha Ostreae) and *Long Gu* (Os Draconis) which also secure the exterior and stop sweating.

3. I have treated a number of cases of both postpartum spontaneous perspiration and night sweats. However, these are not usually the patient's major complaints, although, sometimes, night sweats can be. In any case, abnormal sweating is usually something Chinese medicine deals with quite well, and, if the patient's abnormal perspiration is brought under control, the patient will definitely feel better in other areas of their body and life.

22

Postpartum Constipation

Constipation is a somewhat ambiguous term. It can mean different things to different people. It can mean lack of defecation for more than a day, it can mean hard, dry, bound stools, or it can mean that the act of passing stools is difficult and hesitant. In Chinese medicine, any or all these things can fall under this disease category, and, constipation is a common complaint during the puerperium. As much as 50% of all recently delivered women experience constipation.[1] Some of the causes of postpartum constipation besides the continuation of constipation which developed during pregnancy include the use of some pain pills, such as Vicodin and Percoset, perineal soreness due to tear, episiotomy, and/or hemorrhoids which leads to consciously or unconsciously withholding the stools, atony of the bowels due to cesaraen section, and some iron pills which may be taken for postpartum anemia.

Chinese medical disease categorization

Chan hou da bian nan literally means difficulty passing stools postpartum. This is also referred to in the Chinese gynecology literature as *chan hou da bian bi se bu tong*, postpartum defecation blocked, astringent, and not free-flowing.

Disease causes & disease mechanisms

If there is excessive loss of blood during delivery, the construction and blood may have become vacuous and insufficient. In that case, fluids and humors may also have become consumed and depleted. These then are not able to lubricate and moisten the intestines that are parched and dry. Thus passage of the stools is difficult. In addition, if the qi is too vacuous and weak to move the stools through the intestinal tract, this may complicate blood and fluid dryness and insufficiency.

In women who are chronically or constitutionally yin vacuous, postpartum vacuity may lead to exacerbation of yin vacuity with flourishing of fire. Such fire may internally scorch body fluids and humors. The fluids become scanty and the humors become depleted. The intestinal tract loses its nourishment and moisture, and this likewise leads to the stools being dry and bound.

It is also possible, but less probable in Western patients, that overeating postpartum has caused food damage to the stomach and intestines. Due to accumulation, there is stagnation, and due to stagnation, there is lack of movement.

Patterns common to this condition

Spleen-stomach vacuity weakness, qi & blood dual vacuity
Yin & blood insufficiency
Yin vacuity-internal heat
Food damage bowel binding

Treatment based on pattern discrimination

Spleen-stomach vacuity weakness, qi & blood dual vacuity

Main symptoms: Dry, parched, difficult to precipitate stools postpartum despite normal eating and drinking, a sallow yellow facial complexion, dry skin, no abdominal aching or pain, a pale tongue with thin fur, and a fine, forceless or small, weak pulse

Treatment principles: Fortify the spleen and supplement the qi, nourish the blood and moisten dryness

Guiding formulas:

Ba Zhen Tang Jia Yu Li Ren Huo Ma Ren
(Eight Pearls Decoction plus Prune Pit & Cannabis)
Ren Shen (Radix Ginseng), 3-9g
mix-fried *Gan Cao* (Radix Glycyrrhizae), 6-9g
Bai Zhu (Rhizoma Atractylodis Macrocephalae), 9g
Fu Ling (Poria), 9g
Dang Gui (Radix Angelicae Sinensis), 9g
Bai Shao (Radix Albus Paeoniae Lactiflorae), 9g
Shu Di (cooked Radix Rehmanniae), 12-15g
Chuan Xiong (Radix Ligustici Wallichii), 6-9g
Yu Li Ren (Semen Pruni), 9g
Huo Ma Ren (Semen Cannabis), 9-12g

Ruan Zao Tang **(Moisten Dryness Decoction)**
Ren Shen (Radix Ginseng), 3-9g
Gan Cao (Radix Glycyrrhizae), 3-9g
Dang Gui (Radix Angelicae Sinensis), 9g

Sheng Di (uncooked Radix Rehmanniae), 12-15g
Zhi Ke (Fructus Aurantii), 6g
Huo Ma Ren (Semen Cannabis), 9-12g
Tao Ren (Semen Persicae), 9g
Bing Lang (Semen Arecae), 6-9g

In this case, qi and blood vacuity are complicated by qi stagnation and blood stasis.

Bu Zhong Yi Qi Tang Jia Wei (Supplement the Center & Boost the Qi Decoction with Added Flavors)
Huang Qi (Radix Astragali), 9-18g
Chen Pi (Pericarpium Citri Reticulatae), 6g
Sheng Ma (Rhizoma Cimicifugae), 3-4.5g
Chai Hu (Radix Bupleuri), 3-9g
Dang Gui (Radix Angelicae Sinensis), 9g
mix-fried *Gan Cao* (Radix Glycyrrhizae), 6-9g
Dang Shen (Radix Codonopsitis), 9g
Huo Ma Ren (Semen Cannabis), 9-12g
Yu Li Ren (Semen Pruni), 9g
Shan Yao (Radix Dioscoreae), 9g

If there is abdominal distention, glomus, and fullness, add *Mu Xiang* (Radix Auklandiae), *Zhi Ke* (Fructus Aurantii), *Hou Po* (Cortex Magnoliae Officinalis), and processed *Da Huang* (Radix Et Rhizoma Rhei). If there are heart palpitations and loss of sleep, add *Bai Zi Ren* (Semen Platycladi) and *Yi Zhi Ren* (Fructus Alpiniae Oxyphyllae). If qi and yin are both vacuous with a dry mouth and parched throat, add *Mai Men Dong* (Tuber Ophiopogonis) and *Wu Wei Zi* (Fructus Schisandrae).

Acupuncture & moxibustion: *Tian Shu* (St 25), *Da Chang Shu* (Bl 25), *Pi Shu* (Bl 20), *Zhong Wan* (CV 12), *Zu San Li* (St 36)

If there is concomitant blood vacuity, add *Ge Shu* (Bl 17) and *Gan Shu* (Bl 18).

Yin & blood insufficiency

Main symptoms: This pattern is similar to the above except that there is no particular spleen qi vacuity signs and symptoms and the yin vacuity symptoms are more pronounced. There is unresolved constipation several days after delivery but no distention or pain in the lower abdomen. Food and drink are normal. There is vertigo, dizziness, impaired memory, dry skin, and a flushed red facial complexion. The lips and tongue are dry and pale, but there is heat in the hands, feet, and heart. The pulse is bowstring and fine.

Treatment principles: Enrich yin and supplement the blood, moisten dryness and free the flow of the bowels

Guiding formulas:

Si Wu Tang Jia Wei (Four Materials Decoction with Added Flavors)
Dang Gui (Radix Angelicae Sinensis), 9g
Shu Di (cooked Radix Rehmanniae), 12-15g
Bai Shao (Radix Albus Paeoniae Lactiflorae), 9g
Chuan Xiong (Radix Ligustici Wallichii), 6-9g
Rou Cong Rong (Herba Cistanchis), 9g
Song Ren (Semen Pini), 9g
Hei Zhi Ma (black Semen Sesami Indici), 9-15g

Yi Xue Run Chang Pian (Boost the Blood & Moisten the Intestines Tablets)
Shu Di (cooked Radix Rehmanniae), 12-15g
Xing Ren (Semen Armeniacae), 9g
Huo Ma Ren (Semen Cannabis), 9-12g
Zhi Ke (Fructus Aurantii), 6g
Ju Hong (Exocarpium Citri Erythrocarpae), 6-9g
E Jiao (Gelatinum Corii Asini), 9g
Rou Cong Rong (Herba Cistanchis), 9g
Zi Su Zi (Fructus Perillae Frutescentis), 9g
Dang Gui (Radix Angelicae Sinensis), 9g

If there is lassitude of the spirit, shortness of breath, and spontaneous perspiration, add *Dang Shen* (Radix Codonopsitis), *Huang Qi* (Radix Astragali), and *Shan Yao* (Radix Dioscoreae). If there is epigastric and abdominal distention and fullness, add *Shan Zha* (Fructus Crataegi), *Liu Qu* (Massa Medica Fermentata), *Zhi Ke* (Fructus Aurantii), *Huo Po* (Cortex Magnoliae Officinalis), *Da Huang* (processed Radix Et Rhizoma Rhei), and *Gua Lou* (Fructus Trichosanthis). If there is dry mouth and parched throat with a red tongue and scanty fluids, add *Mai Men Dong* (Tuber Ophiopogonis), *Sheng Di* (uncooked Radix Rehmanniae), *Xuan Shen* (Radix Scrophulariae), *Tian Hua Fen* (Radix Trichosanthis), *Shi Hu* (Herba Dendrobii), *Yu Zhu* (Rhizoma Polygonati Odorati), and *Gua Lou Ren* (Semen Trichosanthis). If there is yin vacuity and fire dryness with vexatious heat in the five hearts and epigastric and abdominal glomus and distention, add *Da Huang* (uncooked Radix Et Rhizoma Rhei), *Huang Lian* (Rhizoma Coptidis), *Zhi Zi* (Fructus Gardeniae), *Sheng Di* (uncooked Radix Rehmanniae), and *Di Gu Pi* (Cortex Lycii) and remove the *Ju Hong* and *Rou Cong Rong*.

Acupuncture & moxibustion: *Tian Shu* (St 25), *Da Chang Shu* (Bl 25), *Ge Shu* (Bl 17), *Gan Shu* (Bl 18), *San Yin Jiao* (Sp 6), *Zhao Hai* (Ki 6)

Yin vacuity-internal heat

Main symptoms: Postpartum constipation with a dry mouth, a full chest, abdominal distention, a red tongue with thin, yellow fur, and a fine, rapid pulse

Treatment principles: Nourish the blood, moisten dryness, and precipitate heat

Guiding formulas:

Yu Li Ren Yin (Prune Pit Drink)
Yu Li Ren (Semen Pruni), 9g
Mang Xiao (Mirabilitum), 3-9g
Dang Gui (Radix Angelicae Sinensis), 9g
Sheng Di (uncooked Radix Rehmanniae), 12-15g

Ma Ren Wan Jia Wei (Cannabis Seed Pills with Added Flavors)
Zhi Ke (Fructus Aurantii), 6g
Ren Shen (Radix Ginseng), 3-9g
Da Huang (Radix Et Rhizoma Rhei), 3-9g
Mi Tang (honey), a suitable amount
Mai Men Dong (Tuber Ophiopogonis), 9-12g
Xuan Shen (Radix Scrophulariae), 9-12g

Yi Xue Ruan Chang Tang
(Boost the Blood & Moisten the Intestines Decoction)
Sheng Di (uncooked Radix Rehmanniae), 12-15g
Dang Gui (Radix Angelicae Sinensis), 9g
Huo Ma Ren (Semen Cannabis), 9-12g
Zhi Ke (Fructus Aurantii), 6g
Gua Lou Ren (Semen Trichosanthis), 9g
Xuan Shen (Radix Scrophulariae), 9-12g
Suo Yang (Herba Cynomorii), 9g

This formula is for use with yin vacuity with only a small amount of internal heat manifesting as a dry, hot throat.

Acupuncture & moxibustion: *Tian Shu* (St 25), *Da Chang Shu* (Bl 25), *Ge Shu* (Bl 17), *Gan Shu* (Bl 18), *San Yin Jiao* (Sp 6), *Zhao Hai* (Ki 6), *He Gu* (LI 4), *Nei Ting* (St 44)

Food damage bowel binding

Main symptoms: Non-smoothly flowing stools or constipation which is not freely flowing, epigastric and abdominal distention and fullness, a foul mouth odor, heart vexation, easy anger, a red tongue with yellow or dry, yellow fur, and a bowstring or bowstring, rapid pulse

Treatment principles: Clear heat, abduct stagnation, and free the flow of the stools

Guiding formulas:

Dang Gui Cheng Qi Tang (Dang Gui Order the Qi Decoction)
Dang Gui (Radix Angelicae Sinensis), 9g
uncooked *Da Huang* (Radix Et Rhizoma Rhei), 3-9g
Mang Xiao (Mirabilitum), 3-6g
Hou Po (Cortex Magnoliae Officinalis), 6-9g

Zhi Ke (Fructus Aurantii), 6g
mix-fried *Gan Cao* (Radix Glycyrrhizae), 6-9g

Postpartum, mostly there is vacuity damage of the fluids. However, in this case, this is mixed with a bowel repletion pattern. Therefore, one must use bitter, cold, harsh, draining medicinals with care. One should not use the above formula for a long time. Once the stools are freely and smoothly flowing, this formula should be stopped and then medicinals should be administered based on the pattern discrimination.

Zhi Shi Dao Zhi Tang (Immature Aurantium Abduct Stagnation Decoction)
Zhi Shi (Fructus Immaturus Aurantii), 6-9g
Hou Po (Cortex Magnoliae Officinalis), 6-9g
Gua Lou Ren (Semen Trichosanthis), 9g
Ji Nei Jin (Endothelium Corneum Gigeriae Galli), 6-9g
scorched *Shan Zha* (Fructus Crataegi), 9g
Shen Qu (Massa Medica Fermentata), 9g
Yu Li Ren (Semen Pruni), 9g
Chen Pi (Pericarpium Citri Reticulatae), 6g
Sha Ren (Fructus Amomi), 3-4.5g

Acupuncture & moxibustion: *Tian Shu* (St 25), *Da Chang Shu* (Bl 25), *Zhong Wan* (CV 12), *Liang Men* (St 21), *He Gu* (LI 4), *Nei Ting* (St 44), *Zu San Li* (St 36), *Zhi Gou* (TB 6)

If fluids have been damaged by heat, add *Zhao Hai* (Ki 6). If there is marked qi stagnation, add *Yang Ling Quan* (GB 34).

Remarks

1. Although postpartum constipation is usually benign and self-limiting, it may be a symptom of something potentially serious. Therefore, practitioners should take special care whenever postpartum constipation is accompanied by severe, constant or worsening abdominal pain, fever above 101.3° F (38.5° C), rash, rectal bleeding, and/or vomiting.

2. Besides the above treatment methods, patients with postpartum constipation should:

   A. Drink plenty of fluids

   B. Eat high fiber foods

   C. Get some exercise, like walking, even though this may be painful at first and especially if there has been a c-section or episiotomy

   D. Relax

3. In general, it is my experience that Chinese medicine treats constipation,

including postpartum constipation, very well as long as the treatment is predicated on the patient's personal pattern(s). Although textbooks such as this divide constipation into several neat categories, real-life patients with constipation typically present complex, multi-pattern scenarios which may include, in addition to the above, qi stagnation, blood stasis, and/or dampness.

4. Although *Da Huang* (Radix Et Rhizoma Rhei) will purge the bowels in almost any person with constipation no matter what their pattern discrimination, it will only create further problems if used in patients not suffering from bowel heat repletion and/or if it is used too long. Therefore, practitioners should not think of this medicinal as a panacea for constipation.

5. While acupuncture may treat food stagnation constipation and aid in cases complicated by internal heat, it is not so effective in yin and blood vacuity patterns of difficult defecation.

Endnote:

[1] www.babycenter.com/refcap/baby/physrecovery/11707.html

23

Postpartum Diarrhea & Dysentery

In Chinese medicine, diarrhea refers to profuse, loose, watery, possible urgent stools with or without cramping which occur up to 10 times per day. Dysentery refers to profuse, loose, watery, possibly urgent stools which occur more than 10 times per day. In this case, there typically is cramping, and there can be either or both blood and mucus in the stools. Because irritable bowel syndrome (a.k.a. mucus colitis) may result in diarrhea with mucus in the stools, and ulcerative colitis and Crohn's disease may also result in blood and/or mucus in the stools, the Chinese category of dysentery often covers these Western conditions. While I know of no statistical evidence of increased incidence of any of these three conditions postpartum, since they are all linked, at least in part, to psychoemotional stress and depression, and since having a new baby is stressful and many postpartum women become variably depressed, it is not unreasonable to think that some women see a worsening of these conditions during the puerperium. In addition, this Chinese disease category also covers both bacterial and amebic dysentery occurring postpartum.

Chinese medical disease categorization

Postpartum diarrhea is referred to as *chan hou xie xie* in Chinese, while postpartum dysentery is referred to as *chan hou xie li*. In this latter case, the word *li* is the Chinese word for dysentery.

Disease causes & disease mechanisms

Postpartum diarrhea and dysentery are mostly due to postpartum qi and blood vacuity. This can result in the spleen losing its governance of movement and transformation. In that case, water and grains are not transformed, nor is their finest essence transported upward. Thus, clear and turbid are not separated, and there is diarrhea.

Postpartum vacuity can also lead to a loss of harmony between the constructive and defensive. In that case, external wind cold evils or summerheat and dampness may take advantage of this vacuity to invade the body, thus causing diarrhea if not too serious or dysentery if more serious. In some cases, evil cold and heat may join together. Contraction of cold and chill leads to a downward discharge of white pus, while contraction of dampness and heat leads to a downward discharge of yellow mucus and red blood, with possible sudden bleeding from the anus. If cold and heat join together, this may lead to the downward discharge of white and red or pus and blood.

Postpartum women are also especially susceptible to damage due to food stagnation. Because of postpartum qi and blood vacuity, their spleens tend to be weaker than usual. However, because many people believe that a postpartum recuperating woman should eat highly nutritious food, she may be fed an excessive amount of such rich, greasy, fatty things. In that case, stagnant food fails to advance, and pure and turbid are not separated. Thus defecation loses its normalcy.

Patterns common to this condition

Spleen vacuity

Cold dampness

Damp heat

Food stagnation

Postpartum red dysentery due to heat damaging the uterine vessel

Postpartum white dysentery due to cold dampness

Postpartum red & white dysentery due to dampness & heat mutually wrestling

Treatment based on pattern discrimination

Spleen vacuity

Main symptoms: Postpartum diarrhea with borborygmus, chest and ductal distention and oppression, lower abdominal aching and pain, inhibited urination, fatigue, no appetite for food and drink, a sallow yellow facial complexion, and a fine, forceless, possibly moderate (*i.e.*, relaxed, slightly slow) pulse

Treatment principles: Fortify the spleen, eliminate dampness, and stop diarrhea

Guiding formulas:

Shen Ling Bai Zhu San (Ginseng, Poria & Atractylodes Powder)
Ren Shen (Radix Ginseng), 3-9g
Bai Zhu (Rhizoma Atractylodis Macrocephalae), 9g
Fu Ling (Poria), 9-12g
Bai Bian Dou (Semen Dolichoris), 9-12g
Chen Pi (Pericarpium Citri Reticulatae), 6g
Shan Yao (Radix Dioscoreae), 9-12g

Gan Cao (Radix Glycyrrhizae), 3-9g
Lian Rou (Semen Nelumbinis), 9g
Sha Ren (Fructus Amomi), 3-4.5g
Yi Yi Ren (Semen Coicis), 15-30g
Sheng Jiang (uncooked Rhizoma Zingiberis), 6g
Da Zao (Fructus Jujubae), 3 pieces

This formula is for spleen vacuity diarrhea complicated by dampness.

Li Zhong Wan (Rectify the Center Pills)
Ren Shen (Radix Ginseng), 3-9g
Bai Zhu (Rhizoma Atractylodis Macrocephalae), 9g
Gan Jiang (dry Rhizoma Zingiberis), 6g
mix-fried *Gan Cao* (Radix Glycyrrhizae), 6-9g

This formula is for spleen vacuity complicated by yang vacuity. If the diarrhea will not stop, add *Rou Gui* (Cortex Cinnamomi) and *Rou Dou Kou* (Fructus Myristicae).

Jia Jian Sheng Hua Tang
(Modified Engendering & Transforming Decoction)
Chuan Xiong (Radix Ligustici Wallichii), 9-15g
Fu Ling (Poria), 9-12g
Dang Gui (Radix Angelicae Sinensis), 9g
Pao Jiang (blast-fried Rhizoma Zingiberis), 6-9g
mix-fried *Gan Cao* (Radix Glycyrrhizae), 6-9g
Tao Ren (Semen Persicae), 9g
Lian Zi (Semen Nelumbinis), 9g

Fu Qing-zhu says to use this formula for spleen vacuity postpartum diarrhea when there is still spoilt blood retained in the uterus as evidenced by clots not yet eliminated from the lochia.

Acupuncture & moxibustion: Zhong Wan (CV 12), Tian Shu (St 25), Da Chang Shu (Bl 25), Pi Shu (Bl 20), Wei Shu (Bl 21), Zu San Li (St 36)

Cold dampness

Main symptoms: Postpartum diarrhea accompanied by chilly abdominal pain, greenish white urination, lack of warmth in the four limbs, a greenish white facial complexion, pale, moist lips and tongue, no oral dryness or thirst, and a deep, moderate (*i.e.*, relaxed, slightly slow) pulse

Treatment principles: Fortify the spleen, warm the middle, and stop diarrhea

Guiding formula:

Tiao Zhong Tang (Regulate the Center Decoction)
Sheng Jiang (uncooked Rhizoma Zingiberis), 6g
Gan Jiang (dry Rhizoma Zingiberis), 6-9g
Dang Gui (Radix Angelicae Sinensis), 9g

Rou Gui (Cortex Cinnamomi), 3-9g
Bai Shao (Radix Albus Paeoniae Lactiflorae), 9g
Chuan Xiong (Radix Ligustici Wallichii), 6-9g
Zhi Fu Zi (Radix Lateralis Praeparatus Aconiti Carmichaeli), 3-9g
Ren Shen (Radix Ginseng), 3-9g
Gan Cao (Radix Glycyrrhizae), 3-9g

Han Bail-ling suggests adding *Bai Zhu* (Rhizoma Atractylodis Macrocephalae) and *Fu Ling* (Poria) to fortify the spleen and seep dampness.

Acupuncture & moxibustion: Same as above, except with moxibustion

Damp heat

Main symptoms: Postpartum diarrhea consisting of yellow water or yellow stools, inhibited urination, a scorching hot anus after defecation, heart vexation, thirst, heat emitted from the four limbs, pain in the front of the abdomen, a bitter taste in the mouth and a dry throat, a desire for cold drinks, a red facial complexion, a red tongue with yellow, possible slimy fur, and a bowstring, slippery, rapid pulse

Treatment principles: Clear heat, disinhibit dampness, and stop diarrhea

Guiding formulas:

Qing Re Zhi Xie Tang (Clear Heat & Stop Diarrhea Decoction)
Huang Qin (Radix Scutellariae), 9-12g
Huang Lian (Rhizoma Coptidis), 3-9g
Bai Shao (Radix Albus Paeoniae Lactiflorae), 9g
Dan Zhu Ye (Herba Lophatheri), 9g
Hua Shi (Talcum), 9-15g
Bai Zhu (Rhizoma Atractylodis Macrocephalae), 9g
Fu Ling (Poria), 9-12g
Ze Xie (Rhizoma Alismatis), 6-9g
Gan Cao (Radix Glycyrrhizae), 3-9g

Ban Xia Xie Xin Tang (Pinellia Drain the Heart Decoction)
Ren Shen (Radix Ginseng), 3-9g
Ban Xia (Rhizoma Pinelliae), 9g
Huang Qin (Radix Scutellariae), 9-12g
Huang Lian (Rhizoma Coptidis), 3-9g
mix-fried *Gan Cao* (Radix Glycyrrhizae), 6-9g
Gan Jiang (dry Rhizoma Zingiberis), 6-9g
Sheng Jiang (uncooked Rhizoma Zingiberis), 6g

This formula is for damp heat diarrhea complicated by more conspicuous spleen qi vacuity.

Acupuncture & moxibustion: *Zhong Wan* (CV 12), *Tian Shu* (St 25), *Da Chang Shu* (Bl 25), *He Gu* (LI 4), *Zu San Li* (St 36), *Nei Ting* (St 44), *Yin Ling Quan* (Sp 9)

Food stagnation

Main symptoms: Abdominal distention and pain, foul breath, loss of appetite, nausea, possible vomiting, a hot body, possible oral dryness, and a rapid, large, slippery pulse

Treatment principles: Disperse food and abduct stagnation

Guiding formulas:

Jia Wei Xiao Cheng Qi Tang **(Added Flavors Minor Order the Qi Decoction)**
Zhi Shi (Fructus Immaturus Aurantii), 6-9g
Hou Po (Cortex Magnoliae Officinalis), 6-9g
Da Huang (Radix Et Rhizoma Rhei), 3-9g
Bing Lang (Semen Arecae), 6-9g
mix-fried *Gan Cao* (Radix Glycyrrhizae), 6-9g
Sheng Jiang (uncooked Rhizoma Zingiberis), 6g

After the food stagnation has been dispersed, follow the above with *Si Jun Zi Tang* (Four Gentlemen Decoction): *Ren Shen* (Radix Ginseng), *Bai Zhu* (Rhizoma Atractylodis Macrocephalae), *Fu Ling* (Poria), and mix-fried *Gan Cao* (Radix Glycyrrhizae).

Zhi Shi Tang (Immature Aurantium Decoction)
Zhi Shi (Fructus Immaturus Aurantii), 6g
Mu Xiang (Radix Auklandiae), 6-9g
Hou Po (Cortex Magnoliae Officinalis), 6-9g
Bing Lang (Semen Arecae), 6-9g
Sheng Jiang (uncooked Rhizoma Zingiberis), 6g

This formula treats a less severe condition than that above. However, after the food stagnation is dispersed, one should likewise use *Si Jun Zi Tang* (Four Gentlemen Decoction) to fortify the spleen and supplement the qi.

Sheng Hua Tang Jia Wei
(Engendering & Transforming Decoction with Added Flavors)
Dang Gui (Radix Angelicae Sinensis), 9g
Chuan Xiong (Radix Ligustici Wallichii), 9g
mix-fried *Gan Cao* (Radix Glycyrrhizae), 6-9g
Pao Jiang (blast-fried Rhizoma Zingiberis), 6-9g
Tao Ren (Semen Persicae), 9g
Shen Qu (Massa Medica Fermentata), 6-9g
Mai Ya (Fructus Germinatus Hordei), 9-15g

This is Fu Qing-zhu's formula for food and drink damage postpartum dysentery when over-eating cereal foods is the cause. If overeating meat is at fault, then *Shen Qu* and *Mai Ya* are removed, and *Sha Ren* (Fructus Amomi) and *Shan Zha* (Fructus Crataegi) are used instead.

Acupuncture & moxibustion: *Zhong Wan* (CV 12), *Liang Men* (St 21), *Tian Shu* (St 25), *Da Chang Shu* (Bl 25), *He Gu* (LI 4), *Zu San Li* (St 36), *Nei Ting* (St 44)

Postpartum red dysentery due to heat damaging the uterine vessel

Main symptoms: Postpartum dysentery with downward discharge of bloody fluids whose color is blackish purple with clots, heavy, downward abdominal pain accompanied by heart vexation, oral thirst, uninhibited urination, a red facial complexion, chapped lips, a red tongue with slightly yellow fur, and a bowstring, slippery, rapid pulse

Treatment principles: Clear heat, cool the blood, and stop dysentery

Guiding formulas:

Huai Lian Si Wu Tang (Sophora & Coptis Four Materials Decoction)
Dang Gui (Radix Angelicae Sinensis), 9g
Bai Shao (Radix Albus Paeoniae Lactiflorae), 9-15g
Sheng Di (uncooked Radix Rehmanniae), 12-15g
Chuan Xiong (Radix Ligustici Wallichii), 9g
Huai Hua Mi (Flos Immaturus Sophorae), 9-15g
Huang Lian (Rhizoma Coptidis), 3-9g
Mi Qiao (rice husks), 15-30g

Han Bai-ling says to add *Di Yu* (stir-fried Radix Sanguisorbae) and *Mai Men Dong* (Tuber Ophiopogonis) to clear heat and engender fluids.

Xiang Lian San Jia Wei (Auklandia & Coptis Powder with Added Flavors)
Huang Lian (Rhizoma Coptidis), 3-9g
Mu Xiang (Radix Auklandiae), 6-9g
Bai Zhu (Rhizoma Atractylodis Macrocephalae), 9g
Bai Shao (Radix Albus Paeoniae Lactiflorae), 9g
Hua Shi (Talcum), 9-15g
Gan Cao (Radix Glycyrrhizae), 3-9g
Ren Shen (Radix Ginseng), 3-9g
Dang Gui (Radix Angelicae Sinensis), 9g
Shen Qu (Massa Medica Fermentata), 6-9g
Hou Po (Cortex Magnoliae Officinalis), 6-9g
Mai Ya (Fructus Germinatus Hordei), 9-15g

Huang Fu-zhong recommends this formula for postpartum dysentery with abdominal pain and tenesmus. It is for a combination of damp heat, spleen vacuity, and stagnant food.

Si Jun Zi Tang Jia Wei (Four Gentlemen Decoction with Added Flavors)
Ren Shen (Radix Ginseng), 3-9g
mix-fried *Gan Cao* (Radix Glycyrrhizae), 6-9g
Bai Zhu (Rhizoma Atractylodis Macrocephalae), 9g
Fu Ling (Poria), 9-12g

Dang Gui (Radix Angelicae Sinensis), 9g
Bai Shao (Radix Albus Paeoniae Lactiflorae), 9g
Shen Qu (Massa Medica Fermentata), 6-9g
Chen Pi (Pericarpium Citri Reticulatae), 6g
Mu Xiang (Radix Auklandiae), 6-9g
Huang Lian (Rhizoma Coptidis), 3-9g

Huang says to use this formula if the disease is chronic and unstoppable.

Acupuncture & moxibustion: See damp heat above

Postpartum white dysentery due to cold dampness

Main symptoms: Postpartum dysentery with discharge of white pus accompanied by heavy, downward abdominal pain, inhibited urination which is greenish white in color, lack of warmth in the four limbs, a white facial complexion, pale, moist lips and tongue, and a fine, forceless, possibly deep, moderate (*i.e.,* relaxed, slightly slow) pulse

Treatment principles: Boost the qi, warm the middle, and stop dysentery

Guiding formulas:

Bu Zhong Yi Qi Tang Jia Wei
(Supplement the Center & Boost the Qi Decoction with Added Flavors)
Huang Qi (Radix Astragali), 9-18g
Ren Shen (Radix Ginseng), 3-9g
Bai Zhu (Rhizoma Atractylodis Macrocephalae), 9g
mix-fried *Gan Cao* (Radix Glycyrrhizae), 6-9g
Chen Pi (Pericarpium Citri Reticulatae), 6g
Dang Gui (Radix Angelicae Sinensis), 9g
Chai Hu (Radix Bupleuri), 3-9g
Sheng Ma (Rhizoma Cimicifugae), 3-4.5g

Han Bai-ling recommends adding *Fu Ling* (Poria) and *Shan Yao* (Radix Dioscoreae) to fortify the spleen and seep dampness.

Ba Wei Di Huang Wan Jia Wei
(Eight Flavors Rehmannia Pills with Added Flavors)
Shu Di (cooked Radix Rehmanniae), 12-15g
Shan Yao (Radix Dioscoreae), 9-12g
Shan Zhu Yu (Fructus Corni), 9g
Fu Ling (Poria), 9-12g
Ze Xie (Rhizoma Alismatis), 6-9g
Dan Pi (Cortex Moutan), 6-9g
Bu Gu Zhi (Fructus Psoraleae), 9-15g
Rou Dou Kou (Semen Myristicae), 9g

This formula is for spleen-kidney yang vacuity dysentery. In this case, urination tends to also be short and frequent or incontinent.

Acupuncture & moxibustion: Same as for cold dampness above. If there is a spleen-kidney dual vacuity, add moxibustion at *Shen Shu* (Bl 23), *Ming Men* (GV 4), and *Guan Yuan* (CV 4).

Postpartum red & white dysentery due to dampness & heat mutually wrestling

Main symptoms: Postpartum dysentery with downward discharge of red blood and white mucus in the stools, heavy pain within the abdomen, inhibited urination, heart vexation, hiccup, fullness and distention of the chest and rib-side, no desire for food or drink, a yellowish white facial complexion, chapped lips, slightly yellow tongue fur, and a bowstring, rapid, slippery pulse

Treatment principles: Clear heat and disinhibit dampness, regulate the qi and stop bleeding

Guiding formulas:

Bai Tou Weng Tang Jia Wei (Pulsatilla Decoction with Added Flavors)
Bai Tou Weng (Radix Pulsatillae), 9-12g
Huang Bai (Cortex Phellodendri), 9g
Huang Lian (Rhizoma Coptidis), 3-9g
Qin Pi (Cortex Fraxini), 9g
E Jiao (Gelatinum Corii Asini), 9g
Huang Qin (Radix Scutellariae), 9-12g
stir-fried *Di Yu* (Radix Sanguisorbae), 9g

For marked pus and inhibited urination, add *Che Qian Zi* (Semen Plantaginis), *Ze Xie* (Rhizoma Alismatis), *Cang Zhu* (Rhizoma Atractylodis), and *Yi Yi Ren* (Semen Coicis).

Huang Lian Wan (Coptis Pills)
Huang Lian (Rhizoma Coptidis), 3-9g
Huang Qin (Radix Scutellariae), 9-12g
Huang Bai (Cortex Phellodendri), 9g
Zhi Zi (Fructus Gardeniae), 6-9g
E Jiao (Gelatinum Corii Asini), 9g
Pu Huang (Pollen Typhae), 9g
Dang Gui (Radix Angelicae Sinensis), 9g

For marked pus and inhibited urination, add *Che Qian Zi* (Semen Plantaginis), *Ze Xie* (Rhizoma Alismatis), *Cang Zhu* (Rhizoma Atractylodis), and *Yi Yi Ren* (Semen Coicis).

Acupuncture & moxibustion: Zhong Wan (CV 12), *Tian Shu* (St 25), *Pi Shu* (Bl 20), *Wei Shu* (Bl 21), *Da Chang Shu* (Bl 25), *Zu San Li* (St 36), *Yin Ling Quan* (Sp 6)

Remarks

Postpartum diarrhea is one of the three postpartum emergencies in Chinese gynecology. Therefore, it should be treated and stopped as quickly as possible. Otherwise the loss of the clear with the turbid will cause even worse postpartum vacuity weakness of the righteous qi. The good news is that Chinese medicine usually treats diarrhea and dysentery quite well, remembering that these Chinese categories may also include irritable bowel syndrome, ulcerative colitis, and Crohn's disease. In my experience, the combination of internally prescribed Chinese medicinals with acupuncture is better than acupuncture alone, especially for spleen and kidney vacuities and for damp heat.

24

Postpartum Urinary Stress Incontinence

Postpartum urinary stress incontinence refers to increased urinary frequency, nocturia, dribbling, urge incontinence, and stress incontinence occurring during the puerperium. Its incidence is approximately 35% of postpartum women.[1] It is referred to as urinary stress incontinence; however, this may be a misnomer. It was previously thought to be due to damage to the perineum during birthing, and vaginal delivery does appear to be a statistical risk factor, but recent studies suggest that this complaint may also be due to changes in the body which occur during pregnancy. In fact, women who had similar problems tend to see these problems continue postpartum.[2] Besides vaginal delivery, other risk factors appear to be advanced age, possibly race, and episiotomy. Typically the symptoms associated with this condition resolve in anywhere from a few weeks to several months. In terms of treatment, Western medicines used for the treatment of urinary incontinence in general are not very effective for postpartum urinary incontinence. In severe, intractable cases, surgery may be advised. However, more conservative treatment is limited to the advice to do Kegel exercises.

Chinese medical disease categorization

Postpartum polyuria is called *chan hou xiao bian pin shu* in Chinese, while postpartum urinary incontinence is called *chan hou xiao bian shi jia*.

Disease causes & disease mechanisms

This condition is, like many other postpartum complaints, mostly due to qi vacuity not securing. This qi vacuity may be either spleen qi or kidney qi vacuity. In either case, if the woman is chronically ill, older in age, or constitutionally vacuous and weak, postpartum vacuity can aggravate any existing tendencies to vacuity weakness.

The spleen is one of the three viscera which control water metabolism according to Chinese medical theory. Its role is to govern the movement and transformation of fluids in the body. If central qi falls downward, since the qi moves the fluids and water follows the qi, urination may become frequent and incontinent.

The kidneys govern the sealing and closing of the two lower yin, *i.e.*, the anus and urethra. Therefore, if the kidney qi becomes vacuous, it may be too weak to properly secure the front yin or urethra. In that case, the urination may also become frequent and incontinent.

If excessive blood loss during labor aggravates any pre-existing tendency to yin vacuity, ministerial fire may flame up internally. This evil heat may scorch and damage the bladder. If this heat is strong enough, it may cause the blood to move frenetically outside its pathways, resulting in hematuria.

Urinary frequency with dribbling and dripping, pain, and even hematuria may also be the result of manual or traumatic injury during birthing. Chinese gynecology texts say that, if the midwife is not careful, she may damage the bladder in the process of delivering the baby.

Patterns common to this condition

Spleen qi vacuity
Kidney vacuity not securing
Vacuity heat in the bladder
Damage & detriment to the bladder

Treatment based on pattern discrimination

Spleen qi vacuity

Main symptoms: Postpartum polyuria and/or incontinence accompanied by dizziness standing up, shortness of breath, spontaneous perspiration, fatigue, lack of strength, no lower abdominal pain or distention but a sensation of downward sagging, a somber white facial complexion, a pale, moist tongue, and a fine, forceless, possibly deep or short, and/or moderate (*i.e.*, relaxed, slightly slow) pulse

Treatment principles: Boost the qi and lift the fallen assisted by securing and astringing

Guiding formulas:

Bu Zhong Yi Qi Tang Jia Wei
(Supplement the Center & Boost the Qi Decoction with Added Flavors)
Huang Qi (Radix Astragali), 9-18g
Ren Shen (Radix Ginseng), 3-9g
Bai Zhu (Rhizoma Atractylodis Macrocephalae), 9g
mix-fried *Gan Cao* (Radix Glycyrrhizae), 6-9g

Chai Hu (Radix Bupleuri), 3-9g
Sheng Ma (Rhizoma Cimicifugae), 3-4.5g
Dang Gui (Radix Angelicae Sinensis), 9g
Chen Pi (Pericarpium Citri Reticulatae), 6g
Shan Zhu Yu (Fructus Corni), 9-18g
Yi Zhi Ren (Fructus Alpiniae Oxyphyllae), 9-15g

This formula also treats a lochia which will not cease. A variation of this formula uses *Jin Ying Zi* (Fructus Rosae Laevigatae) instead of *Shan Zhu Yu*.

Yi Qi Suo Quan Yin (Boost the Qi & Shrink the Spring Drink)
Huang Qi (Radix Astragali), 9-18g
Dang Shen (Radix Codonopsitis), 9-18g
Bai Zhu (Rhizoma Atractylodis Macrocephalae), 9g
Jin Ying Zi (Fructus Rosae Laevigatae), 9g
Qian Shi (Semen Euryalis), 9g
Sang Piao Xiao (Ootheca Mantidis), 9g
Shan Yao (Radix Dioscoreae), 9g
Wu Yao (Radix Linderae), 9g

This formula treats a dual spleen and kidney qi vacuity.

Acupuncture & moxibustion: *Zu San Li* (St 36), *San Yin Jiao* (Sp 6), *Pi Shu* (Bl 20), *Wei Shu* (Bl 21), *Qi Hai* (CV 6), *Guan Yuan* (CV 4), *Bai Hui* (GV 20)

Kidney vacuity not securing

Main symptoms: Frequent postpartum urination or incontinence accompanied by vertigo, impaired memory, low back and knee soreness and limpness, lack of warmth in the four limbs, and a dark, dusky facial complexion, a pale, moist tongue, and a deep, weak pulse

Treatment principles: Warm and supplement kidney yang assisted by securing and astringing

Guiding formulas:

Shen Qi Wan Jia Wei (Kidney Qi Pills with Added Flavors)
Shu Di (cooked Radix Rehmanniae), 9-12g
Shan Yao (Radix Dioscoreae), 9g
Shan Zhu Yu (Fructus Corni), 9g
Ze Xie (Rhizoma Alismatis), 6-9g
Dan Pi (Cortex Moutan), 6-9g
Fu Ling (Poria), 9g
Rou Gui (Cortex Cinnamomi), 3-9g
Zhi Fu Zi (Radix Lateralis Praeparatus Aconiti Carmichaeli), 3-9g
Sang Piao Xiao (Ootheca Mantidis), 9g
Fu Pen Zi (Fructus Rubi), 9g
Bu Gu Zhi (Fructus Psoraleae), 9g

Mu Li San (Oyster Shell Powder)

Mu Li (Conchae Ostreae), 9-18g
Chuan Xiong (Radix Ligustici Wallichii), 6-9g
Fu Ling (Poria), 9-12g
Shu Di (cooked Radix Rehmanniae), 12-15g
Long Gu (Os Draconis), 9-18g
Xu Duan (Radix Dipsaci), 9g
Dang Gui (Radix Angelicae Sinensis), 9g
Ai Ye (Folium Artemesiae Argyii), 9g
Ren Shen (Radix Ginseng), 3-9g
Wu Wei Zi (Fructus Schisandrae), 9g
Di Yu (Radix Sanguisorbae), 9g
Gan Cao (Radix Glycyrrhizae), 3-9g
Sheng Jiang (uncooked Rhizoma Zingiberis), 6g
Da Zao (Fructus Jujubae), 3 pieces

Huang Fu-zhong recommends this formula for loss of securing due to vacuity with lack of strength of the four limbs and no desire for food and drink. In this case, both the spleen and kidneys are vacuous and weak.

Acupuncture & moxibustion: *San Yin Jiao* (Sp 6), *Tao Xi* (Ki 3), *Guan Yuan* (CV 4), *Qi Hai* (CV 6), *Shen Shu* (Bl 23), *Pang Guang Shu* (Bl 28)

Vacuity heat in the bladder

Main symptoms: Postpartum polyuria or even possible hematuria with hot pain on urination in the urethra, heart vexation, lack of tranquility, heat emitted from the four limbs, a flushed red facial complexion, dry, red lips, a dry mouth with no particular desire to drink, little or no tongue fur, and a bowstring, fine, rapid pulse

Treatment principles: Enrich yin, cool the blood, and clear heat

Guiding formulas:

Zhi Bai Di Huang Tang Jia Wei (Anemarrhena & Phellodendron Rehmannia Decoction with Added Flavors)

Sheng Di (uncooked Radix Rehmanniae), 12-15g
Dan Pi (Cortex Moutan), 9g
Shan Zhu Yu (Fructus Corni), 9g
Shan Yao (Radix Dioscoreae), 9g
Fu Ling (Poria), 9-12g
Ze Xie (Rhizoma Alismatis), 6-9g
Zhi Mu (Rhizoma Anemarrhenae), 9g
Huang Bai (Cortex Phellodendri), 9g
Bai Mao Gen (Rhizoma Imperatae), 9-15g
Xiao Ji (Herba Cephalanoploris), 9-12g

Dao Chi San Jia Wei (Abduct the Red Powder with Added Flavors)
Sheng Di (uncooked Radix Rehmanniae), 12-15g
Mu Tong (Caulis Akebiae), 6-9g
Dan Zhu Ye (Herba Lophatheri), 9g
Gan Cao (Radix Glycyrrhizae), 3-9g
Niu Xi (Radix Achyranthis Bidentatae), 9-12g
Xiao Ji (Herba Cephalanoploris), 9-12g
Bai Mao Gen (Rhizoma Imperatae), 9-15g
Dan Pi (Cortex Moutan), 9g

Acupuncture & moxibustion: *San Yin Jiao* (Sp 6), *Yin Ling Quan* (Sp 9), *Tai Xi* (Ki 3), *Zhong Ji* (CV 3), *Guan Yuan* (CV 4), *Shen Shu* (Bl 23), *Pang Guang Shu* (Bl 28)

If there is hematuria, add *Xue Hai* (Sp 10).

Damage & detriment to the bladder

Main symptoms: Postpartum urinary dribbling and dripping with aching and pain or hematuria and terminal dribbling which is unable to stop by itself. The six pulses are harmonious and moderate, *i.e.*, normal.

Treatment principles: Boost the qi, secure the bladder, and stop bleeding

Guiding formula:

Sheng Hua Tang Jia Wei
(Engendering & Transforming Decoction with Added Flavors)
Dang Gui (Radix Angelicae Sinensis), 9g
Chuan Xiong (Radix Ligustici Wallichii), 9g
Pao Jiang (blast-fried Rhizoma Zingiberis), 6-9g
Tao Ren (Semen Persicae), 9g
mix-fried *Gan Cao* (Radix Glycyrrhizae), 6-9g
Hai Piao Xiao (Os Sepiae Seu Sepiellae), 9-15g
Yi Zhi Ren (Fructus Alpiniae Oxyphyllae), 9-15g

Acupuncture & moxibustion: *San Yin Jiao* (Sp 6), *Zu San Li* (St 36), *Zhong Ji* (CV 3), *Guan Yuan* (CV 4), *Shen Shu* (Bl 23), *Pang Guang Shu* (Bl 28)

Representative case histories

Case 1: The patient was a 25 year-old female who had given birth to a son in the 38th week plus five days of her pregnancy. She had to have an episiotomy, and the child was delivered by fetal head vacuum extraction. Postpartum, she lost about 400ml of blood from her vaginal tract injuries and experienced loss of control of urination. Her temperature was 37.3° C, and her heartbeat was 84 beats per minute. Her heart and lungs were normal, her abdomen was soft, her bladder was full, and there was not much bleeding from her vaginal tract. The wound in her perineum was not red or swollen. The patient had already been treated with several kinds of medicinals, but she was still not able to discharge urine with normal self-control. Her facial complexion was somber white, she had diminished qi, was disinclined to speak, her spirit was fatigued, and she lacked strength. Her low back and knees were sore and limp, her tongue was pale with white fur, and her pulse was deep, fine, and slow.

Based on the above signs and symptoms, the patient's pattern was categorized as postpartum detriment and damage of qi and blood due to extreme use of force during labor. This had led to non-securing of kidney qi with loss of duty of the bladder's qi transformation. Therefore, treatment was in order to fortify and secure the kidney qi, strengthen the bladder or, in other words, supplement the qi and secure the bladder. Hence the points chosen were: *Guan Yuan* (CV 4), *Zhong Ji* (CV 3), *Zu San Li* (St 36), *San Yin Jiao* (Sp 6), *Shen Shu* (Bl 23), *Pang Guang Shu* (Bl 28), *San Jiao Shu* (Bl 22). *Shen Shu, Pang Guang Shu,* and *San Jiao Shu* were needled with 0.5-1.0 inch needles with supplementing technique producing a warm sensation in the birthing area. These needles were retained for 20 minutes. *Guan Yuan* and *Zhong Ji* were needled with 2.5-3.0 inch needles with supplementing technique causing the needle sensation to be propagated to the vaginal area. *Zu San Li* and *San Yin Jiao* were needled with 1.5-2.0 inch needles also with supplementing technique. All these needles were retained for 30 minutes. Every 10 minutes, the needles were stimulated with supplementing technique once.

After needling once, the woman could control her urination. However, her urination was still urgent. After needling the second day, her urinary discharge returned to normal and her face became moist again, but she still experienced lassitude of the spirit and lack of strength, low back and knee soreness and limpness, etc. After needling the third day, the patient was back to normal. On follow-up after one year, the patient's body was strong and normal.

Case 2: The patient was a 25 year-old female who was first seen on June 8, 1993. On June 6, this patient had given birth normally. However, two days after delivery, her urination had become incontinent. Her lochia was not profuse. Prior to delivery, she had had no history of urinary disease. Based on the above, the patient's pattern was categorized as damage of the bladder during delivery, and she was administered the following medicinals: *Dang Gui* (Radix Angelicae Sinensis), 12g, *Chuan Xiong* (Radix Ligustici Wallichii), 6g, blast-fried *Pao Jiang* (Rhizoma Zingiberis), 5g, *Tao Ren* (Semen Persicae), 6g, mix-fried *Gan Cao* (Radix Glycyrrhizae), 3g, *Hai Piao Xiao* (Os Sepiae Seu Sepiellae), 9g, and *Yi Zhi Ren* (Fructus Alpiniae Oxyphyllae), 9g. After taking four packets of these medicinals, the patient's condition was cured and she did not need to receive acupuncture in addition to this therapy.

Remarks

Spleen and kidney qi vacuity types of postpartum polyuria and urinary incontinence are usually well treated with Chinese medicinals, with or without the addition of acupuncture. Vacuity heat may be more difficult to treat, because it does not respond so well to acupuncture, but can typically be brought under control with Chinese medical treatment.

Endnotes:

[1] www.icsoffice.org/publications/2000/POSTERS/PELVIC%20FLOOR/98.htm

[2] www.babycenter.com/refcap/baby/physrecovery/1152241.html

25

Postpartum
Urinary Retention

Acute, nonobstructive postpartum urinary retention is a frequent phenomenon in the first few days postpartum for a number of reasons. During the second stage of labor, the fetal head puts pressure on the bladder and urethra, possibly resulting in their becoming edematous. Lacerations and pain of the vulvar region may inhibit urination. Changed lower abdominal anatomy may reduce bladder sensation at the same time that the body's production of urine is increased. Postpartum, the body begins eliminating the excess fluids it accumulated during pregnancy. If the bladder becomes overdistended, this may lead to further lack of bladder sensation and impairment of bladder muscles.[1] This is why women are encouraged to get up and urinate as soon as possible after delivery. Epidurals also increase the risk of postpartum urinary retention.[2] Western medicine treats acute, nonobstructive postpartum urinary retention via catheterization. Medications, such as Urecholine (bethanechol chloride) are also reported to be effective for this condition.

Chinese medical disease categorization

In Chinese, postpartum urinary retention is referred to as *chan hou xiao bian bu tong*, postpartum urination not freely flowing. It is also referred to in the most modern Chinese literature as *chan hou niao zhu liu*, postpartum urinary retention.

Disease causes & disease mechanisms

In postpartum women, this condition is most often due to insufficiency of kidney qi. If, during the puerperium, the kidney qi is vacuous, the lifegate fire may become debilitated. Since it is kidney yang which provides the motivating force in the lower burner, the bladder may not transform liquids properly and thus urination is inhibited.

The other two viscera which Chinese medical theory posits as playing a major role in water metabolism are the lungs and spleen. If qi and blood are damaged and consumed postpartum from excessive blood loss, then the lungs and spleen may both become vacuous. In that case, the lungs lose their control over the downbearing and diffusion of fluids, while the spleen loses its control over movement and transformation of water. Therefore, water fluids are not sent down to the bladder and thus fluids and humors in the bladder wither and dry up. Hence the urination is inhibited or absent.

It is also possible for emotional damage by the seven affects and especially anger and depression which are unresolved to cause loss of normalcy in the qi mechanism. The liver is responsible for coursing and discharge. If liver qi becomes stagnant, since it is the qi that moves water fluids in the body, these yin fluids may also not move, and this may thus cause inhibited urination.

In addition, damp heat associated with postpartum infection may also inhibit urination during the puerperium.

Patterns common to this condition

Kidney yang vacuity
Lung-spleen dual vacuity
Qi stagnation
Damp heat

Treatment based on pattern discrimination

Kidney yang vacuity

Main symptoms: Postpartum inhibited urination or even anuria, lower abdominal distention and pain, heart vexation, lack of calm, low back and knee soreness and limpness, lack of warmth in the four limbs, a dark, dusky facial complexion, a pale, moist tongue with white, slimy fur, and a deep, weak pulse

Treatment principles: Warm the kidneys, boost fire, and move water

Guiding formulas:

Shen Qi Wan Jia Wei (Kidney Qi Pills with Added Flavors)
Shu Di (cooked Radix Rehmanniae), 9-15g
Shan Yao (Radix Dioscoreae), 9g
Shan Zhu Yu (Fructus Corni), 9g
Rou Gui (Cortex Cinnamomi), 3-9g
Zhi Fu Zi (Radix Lateralis Praeparatus Aconiti Carmichaeli), 3-9g
Fu Ling (Poria), 9-12g
Dan Pi (Cortex Moutan), 6-9g

Ze Xie (Rhizoma Alismatis), 6-9g
Bu Gu Zhi (Fructus Psoraleae), 9-15g
Yi Zhi Ren (Fructus Alpiniae Oxyphyllae), 9-15g
Tu Si Zi (Semen Cuscutae), 9g
Ba Ji Tian (Radix Morindae), 9g

Zi Shen Tang (Enrich the Kidneys Decoction)
Huang Bai (Cortex Phellodendri), 9g
Zhi Mu (Rhizoma Anemarrhenae), 9g
Che Qian Zi (Semen Plantaginis), 6-9g
Zhu Ling (Polyporus), 9-12g
Fu Ling (Poria), 9-12g
Rou Gui (Cortex Cinnamomi), 3-9g
Jie Gen (Radix Platycodi), 6-9g
Mu Tong (Caulis Akebiae), 6-9g
Hua Shi (Talcum), 9-15g

This formula is for a kidney yin and yang dual vacuity. If there is also qi vacuity, add *Dang Shen* (Radix Codonopsitis) and *Huang Qi* (Radix Astragali). If the pulse is rapid and there is fever with obvious inflammation, add *Pu Gong Ying* (Herba Taraxaci) and *Jin Yin Hua* (Flos Lonicerae). If the stools are constipated and bound, add *Da Huang* (Radix Et Rhizoma Rhei).

Acupuncture & moxibustion: San Yin Jiao (Sp 6), Tai Xi (Ki 3), Yin Ling Quan (Sp 9), Zhong Ji (CV 3), Guan Yuan (CV 4), Shen Shu (Bl 23), Pang Guang Shu (Bl 28)

Lung-spleen dual vacuity

Main symptoms: Inhibited postpartum urination and even anuria, no lower abdominal distention or pain, but dizziness, shortness of breath, spontaneous perspiration, disinclination to speak and a weak voice, lack of strength, fatigue, lassitude of the spirit, a pale facial complexion, a pale, moist tongue with thin fur, and a fine, forceless, possibly weak, deep, short, or moderate (*i.e.*, relaxed, slightly slow) pulse

Treatment principles: Boost the qi and engender fluids

Guiding formulas:

Bu Zhong Yi Qi Tang Jia Wei
(Supplement the Center & Boost the Qi Decoction with Added Flavors)
Huang Qi (Radix Astragali), 9-18g
Ren Shen (Radix Ginseng), 3-9g
Bai Zhu (Rhizoma Atractylodis Macrocephalae), 9g
Dang Gui (Radix Angelicae Sinensis), 9g
mix-fried *Gan Cao* (Radix Glycyrrhizae), 6-9g
Sheng Ma (Rhizoma Cimicifugae), 3-4.5g
Chai Hu (Radix Bupleuri), 3-9g

Chen Pi (Pericarpium Citri Reticulatae), 6g
Jie Geng (Radix Platycodi), 6-9g
Tong Cao (Medulla Tetrapanacis), 9g
Fu Ling (Poria), 9-12g

Yi Qi Dao Ni Tang (Boost the Qi & Abduct the Urine Decoction)
Dang Shen (Radix Codonopsitis), 9-18g
Bai Zhu (Rhizoma Atractylodis Macrocephalae), 9g
Bai Bian Dou (Semen Dolichoris), 9g
Fu Ling (Poria), 9-12g
Gui Zhi (Ramulus Cinnamomi), 6-9g
Sheng Ma (Rhizoma Cimicifugae), 3-4.5g
Jie Geng (Radix Platycodi), 6-9g
Tong Cao (Medulla Tetrapanacis), 9g
Wu Yao (Radix Linderae), 9g

If there is concomitant kidney yin vacuity, add *Liu Wei Di Huang Wan* (Six Flavors Rehmannia Pills). If there is yang vacuity, add *Zhi Fu Zi* (Radix Lateralis Praeparatus Aconiti Carmichaeli). If there is also infection, add *Jin Yin Hua* (Flos Lonicerae) and *Pu Gong Ying* (Herba Taraxaci).

This formula boosts the qi and raises prolapse, opens the yang and disinhibits urination. It takes the connection of the lungs and urination into account through the use of *Jie Geng* at the same time as it regulates the qi through the inclusion of *Wu Yao*.

Gui Fu Zhi Long Tang
(Cinnamon & Poria Stop Urinary Dribbling Decoction)
Gui Zhi (Ramulus Cinnamomi), 9g
Bai Zhu (Rhizoma Atractylodis Macrocephalae), 9g
Zhu Ling (Polyporus), 9-12g
Fu Ling (Poria), 9-12g
Ze Xie (Rhizoma Alismatis), 9g
Bai Shao (Radix Albus Paeoniae Lactiflorae), 9g
Huang Bai (Cortex Phellodendri), 9g
Shi Chang Pu (Rhizoma Acori Tatarinowii), 6-9g
Cang Zhu (Rhizoma Atractylodis), 9g
mix-fried *Gan Cao* (Radix Glycyrrhizae), 6-9g

This formula frees the flow of yang and boosts the qi, disinhibits urination and resolves dribbling urinary block. If there is yang vacuity, add *Zhi Fu Zi* (Radix Lateralis Praeparatus Aconiti Carmichaeli). If there is qi vacuity, add *Dang Shen* (Radix Codonopsitis) and *Huang Qi* (Radix Astragali). If the condition is mixed with dampness, add *Bai Dou Kou* (Fructus Cardamomi) and *Tong Cao* (Medulla Tetrapanacis). If there is abdominal distention and fullness, add *Wu Yao* (Radix Linderae) and *Xiao Hui Xiang* (Fructus Foeniculi). If the urine is yellowish red, add *Bai Mao Gen* (Rhizoma Imperatae) and *Pu Gong Ying* (Herba Taraxaci).

Li Niao Tong Qiao Tang
(Disinhibit Urination & Free the Flow of the Orifices Decoction)
Dang Gui (Radix Angelicae Sinensis), 9g
Huang Qi (Radix Astragali), 9-18g
Fu Ling (Poria), 9-12g
Ze Xie (Rhizoma Alismatis), 9g
Bai Zhu (Rhizoma Atractylodis Macrocephalae), 9g
Gui Zhi (Ramulus Cinnamomi), 6-9g
Zhu Ling (Polyporus), 9-12g
Xing Ren (Semen Armeniacae), 9g
Mu Tong (Caulis Akebiae), 6-9g
Zao Jiao Ci (Spina Gleditschiae Chinensis), 6-9g
Gan Cao (Radix Glycyrrhizae), 3-9g

If there is damp heat, add *Cang Zhu* (Rhizoma Atractylodis), *Yi Yi Ren* (Semen Coicis), *Huo Xiang* (Herba Pogostemonis), *Hua Shi* (Talcum), and *Huang Lian* (Rhizoma Coptidis). If there is lung heat, add *Sang Bai Pi* (Cortex Mori), *Huang Qin* (Radix Scutellariae), *Chai Hu* (Radix Bupleuri), *Bo He* (Herba Menthae Haplocalycis), and *Gua Lou Pi* (Pericarpium Trichosanthis). If there is qi insufficiency, double the *Huang Qi* and add *Dang Shen* (Radix Codonopsitis) or add *Tai Zi Shen* (Radix Pseudostellariae) and *Huang Jing* (Rhizoma Polygonati). Choose the first two if there is only qi insufficiency and the last two if there is also fluid dryness of the lungs. If there is yin vacuity, add *Sheng Di* (uncooked Radix Rehmanniae), *Nu Zhen Zi* (Fructus Ligustri Lucidi), *Han Lian Cao* (Herba Ecliptae), *Gou Qi Zi* (Fructus Lycii), and *Di Gu Pi* (Cortex Lycii). If the area around the genitalia is cut or torn or the vaginal meatus is swollen and painful, add *Jin Yin Hua* (Flos Lonicerae), *Pu Gong Ying* (Herba Taraxaci), *Hong Teng* (Caulis Sargentodoxae), and *Bai Jiang Cao* (Herba Patriniae).

Acupuncture & moxibustion: *San Yin Jiao* (Sp 6), *Zu San Li* (St 36), *Pi Shu* (Bl 20), *Wei Shu* (Bl 21), *Pang Guang Shu* (Bl 28), *Zhong Ji* (CV 3), *Guan Yuan* (CV 4)

Qi stagnation

Main symptoms: Postpartum inhibited urination or even anuria, dizziness and vertigo, distention and fullness of the chest and rib-sides, heaviness and distention in the lower abdomen, a dark, stagnant facial complexion, slightly yellow tongue fur, and a bowstring, moderate (*i.e.*, relaxed, slightly slow) pulse

Treatment principles: Regulate the liver, rectify the qi, and disinhibit urination

Guiding formulas:

Xiao Yao San Jia Wei (Rambling Powder with Added Flavors)
Chai Hu (Radix Bupleuri), 9g
Dang Gui (Radix Angelicae Sinensis), 9g
Bai Shao (Radix Albus Paeoniae Lactiflorae), 9g

Bai Zhu (Rhizoma Atractylodis Macrocephalae), 9g
Fu Ling (Poria), 9-12g
Bo He (Herba Menthae Haplocalycis), 3-6g
mix-fried *Gan Cao* (Radix Glycyrrhizae), 6-9g
Sheng Jiang (uncooked Rhizoma Zingiberis), 6g
Hua Shi (Talcum), 9-15g
Dan Zhu Ye (Herba Lophatheri), 9g
Niu Xi (Radix Achyranthis Bidentatae), 9-12g
Che Qian Zi (Semen Plantaginis), 9g

Mu Tong San (Akebia Powder)
Mu Tong (Caulis Akebiae), 9g
Hua Shi (Talcum), 9-15g
Dong Kui Zi (Semen Benincasae), 9-15g
Bing Lang (Semen Arecae), 6-9g
 Zhi Ke (Fructus Aurantii), 6-9g
Gan Cao (Radix Glycyrrhizae), 3-9g

This formula courses the liver and regulates the qi, clears heat and disinhibits dampness. It is for the treatment of liver qi depression and stagnation with damp heat accumulating internally. Huang Fu-zhong includes *Huo Ma Ren* (Semen Cannabis) in his version of this formula. In addition, if there is qi vacuity, add *Dang Shen* (Radix Codonopsitis) and *Huang Qi* (Radix Astragali). If there is yin and blood vacuity, add *Dang Gui* (Radix Angelicae Sinensis) and *Mai Men Dong* (Tuber Ophiopogonis). If urination is not smoothly flowing, add *Fu Ling* (Poria) and *Ze Xie* (Rhizoma Alismatis).

Si Wu Tang Jia Wei (Four Materials Decoction with Added Flavors)
Shu Di (cooked Radix Rehmanniae), 9-15g
Dang Gui (Radix Angelicae Sinensis), 9g
Chuan Xiong (Radix Ligustici Wallichii), 9g
Bai Shao (Radix Albus Paeoniae Lactiflorae), 9g
Pu Huang (Pollen Typhae), 9g
Qu Mai (Herba Dianthi), 9g
Tao Ren (Semen Persicae), 9g
Niu Xi (Radix Achyranthis Bidentatae), 9g
Hua Shi (Talcum), 9-15g
Gan Cao Shao (Extremitas Radicis Glycyrrhizae), 6-9g
Mu Xiang (Radix Auklandiae), 6-9g
Mu Tong (Caulis Akebiae), 6-9g

This formula is for use if blood stasis complicates qi stagnation. In this case, postpartum dribbling and dripping is combined with heat evils forcing the blood to ooze into the bladder with abdominal distention and pain.

Acupuncture & moxibustion: *Tai Chong* (Liv 3), *San Yin Jiao* (Sp 6), *Yin Ling Quan* (Sp 9), *He Gu* (LI 4), *Zhong Ji* (CV 3), *Qi Hai* (CV 6), *Pang Guang Shu* (Bl 28)

Damp heat

Main symptoms: If the external genitalia have been injured, cut, or torn, signs and symptoms of damp heat may arise postpartum with consequent inhibition of urination. This may manifest as frequent and painful urination with scanty or obstructed flow, abdominal distention, a dry throat and mouth, reddish yellow urine, a red tongue with yellow fur, and a rapid, slippery, forceful pulse.

Treatment principles: Clear heat and drain fire, disinhibit dampness and free the flow of strangury

Guiding formula:

Ba Zheng Tong Lin Yin
(Eight [Ingredients] Correcting & Freeing the Flow of Strangury Drink)
Bian Xu (Herba Polygoni Avicularis), 9g
Qu Mai (Herba Dianthi), 9g
Tong Cao (Medulla Tetrapanacis), 9g
Che Qian Zi (Semen Plantaginis), 9g
Hua Shi (Talcum), 9-15g
Zhi Zi (Fructus Gardeniae), 6-9g
Gan Cao Shao (Extremitas Radicis Glycyrrhizae), 6-9g
Huang Bai (Cortex Phellodendri), 9g

If there is qi vacuity, add *Dang Shen* (Radix Codonopsitis), *Huang Qi* (Radix Astragali), and/or *Ren Shen* (Radix Ginseng). If the stools are constipated and bound, add *Da Huang* (Radix Et Rhizoma Rhei). If there is insomnia, add *Hu Po* (Succinum).

Acupuncture & moxibustion: Yin Ling Quan (Sp 9), Yang Ling Quan (GB 34), San Yin Jiao (Sp 6), Zhong Ji (CV 3), Guan Yuan (CV 4), Pang Guang Shu (Bl 28), Ci Liao (Bl 32)

Abstracts of representative Chinese research

From "The Treatment of 15 Cases of Postpartum Urinary Retention with Self-composed *Huang Qi Tong Cao Tang* (Astragalus & Tetrapanax Decoction)" by Zhou Long-mei, *Shang Hai Zhong Yi Yao Za Zhi (Shanghai Journal of Chinese Medicine & Medicinals)*, #4, 1995, p. 7

Cohort description:

Since 1990, the author has treated 15 cases of postpartum urinary retention with self-composed *Huang Qi Tong Cao Tang* with good results. Of these 15 patients, the oldest was 35 and the youngest was 23 years old. Five cases delivered by cesarean section, and 10 cases delivered normally. The shortest course of disease was five days and the longest was 10 days.

Treatment method:

Huang Qi Tong Cao Tang was composed of: *Huang Qi* (Radix Astragali), 20g, *Tong*

Cao (Medulla Tetrapanacis), 12g, *Dang Gui* (Radix Angelicae Sinensis), 12g, *Mu Tong* (Caulis Akebiae), 10g, *Che Qian Zi* (Semen Plantaginis), 12g, *Fu Ling* (Poria), 12g, *Wang Bu Liu Xing* (Semen Vaccariae), 12g, blast-fried *Chuan Shan Jia* (Squama Manitis), 10g, and uncooked *Gan Cao* (Radix Glycyrrhizae), 10g. One packet was administered per day taken in two divided doses. If there was qi vacuity, *Dang Shen* (Radix Codonopsitis), 12g, and *Bai Zhu* (Rhizoma Atractylodis Macrocephalae), 10g, were added. If the appetite was poor, scorched *Shan Zha* (Fructus Crataegi), 12g, and *Shen Qu* (Massa Medica Fermentata), 12g, were added.

Treatment outcomes:

Complete cure meant that all generalized symptoms disappeared and that the urination returned to normal. Marked improvement meant that the main symptoms were markedly improved. Some improvement meant that symptoms of the main condition ameliorated and became stabilized, but there was no marked improvement in the other generalized symptoms. No results meant that there was no improvement in either the symptoms of the main condition or the accompanying generalized symptoms. Based on these criteria, 13 cases were cured, one case got marked improvement, and one case got no result. Thus the total amelioration rate was 93.4%.

From "The Treatment of 52 Cases of Postpartum Urinary Retention by Boosting the Qi, Warming Yang & Disinhibiting Water" by Peng Mei-yu, *Shang Hai Zhong Yi Yao Za Zhi (Shanghai Journal of Chinese Medicine & Medicinals)*, #2, 1994, p. 32

Cohort description:

Since 1986, the authors of this study have treated 52 cases of postpartum urinary retention with the methods of boosting the qi, warming yang, and disinhibiting water with good results. All 52 of these women were inpatients in the obstetrical department of a hospital. Five women were between 23-25 years old, 31 were between 26-30, 12 were between 31-35, and four women were over 35 years old. There were 14 cases of normal birth, 12 cases of forceps delivery, two cases of vacuum extraction of the fetal head, and 24 cesarean deliveries. In four cases, birthing took 14 hours; in 18 cases, 20 hours of more; in two cases, 24 hours; and in four cases, the particulars were not known. In the rest of the cases, delivery was normal. Thirty-six of the women in the hospital were not able to urinate on their own, while 16 were able to urinate by dribbles and drips but not smoothly. In 30 cases, the tongue fur was thin and white; in 18 cases, white and slimy; and in four cases, thin and yellow. The pulse images were mostly soggy, fine, and slippery.

Treatment method:

The medicinal formula consisted of: *Huang Qi* (Radix Astragali), *Rou Gui* (Cortex Cinnamomi), *Bai Zhu* (Rhizoma Atractylodis Macrocephalae), *Fu Ling* (Poria), *Jie Geng* (Radix Platycodi), *Ze Xie* (Rhizoma Alismatis), *Chen Xiang* (Lignum Aquilariae), and mix-fried *Sheng Ma* (Rhizoma Cimicifugae), doses unstated.

If there was serious yang qi vacuity, the amount of *Huang Qi* was doubled and *Dang Shen* (Radix Codonopsitis) was added. If central qi was fallen downward, *Chai Hu*

(Radix Bupleuri) was added. If the perineum was obviously swollen and hyper-emic, then *Zhi Zi* (Fructus Gardeniae) and *Jin Yin Hua* (Flos Lonicerae) were added.

Treatment outcomes:

Marked improvement was defined as smooth and free-flowing urination after one packet of the above medicinals with disappearance of lower abdominal distention and pain. Some improvement was defined as smooth and free-flowing urination after taking two packets of the above medicinals. While no improvement meant that the urine was still not smooth and free-flowing after taking three packets of the above medicinals but still came in dribbles and drips. Based on the above criteria, 31 cases experienced marked improvement, 18 cases got some improvement, and three cases registered no improvement. Thus the total amelioration rate was 94.3%.

From "The Treatment of Postpartum Urinary Retention with Semen Plantaginis [*Che Qian Zi*] Applied to Point Locations" by Qing Li, *Si Chuan Zhong Yi (Sichuan Chinese Medicine)*, #6, 2001, p. 22

Cohort description:

Thirty women with postpartum urinary retention were included in this study. The oldest was 32 and the youngest was 21 years old. The average age was 24. Twenty-seven of these women were primiparas. Three women had already given birth at least once before.

Treatment method:

Thirty grams of *Che Qian Zi* (Semen Plantaginis) and three grams of table salt were ground up together into a mash. While each woman was lying down on her back, a disk of this mash 10cm x 10cm was applied to either the *Qi Hai* (CV 6) or *Guan Yuan* (CV 4) areas. If there was no obvious stimulatory reaction after applying one such disk, the treatment was repeated 2-3 times.

Treatment outcomes:

Fifteen of the 30 women in this study (*i.e.*, 50%) urinated within 20 minutes of the medicinals being applied to their lower abdomens. Another eight women (24%) urinated within 20-30 minutes of application. Six cases (18%) urinated after 30-40 minutes, while one case (8%) urinated after 40 minutes. Thus this treatment was effective in promoting urination in all 30 cases included in this study.

From "The Treatment of 62 Cases of Postpartum Urinary Retention with *Yi Qi Pai Niao Tang* (Boost the Qi & Expel Urine Decoction)" by Wu Chun-he & Ye Le-zhen, *Fu Jian Zhong Yi Yao (Fujian Chinese Medicine & Medicinals)*, #6, 1995, p. 25

Cohort description:

Of the 62 patients in this study, 47 (75.6%) were between 20-30 years of age and 15 (24.4%) were over 30. Fifty-three (85.5%) were primiparas, and nine (14.5%)

were multiparas. Eleven gave birth normally, 42 had some complications, and nine had cesarean deliveries.

Treatment method:

The formula consisted of: *Huang Qi* (Radix Astragali), 30g, *Mai Men Dong* (Tuber Ophiopogonis), 10g, *Shan Yao* (Radix Dioscoreae), 15g, *Che Qian Zi* (Semen Plantaginis), 15g, *Gan Cao Shao* (Extremitas Radicis Glycyrrhizae), 6g, *Tong Cao* (Medulla Tetrapanacis), 9g, *Fu Ling Pi* (Cortex Sclerotii Poriae Cocos), 10g, and *Rou Gui* (Cortex Cinnamomi), 3g. If there was a tendency to kidney yang vacuity, six grams of *Zhi Fu Zi* (Radix Lateralis Praeparatus Aconiti Carmichaeli) and 10 grams of *Wu Zhu Yu* (Fructus Evodiae) were added and the *Rou Gui* was increased to six grams. If there was a tendency to kidney yin vacuity, 15 grams of *Gui Ban* (Plastrum Testudinis) and 12 grams each of *Shu Di* (cooked Radix Rehmanniae) and *Gou Qi Zi* (Fructus Lycii) were added. If there was liver depression qi stagnation, eight grams of (Radix Bupleuri) and 10 grams each of *Zhi Ke* (Fructus Aurantii) and *Yi Mu Cao* (Herba Leonuri) were added. One packet of these medicinals was decocted in water and administered orally per day.

Treatment outcomes:

Fifty-nine patients (95%) were judged to have been cured using this protocol, meaning that their urination spontaneously resolved and there were no accompanying symptoms. The other three patients were judged to have gotten a marked effect, meaning that they were able to urinate but that there was still some lower abdominal distention and fullness or other accompanying symptoms. Thus the total amelioration rate was 100%. The shortest length of treatment was two days and the longest was eight days.

From "A Clinical Audit of the Treatment of 30 Cases of Postpartum Urinary Retention with *Bu Zhong Yi Qi Tang* (Supplement the Center & Boost the Qi Decoction)" by Ya Chun-xiang, *Fu Jian Zhong Yi Yao (Fujian Chinese Medicine & Medicinals)*, # 2, 1996, p. 41

Cohort description:

All the women in this study were postpartum. The youngest was 18 and the oldest was 48 years old. The shortest course of disease was one day and the longest was 10 days. Eighteen patients were primiparas, eight patients had had two children, and four had had three. All had urinary retention, lower abdominal distention and fullness, low back pain, and/or restless sleep.

Treatment method:

The formula consisted of: *Dang Shen* (Radix Codonopsitis), 30g, *Huang Qi* (Radix Astragali), 15g, *Dang Gui* (Radix Angelicae Sinensis), 10g, *Sheng Ma* (Rhizoma Cimicifugae), 5g, *Chai Hu* (Radix Bupleuri), 9g, *Fu Ling* (Poria), 20g, *Bai Zhu* (stir-fried Rhizoma Atractylodis Macrocephalae), 10g, *Shi Chang Pu* (Rhizoma Acori Tatarinowii), 5g, *Chen Pi* (Pericarpium Citri Reticulatae), 5g, and mix-fried *Gan Cao* (Radix Glycyrrhizae), 6g. If there was simultaneous external contraction, *Jing*

Jie (Herba Schizonepetae), *Fang Feng* (Radix Sapshnikoviae), and *Ai Ye* (Folium Artemisiae Argyii) were added. If there was simultaneous cough with white phlegm, processed *Ban Xi* (Rhizoma Pinelliae) and *Kuan Dong Hua* (Flos Farfarae) were added. If there was thick, yellow, sticky phlegm, *Huang Qin* (Radix Scutellariae), *She Gan* (Rhizoma Belamcandae), and *Yu Xing Cao* (Herba Houttuyniae) were added. If there was chest and rib-side distention and pain, *Yu Jin* (Tuber Curcumae), *Chuan Lian Zi* (Fructus Toosendan), and *Xiang Fu* (Rhizoma Cyperi) were added. If there was kidney vacuity, *Xu Duan* (Radix Dipsaci), *Tu Si Zi* (Semen Cuscutae), and *Ba Ji Tian* (Radix Morindae) were added. One packet of these medicinals was decocted each day and administered internally.

Treatment outcomes:

All 30 patients were judged to have been cured by this protocol. This meant that their urinary retention and lower abdominal distention and fullness disappeared. The smallest number of packets administered was one and the largest was five, with an average of three. Thus the total amelioration rate using this protocol was 100%.

Representative case histories

Case 1: The patient was a 25 year-old female who had given birth normally on March 3, 1992. At that time, she discharged a lot of blood relatively . For the following five days, she experienced dribbling block urination. She was administered some Western medication by injection but without effect. When she was examined, her urination only dribbled and dripped and was not free-flowing. She had lower abdominal distention, cramping, and pain, and a somber white facial complexion. Movement resulted in sweating. There were also heart palpitations, dizziness, lassitude of the spirit, devitalized appetite, a pale tongue with thin, white fur, and a fine, weak pulse. Her pattern was categorized as qi and blood vacuity and deficiency with upbearing of the clear and downbearing of the turbid not regulated. She was treated with: *Huang Qi* (Radix Astragali), 20g, *Tong Cao* (Medulla Tetrapanacis), 12g, *Dang Gui* (Radix Angelicae Sinensis), 12g, *Wang Bu Liu Xing* (Semen Vaccariae), 12g, *Dang Shen* (Radix Codonopsitis), 12g, *Fu Ling* (Poria), 12g, *Che Qian Ren* (Semen Plantaginis), 10g, and uncooked *Gan Cao* (Radix Glycyrrhizae), 12g. After taking two packets, the patient was examined again. At that time, urinary urgency was relaxed, but her urinary dribbling and dripping were still not smoothly flowing. Therefore, she was given two more packets of the original formula, after which her urination became normal and she was discharged from the hospital.

Case 2: The patient was a 41 year-old postpartum woman. This woman had to have a cesarean section delivery. Twenty-four hours later, her postpartum urinary tract catheter was removed. Five hours later, she was not able to discharge urine on her own, and her lower abdomen was so distended and full it was difficult to bear. Pressure on her bladder revealed that it was full. Her body constitution was vacuous and weak. She experienced dizziness and shortness of breath. Her tongue fur was thin, white, and slimy. Her pulse was fine and weak. Therefore, her condition was categorized as qi vacuity and blood weakness with kidney yang vacuity detriment not able to transform the qi. Thus it was appropriate to mainly boost the qi and supplement the kidneys, transform the qi and move water.

Her prescription was: *Huang Qi* (Radix Astragali), 30g, *Bai Zhu* (Rhizoma Atractylodis Macrocephalae), *Shan Yao* (Radix Dioscoreae), *Fu Ling Pi* (Cortex Sclerotii Poriae Cocos), stir-fried *Du Zhong* (Cortex Eucommiae), *Ze Xie* (Rhizoma Alismatis), and *Niu Xi* (Radix Achyranthis Bidentatae), 12g each, *Jie Geng* (Radix Platycodi), 6g, mix-fried *Sheng Ma* (Rhizoma Cimicifugae), 9g, *Rou Gui* (Cortex Cinnamomi), 3g, *Tong Cao* (Medulla Tetrapanacis), 6g, *Wu Yao* (Radix Linderae), 9g, and *Che Qian Zi* (Semen Plantaginis), 30g. Three hours after taking one packet of the above medicinals, the patient was able to urinate, and, after that, her urination was that of a normal person.

Case 3: The patient was a 23 year-old female who was admitted to the hospital on Jan. 23, 1980. The patient was 19 days postpartum and was not able to urinate. The woman had had an episiotomy at the time of delivery and had not been able to urinate. She had been catheterized numerous times since then and had taken various types of antibiotics but was still not able to urinate on her own. She had also been treated with *Bu Zhong Yi Qi Tang Jia Jian* (Supplement the Center & Boost the Qi Decoction with Additions & Subtractions) as well as with acupuncture, all without result. The patient's affect was good, her temperature was normal, her uterus was not hard, and her lower abdomen was soft and pliable. In fact, the bladder was not full, and she had no sensation of needing to urinate. The episiotomy incision had closed but then a fissure had opened, and a small amount of pus was secreted. The patient's urethra was catheterized, and there was a small amount of lochia coming from the vaginal meatus. Her facial complexion was lusterless, her tongue was pale with thin, white fur, and her pulse was fine and forceless.

Based on the above signs and symptoms, the patient's condition was diagnosed as postpartum urinary retention with incision infection. Her pattern was discriminated as qi and yin dual depletion. Therefore, she was prescribed *Huang Qi Gan Cao Tang* (Astragalus & Licorice Decoction) plus *Zi Shen Tong Guan Wan* (Enrich the Kidneys & Free the Flow of the Bar Pills): *Huang Qi* (Radix Astragali), 60g, *Gan Cao* (Radix Glycyrrhizae), 10g, *Rou Gui* (Cortex Cinnamomi), 6g, *Huang Bai* (Cortex Phellodendri), 6g, and *Zhi Mu* (Rhizoma Anemarrhenae), 6g. After two packets of these medicinals, she could feel the sensation of having to urinate. After three more packets, the woman was able to urinate freely and she was discharged from the hospital.

Case 4: The patient was a 26 year-old female who had had postpartum urinary retention for five days after giving birth to her first child on Nov. 12, 1979. This child had been relatively large, and the woman had had to have surgery, during which she had lost a lot of blood. When later she had tried to urinate, the urine had only dribbled and dripped and would not exit. The patient's lower abdomen was distended and painful. She had been catheterized and administered diuretics and acupuncture. In addition, warm applications were applied to her abdomen, all without result. When examined, the patients facial complexion was pale white. There was fatigue, lack of strength, occasional spontaneous perspiration, heart palpitations, occasional low back soreness, a profuse lochia, a pale tongue, and a fine, forceless pulse.

Based on these signs and symptoms, it was determined that the woman's kidney had suffered detriment postpartum and that there was central qi downward falling. Hence the bladder qi transformation was inhibited. In order to boost the qi and upbear yang, transform the qi and move water, the patient was administered six packets of *Bu Zhong Yi Qi Tang* (Supplement the Center & Boost the Qi Decoction) plus *Wu Ling San* (Five [Ingredients] Poria Powder) with additions and subtractions: *Huang Qi* (Radix Astragali), 20g, *Dang Shen* (Radix Codonopsitis), 15g, *Bai Zhu* (Rhizoma Atractylodis Macrocephalae), 12g, mix-fried *Sheng Ma* (Rhizoma Cimicifugae), 6g, *Fu Ling* (Poria), 10g, *Zhu Ling* (Polyporus), 10g, *Ze Xie* (Rhizoma Alismatis), 10g, *Che Qian Zi* (Semen Plantaginis), 10g, *Chai Hu* (Radix Bupleuri), 10g, *Gou Qi Zi* (Fructus Lycii), 12g, *Gui Zhi* (Ramulus Cinnamomi), 10g, and *Gan Cao* (Radix Glycyrrhizae), 3g. After taking these medicinals, the patient's urine was freely and easily flowing. Therefore, she was switched to *Shi Quan Da Bu Wan* (Ten [Ingredients] Completely & Greatly Supplementing Pills) in order to supplement the qi and blood and secure the root.

Case 5: The patient was a 25 year-old female who was initially seen on Feb. 25, 1980. After giving birth, this patient's urination was not freely flowing. It was now four days postpartum and her urine only dribbled and dripped. The patient's lower abdomen was hard and slightly distended. Her facial complexion was sallow yellow. There was lassitude of the spirit, lack of strength, profuse perspiration, reduced appetite, a faint voice and disinclination to speak, a pale tongue with thin fur, and a fine, weak pulse. Based on these signs and symptoms, the woman's pattern was categorized as central qi insufficiency. Therefore, she was prescribed one packet of modified *Bu Zhong Yi Qi Tang* (Supplement the Center & Boost the Qi Decoction): *Dang Shen* (Radix Codonopsitis), 12g, mix-fried *Huang Qi* (Radix Astragali), 9g, *Bai Zhu* (Rhizoma Atractylodis Macrocephalae), 9g, vinegar stir-fried *Chai Hu* (Radix Bupleuri), 4.5g, mix-fried *Sheng Ma* (Rhizoma Cimicifugae), 3g, *Dang Gui* (Radix Angelicae Sinensis), 9g, *Chen Pi* (Pericarpium Citri Reticulatae), 9g, *Gan Cao* (Radix Glycyrrhizae), 3g, *Rou Gui* (Cortex Cinnamomi), 2g, and *Jie Geng* (Radix Platycodi), 9g. The patient was seen again the next day, and she reported that she had urinated six times. Her urine was now freely and smoothly flowing. Therefore, she was administered one more packet of the original formula and was cured.

Case 6: The patient was a married female of undisclosed age who was first seen on June 29, 1959 and was nine days postpartum after her first delivery. After giving birth, this woman's urination had become inhibited. After a number of attmepts to urinate, she was not able to. There was abdominal distention, low back pain, dry, bound stools, poor sleep, slimy, white tongue fur, and a fine, bowstring pulse. Therefore, in order to course and disinhibit the three burners, and warm and free the flow of the bladder, the patient was prescribed three packets of the following medicinals: *Dang Gui* (Radix Angelicae Sinensis), 9g, *Chai Hu* (Radix Bupleuri), 4.5g, *Chuan Xiong* (Radix Ligustici Wallichii), 4.5g, *Bai Zhu* (Rhizoma Atractylodis Macrocephalae), 9g, *Fu Ling* (Poria), 9g, mix-fried *Gan Cao* (Radix Glycyrrhizae), 3g, processed *Xiang Fu* (Rhizoma Cyperi), 6g, *Xiao Hui Xiang* (Fructus Foeniculi), 3g, and *Chen Pi* (Pericarpium Citri Reticulatae), 3g. In addition, she was also prescribed: *Rou Gui* (powdered Cortex Cinnamomi), 2.7g, powdered *Chen Xiang* (Lignum Aquliariae), 1.8g, and powdered *Hu Po* (Succinum), 6g. These three powders were mixed together and divided into six packets. Each day, the patient was instructed to drink one packet each time, two times per day.

The second examination occurred on July 1. After taking the above medicinals, the patient's urination had become relatively more freely flowing. However, there was still lower abdominal distention, low back soreness, dry stools, and a profuse lochia that was red in color. The woman also had spontaneous perspiration, scanty sleep, devitalized intake of food, and thin, white tongue fur that was slightly yellow in the center. Her pulse was still fine and bowstring.Therefore she was prescribed: *Dang Gui* (Radix Angelicae Sinensis), 9g, *Chuan Xiong* (Radix Ligustici Wallichii), 6g, mix-fried *Gan Cao* (Radix Glycyrrhizae), 3g, processed *Xiang Fu* (Rhizoma Cyperi), 6g, *Xiao Hui Xiang* (Fructus Foeniculi), 3g, *Chen Pi* (Pericarpium Citri Reticulatae), 3g, *Fu Ling* (Poria), 9g, *Tao Ren* (Semen Persicae), 6g, *Jiang Huang* (Rhizoma Curcumae Longae), 3g, *Ze Xie* (Rhizoma Alismatis), 9g, *Mu Tong* (Caulis Akebiae), 3g, and *Huai Xiao Mai* (Fructus Tritici Aestivi), 9g. Additionally, the woman was given four bags made from powdered *Rou Gui* (Cortex Cinnamomi), 2.4g, and powdered *Hu Po* (Succinum), 3.6g. Each day, she was advised to drink one packet each time, morning and night. After taking these two packets of medicinals, the patient's urination was completely, freely and smoothly flowing.

Case 7: The patient was a married female of undisclosed age who was first seen on April 8, 1959 after her second birth whose course had been long. After delivery, the woman was not able to urinate, and, when she was seen by the original author of this history, it was eight days postpartum. She had been catheterized as well as treated with acupuncture and Chinese medicinals. However, she was still not able to urinate on her own. Her lower abdomen was distended and painful and her intake was devitalized. Her stools were dry and bound, her tongue was crimson with yellow fur and peeled edges, and her pulse on the left was fine, bowstring, and rapid though weak in the cubit. On the left, it was slippery and rapid. Therefore, in order to nourish the blood and clear heat, free the flow and disinhibit the bladder, the patient was prescribed: uncooked *Sheng Di* (Radix Rehmanniae), 12g, *Tong Cao* (Medulla Tetrapanacis), 3g, *Gan Cao Shao*

(Extremitas Radicis Glycyrrhizae), 3g, *Chi Xiao Dou* (Semen Phaseoli), 12g, *Hua Shi* (Talcum), 12g, *Che Qian Zi* (Semen Plantaginis), 12g, *Ze Xie* (Rhizoma Alismatis), 9g, *Fu Ling Pi* (Cortex Sclerotii Poriae Cocos), 12g, and *Jie Geng* (Radix Platycodi), 6g. In addition, the patient was prescribed powdered *Hu Po* (Succinum), 2.4g and powdered *Chen Xiang* (Lignum Aquilariae), 1.2g. These two medicinals were mixed together, put in gelatin capsules, and these capsules were divided into two doses.

The second visit occurred on April 10 after the patient had taken the above medicinals. Now the woman was able to urinate on her own. However, she had some pain on urination, and her appetite was only slightly increased. Her tongue fur was thin and white, and her pulse was bowstring and rapid. Therefore, she was prescribed: *Qu Mai* (Herba Dianthi), 9g, *Bian Xu* (Herba Polygoni Avicularis), 9g, *Gan Cao Shao* (Extremitas Radicis Radix Glycyrrhizae), 3g, *Hua Shi* (Talcum), 12g, *Che Qian Zi* (Semen Plantaginis), 12g, *Mu Tong* (Caulis Akebiae), 1.8g, and *Yi Yi Ren* (Semen Coicis), 12g. In addition, she was prescribed powdered *Hu Po* (Succinum), 1.8g, and powdered *Chen Xiang* (Lignum Aquilariae), 1.2g, mixed together and placed in gelatin capsules to be taken in two divided doses per day.

On April 13, the patient reported that she had taken three packets of the above medicinals and that the amount of her urine had gradually increased. There was no pain when she urinated, and her eating and sleeping were OK. Her tongue had slimy, yellow fur, and her pulse was slippery and rapid, so she was administered three more packets of the last formula, after which the patient was considered cured.

Remarks

Acupuncture is typically very effective for postpartum urinary retention due to qi vacuity, yang vacuity, and qi stagnation. Frequently, only a single treatment is necessary, with patient's having to urinate while the treatment is still taking place or shortly thereafter. Acupuncture is also effective for damp heat. However, in that case, it should be combined with internally administered Chinese medicinals for best effect.

Endnotes:

1 www.who.int/reproductive-health/publications/MSM_98_3/MSM_98_3chapter3.en.html

2 www.kimjames.net/epidural_risks_and_side_effects.htm

26

Postpartum Fatigue & Exhaustion

It is extremely common for newly delivered mothers to be fatigued during the puer-perium. Fatigue is not considered a disease in modern Western medicine and, unless associated with some other identifiable pathology, there is no treatment for it in Western medicine. Postpartum fatigue is a disease category in Chinese medicine which typically Chinese medicine excels at treating.

Chinese medical disease categorization

Literally, *chan hou ru lao* means postpartum straw mat taxation. This refers to the fact that, in premodern times, Chinese women gave birth on a straw mat which was then disposed of by burning. This disease category covers fatigue and exhaustion after delivery and failure to recuperate spontaneously.

Disease causes & disease mechanisms

Although postpartum fatigue and exhaustion are essentially a vacuity waning of the five viscera, nonetheless, three main viscera are involved, *i.e.*, the lungs, spleen, and kidneys. The lungs rule the qi of the entire body and govern the hundreds of vessels. They convey the finest essence to and nourish and moisten the entire body. If lung qi is insufficient, depurative downbearing loses its normalcy, and water and essence lose their dissemination. It is also possible for an external contraction of wind cold to enter the body and disturb lung function. In either case, damage to the lung qi leads to postpartum straw mat taxation.

The spleen is the latter heaven root of the engenderment and transformation of qi and blood. The spleen nourishes the viscera and bowels and the four extremities. If spleen qi is insufficient, movement and transformation do not perform their duty, and water and grains are not transformed. In that case, qi and blood are not engendered, and this may also lead to postpartum straw mat taxation.

The kidneys, on the other hand, are the former heaven root. They rule the treasuring of the essence qi, and the essence gives rise to the engenderment and transformation of marrow. If kidney qi is insufficient, yin essence is not transformed, and yin and yang do not counterbalance each other. This then leads to postpartum straw mat taxation. In the case of the kidneys, this may involve either yin or yang vacuity depending upon the patient's age, bodily constitution, diet, and lifestyle.

Patterns common to this condition

Spleen-stomach vacuity weakness
Lung qi vacuity detriment
Kidney yin vacuity
Kidney yang vacuity

Treatment based on pattern discrimination

Spleen-stomach vacuity weakness

Main symptoms: Postpartum loss of appetite, bodily fatigue, relative emaciation, somnolence, abdominal distention after meals, loose stools, swollen and edematous face and limbs, lack of warmth in the hands and feet, dizziness standing up, spontaneous perspiration, a sallow yellow facial complexion, a pale, moist tongue, and a fine, forceless, possibly soggy pulse

Treatment principles: Fortify the spleen and boost the qi, harmonize the stomach and restore the appetite

Guiding formulas:

***Xiang Sha Liu Jun Zi Tang Jia Wei* (Auklandia & Amomum Six Gentlemen Decoction with Added Flavors)**
Mu Xiang (Radix Auklandiae), 6-9g
Chen Pi (Pericarpium Citri Reticulatae), 6g
Chen Pi (Fructus Amomi), 3-4.5g
Ren Shen (Radix Ginseng), 3-9g
Bai Zhu (Rhizoma Atractylodis Macrocephalae), 9g
Fu Ling (Poria), 9-12g
mix-fried *Gan Cao* (Radix Glycyrrhizae), 6-9g
Ban Xia (Rhizoma Pinelliae), 9g
Dang Gui (Radix Angelicae Sinensis), 9g
Bai Shao (Radix Albus Paeoniae Lactiflorae), 9g

***Gui Pi Tang* (Restore the Spleen Decoction)**
Bai Zhu (Rhizoma Atractylodis Macrocephalae), 9g

Ren Shen (Radix Ginseng), 3-9g
Huang Qi (Radix Astragali), 9-18g
Dang Gui (Radix Angelicae Sinensis), 9g
Fu Shen (Sclerotium Pararadicis Poriae Cocos), 9-15g
Yuan Zhi (Radix Polygalae), 6-9g
Suan Zao Ren (Semen Zizyphi Spinosae), 9-15g
Long Yan Rou (Arillus Euphoriae Longanae), 9g
Mu Xiang (Radix Auklandiae), 6-9g
Gan Cao (Radix Glycyrrhizae), 3-9g

Acupuncture & moxibustion: *Zu San Li* (St 36), *San Yin Jiao* (Sp 6), *Guan Yuan* (CV 4), *Qi Hai* (CV 6), *Pi Shu* (Bl 20), *Wei Shu* (Bl 21)

If there's orthostatic hypotension, moxa *Bai Hui* (GV 20) and *Da Zhui* (GV 14).

Lung qi vacuity detriment

Main symptoms: Before delivery, the mother has a slight cough. After delivery, this cough becomes more serious. There is shortness of breath, spontaneous perspiration, fever, aversion to cold, joint aching and pain, withered and wan skin and hair, chest oppression, panting, inability to breath lying down, a puffy, white facial complexion, a pale, moist tongue, and a floating, slippery, forceless pulse.

Treatment principles: Supplement the lungs, boost the qi, and stop coughing

Guiding formulas:

**Bu Zhong Yi Qi Tang Jia Wei
(Supplement the Center & Boost the Qi Decoction with Added Flavors)**
Huang Qi (Radix Astragali), 9-18g
Ren Shen (Radix Ginseng), 3-9g
Bai Zhu (Rhizoma Atractylodis Macrocephalae), 9g
mix-fried *Gan Cao* (Radix Glycyrrhizae), 6g
Dang Gui (Radix Angelicae Sinensis), 9g
Chen Pi (Pericarpium Citri Reticulatae), 6g
Sheng Ma (Rhizoma Cimicifugae), 3-4.5g
Chai Hu (Radix Bupleuri), 3-9g
Mai Men Dong (Tuber Ophiopogonis), 9-12g
Wu Wei Zi (Fructus Schisandrae), 9g

This formula also treats qi vacuity not securing postpartum lochia which will not stop.

Ren Shen Bie Jia San (Ginseng & Mud Turtle Carapax Powder)
Huang Qi (Radix Astragali), 9-18g
Bie Jia (Carapax Amydae Sinensis), 9-15g
Niu Xi (Radix Achyranthis Bidentatae), 9-12g
Ren Shen (Radix Ginseng), 3-9g
Fu Ling (Poria), 9-12g

Dang Gui (Radix Angelicae Sinensis), 9g
Bai Shao (Radix Albus Paeoniae Lactiflorae), 9g
Sang Ji Sheng (Herba Taxilli), 9-12g
Mai Men Dong (Tuber Ophiopogonis), 9-12g
Shu Di (cooked Radix Rehmanniae), 12-15g
Tao Ren (Semen Persicae), 9g
Rou Gui (Cortex Cinnamomi), 3-9g
Gan Cao (Radix Glycyrrhizae), 3-9g
Xu Duan (Radix Dipsaci), 9g

Huang Fu-zhong says to use *Chuan Niu Xi* (Radix Cyathulae) instead of *Niu Xi*. He recommends this formula for straw mat fatigue with great qi and blood vacuity, spontaneous perspiration, indigestion of food and drink, occasional cough, and hot and cold similar to malaria. This formula is to be cooked as a soup with pig kidneys. The broth should be drunk and the kidneys eaten.

Acupuncture & moxibustion: Same as above plus *Fei Shu* (Bl 13) and *Tai Yuan* (Lu 9).

Kidney yin vacuity

Main symptoms: Postpartum coming and going of hot and cold sensations, spontaneous perspiration, night sweats, vertigo, impaired memory, low back and knee soreness and limpness, heat in the hands, feet, and heart, a red facial complexion with flushed cheeks, a dry, red tongue with no fur, and a bowstring, fine, rapid pulse

Treatment principles: Enrich yin and supplement the kidneys

Guiding formula:

Liu Wei Di Huang Wan Jia Wei
(Six Flavors Rehmannia Pills with Added Flavors)
Shu Di (cooked Radix Rehmanniae), 12-15g
Shan Yao (Radix Dioscoreae), 9g
Shan Zhu Yu (Fructus Corni), 9g
Fu Ling (Poria), 9-12g
Ze Xie (Rhizoma Alismatis), 6-9g
Dan Pi (Cortex Moutan), 6-9g
Gui Ban (Plastrum Testudinis), 9-15g
Mu Li (Concha Ostreae), 9-18g
Nu Zhen Zi (Fructus Ligustri Lucidi), 9-15g
Bai Shao (Radix Albus Paeoniae Lactiflorae), 9g

This formula also treats liver-kidney yin vacuity postpartum rib-side pain.

Acupuncture & moxibustion: *San Yin Jiao* (Sp 6), *Tai Xi* (Ki 3), *Zhao Hai* (Ki 6), *Guan Yuan* (CV 4), *Shen Shu* (Bl 23)

Kidney yang vacuity

Main symptoms: A dark, dusky facial complexion while the tongue is pale and moist, lack of warmth in the four limbs, low back weakness, cold feet, frequent urination, nocturia, and a deep, weak pulse

Treatment principles: Warm the kidneys and support yang

Guiding formula:

Ba Wei Di Huang Wan Jia Wei
(Eight Flavors Rehamnnia Pills with Added Flavors)
Shu Di (cooked Radix Rehmanniae), 12-15g
Shan Zhu Yu (Fructus Corni), 9g
Shan Yao (Radix Dioscoreae), 9g
Fu Ling (Poria), 9-12g
Rou Gui (Cortex Cinnamomi), 3-9g
Zhi Fu Zi (Radix Lateralis Praeparatus Aconiti Carmichaeli), 3-9g
Ze Xie (Rhizoma Alismatis), 6-9g
Dan Pi (Cortex Moutan), 6-9g
Niu Xi (Radix Achyranthis Bidentatae), 9-12g
Ba Ji Tian (Radix Morindae), 9g

This formula also treats kidney vacuity postpartum polyuria and incontinence.

Acupuncture & moxibustion: San Yin Jiao (Sp 6), *Tai Xi* (Ki 3), *Fu Liu* (Ki 7), *Guan Yuan* (CV 4), *Shen Shu* (Bl 23), *Ming Men* (GV 4)

Remarks

Postpartum fatigue is generally best treated with herbal medicinals administered internally, although acupuncture and especially moxibustion may be a useful adjunct. Most women are grateful for the ability of Chinese medicine to give them more energy and vigor, both physical and mental. In fact, based on the nondualistic point of view of Chinese medicine, strengthening the bodily qi helps construct and nourish the heart spirit, thus promoting a better, more relaxed mental-emotional mood.

27

Postpartum
Insufficient Lactation

Human milk is specific to human infants and confers many benefits on the newborn, including antiviral, antibacterial, antifungal, and antiporotozoal factors as well as antibodies to many specific disease organisms. Breast-fed babies have a lower incidence of infections, anemia, diarrhea, meningitis, diabetes, gastroenteritis, asthma, constipation, allergies, celiac disease, Crohn's disease, dental and speech problems, childhood cancer, pulmonary disease, cataracts, and high cholesterol. Artificially fed babies are 3-4 times more likely to suffer from ear infections and respiratory infections and 16 times more likely to be sick in the first two months of life. As for maternal benefits, breastfeeding stimulates the release of oxytocin which makes the uterus contract, thus minimizing blood loss, promotes the secretion of prolactin which, in turn, promotes relaxation, uses up extra calories and, therefore, helps the postpartum woman lose weight, and lowers the lifetime risks of breast and ovarian cancer and osteoporosis. Given all these benefits to both mother and child, it is no wonder 50% of American mothers are now breastfeeding as compared to less than half that number during the 1960s and 70s.[1]

Although insufficient milk is considered a relatively rare condition in the West, it does occur. When this causes retardation of growth and development in the child due to insufficient nourishment, it is referred to as neonatal insufficient milk syndrome (NIMS). When insufficient milk does occur, it usually manifests during the first six weeks postpartum. Inadequate milk supply is indicated by the baby's output of urine and feces and by his or her pattern of weight gain. During the first 5-6 weeks of life, the baby should wet 6-8 diapers per day and have 2-3 bowel movements per day. Output of less than these amounts may indicate insufficient milk intake. In terms of weight gain, after the first two weeks, the baby should have regained his or her original birth weight and be adding 4-8 ounces per week, while at 6-12 months, the baby should be gaining 1.5-3 ounces per week.[2]

Mammogenesis is completed during pregnancy, with the gland becoming competent to secrete milk sometime after midpregnancy. The onset of copious milk secretion or lactogenesis is held in check until after parturition. In humans, lactogenesis (referred to as the time when the milk "comes in") starts about 40 hours after birth of the infant and is largely complete within five days. Milk secreted during the period between colostrum secretion and mature milk is called transition milk. Full lactation, or the secretion of mature milk, continues as long as the infant receives substantial quantities of milk from his mother, up to 3-4 years in some cultures. When nursing has ceased, the gland undergoes partial involution, a process which is only completed after menopause.[3]

There is growing evidence that the volume of milk produced by women is primarily a function of infant demand and is unaffected by maternal factors such as nutrition, age, and parity (except at very high parities). There appears to be no direct relation between prolactin levels and milk production, and, therefore, it is thought that the rate of milk production depends on control mechanisms localized within the mammary gland. The milk itself contains an inhibitor of milk production (feedback inhibitor of lactation [FIL]) that builds up if the milk remains in the gland over a prolonged period of time. Adequate milk removal from the breast is absolutely necessary for continued milk production. It is becoming increasingly clear that maternal nutrition and other maternal factors play a surprisingly small role in the regulation of human milk production.[4] Based on this new research on lactation, when insufficient lactation is suspected, it is important that the mother be taught how to correctly breastfeed.

That being said, suckling does initiate a neuroendocrine reflex. Afferent impulses travel via sensory neurons from the areola to the hypothalamus. Here they stimulate special neurons to fire, sending an impulse down their axons into the posterior pituitary where the hormone, oxytocin, is released. The oxytocin flows to the breast via the blood and causes contraction of the myoepithelial cells and, thus ejection of the milk. The activity of these neurons can be profoundly influenced by higher brain centers. Therefore, emotional distress can most definitely inhibit milk-ejection.[5] Other factors which are known to decrease milk production are birth control pills, antihistamines, sedatives, smoking tobacco, and excessive caffeine (*i.e.*, more than five cups per day). Hormonal problems and fatigue are also believed to negatively affect the quantity of milk produced.[6] Modern Western medicine currently offers no treatment for women with insufficient milk.

Chinese medical disease categorization

Que ru in Chinese literally means shortness of breast (milk). More traditional terms for this condition found in premodern gynecology texts are *ru ye bu zu*, insufficiency of breast milk, *ru ye bu tong*, breast milk not freely flowing, and *ru ye bu xing*, breast milk not moving. Another contemporary name for this disease category is *chan hou ru ye guo shao*, excessively scanty postpartum breast milk.

Disease causes & disease mechanisms

In Chinese medicine, there are two basic mechanisms responsible for insufficient lactation. Either not enough milk is being engendered or the flow of milk is obstructed and not freely flowing. In the first case, it should be remembered that milk is transformed from blood. If the woman is constitutionally vacuous and weak with less yin and blood and has lost much blood and fluids during delivery or is malnourished, there may not be enough blood from which to engender and transform milk. On the other hand, if the woman's qi is weak, it may be insufficient to engender and transform the blood in order to produce milk.

In the second case, it should be remembered that the liver channel homes to the nipple via an internal pathway and that the flow of qi through the breast is largely dependent on the liver's control over coursing and discharge of the qi horizontally through the chest. If a woman suffers from stress, frustration, anger, or jealousy, this may cause liver depression qi stagnation. Since the qi moves blood and fluids, if the qi does not move, the milk may likewise be stuck within the breast.

Although all Chinese gynecology texts of which I am aware only discuss the above two mechanisms, it is also possible for wind cold external contraction to cause agalactia. In that case, the patient's condition is more likely to be diagnosed as mastitis. Nonetheless, this can also cause agalactia.

Patterns common to this condition

Qi & blood vacuity weakness
Liver depression qi stagnation
Wind cold external contraction

Treatment based on pattern discrimination

Qi & blood vacuity weakness

Main symptoms: Scanty or absent lactation, thin, watery milk, atonic breast tissue, absence of distention or pain, a lusterless facial complexion, heart palpitations, shortness of breath, a pale red tongue, and a fine, forceless pulse. If yin vacuity is more pronounced, there may be night sweats, heat in the hands, feet, and heart, facial flushing, a red tongue with scanty fur, and a fine, rapid pulse.

Treatment principles: Supplement the blood and boost the qi assisted by freeing the flow of the breast milk

Guiding formulas:

Huang Qi Ba Zhen Tang Jia Wei
(Astragalus Eight Pearls Decoction with Added Flavors)
Huang Qi (Radix Astragali), 9-18g

Dang Gui (Radix Angelicae Sinensis), 9g
Bai Shao (Radix Albus Paeoniae Lactiflorae), 9g
Shu Di (cooked Radix Rehmanniae), 9-15g
Chuan Xiong (Radix Ligustici Wallichii), 6-9g
Dang Shen (Radix Codonopsitis), 9-18g
Bai Zhu (Rhizoma Atractylodis Macrocephalae), 9g
Fu Ling (Poria), 9-12g
Gan Cao (Radix Glycyrrhizae), 3-9g
Chi Xiao Dou (Semen Phaseoli), 15-60g
Wang Bu Liu Xing (Semen Vaccariae), 9g

Wang Mi-zhai's Jia Wei Si Wu Tang
(Added Flavors Four Materials Decoction)
Dang Gui (Radix Angelicae Sinensis), 9g
Ren Shen (Radix Ginseng), 3-9g
Chuan Xiong (Radix Ligustici Wallichii), 6-9g
Chi Shao (Radix Rubrus Paeoniae Lactiflorae), 9g
Sheng Di (uncooked Radix Rehmanniae), 9-15g
Jie Geng (Radix Platycodi), 6-9g
Gan Cao (Radix Glycyrrhizae), 3-9g
Mai Men Dong (Tuber Ophiopogonis), 9-12g
Bai Zhu (Rhizoma Atractylodis Macrocephalae), 9g

If the body is hot and the chest and diaphragm are distended and oppressed with dizziness and vertigo of the head and eyes, add *Mu Tong* (Caulis Akebiae) and *Hua Shi* (Talcum).

Tong Ru Dan (Free the Flow of the Breast [Milk] Elixir)
Ren Shen (Radix Ginseng), 3-9g
Huang Qi (Radix Astragali), 9-18g
Dang Gui (Radix Angelicae Sinensis), 9g
Mai Men Dong (Tuber Ophiopogonis), 9-12g
Tong Cao (Medulla Tetrapanacis), 4.5-9g
Jie Geng (Radix Platycodi), 6-9g

Bu Ru Fang (Supplement the Breast [Milk] Formula)
Dang Shen (Radix Codonopsitis), 9-18g
Fu Ling (Poria), 9-12g
Bai Zhu (Rhizoma Atractylodis Macrocephalae), 9g
Dang Gui (Radix Angelicae Sinensis), 9g
Jie Geng (Radix Platycodi), 6-9g
Mu Tong (Caulis Akebiae), 6-9g
Tong Cao (Medulla Tetrapanacis), 4.5-9gg
Chuan Shan Jia (Squama Manitis), 9-12g
Wang Bu Liu Xing (Semen Vaccariae), 9g
Lu Lu Tong (Fructus Liquidambaris Taiwaniae), 9g

Acupuncture & moxibustion: *Ru Gen* (St 18), *Shan Zhong* (CV 17), *Shao Ze* (SI 1), *Pi Shu* (Bl 20), *Zu San Li* (St 36)

Ear points: Chest, Internal Secretion, Liver, Spleen, Kidneys, Triple Burner

Liver depression qi stagnation

Main symptoms: Nonfreely flowing breast milk, breast distention and pain, chest and rib-side distention and fullness, belching, burping, headache, distention of the head and, if serious, fear of cold and slight fever, emotional depression or frustration, a normal tongue with thin, yellow fur, and a bowstring, fine, and/or rapid pulse

Treatment principles: Course the liver and resolve depression, free the flow of the network vessels and precipitate the milk

Guiding formulas:

Shu Gan Tong Ru Tang
(Course the Liver & Free the Flow of the Breast [Milk] Decoction)
Chai Hu (Radix Bupleuri), 9g
Qing Pi (Fructus Citri Reticulatae Viride), 6-9g
Chuan Shan Jia (Squama Manitis), 9-12g
Dan Shen (Radix Salviae Miltiorrhizae), 9-15g
Wang Bu Liu Xing (Semen Vaccariae), 9g
Bai Zhu (Rhizoma Atractylodis Macrocephalae), 9g
Tong Cao (Medulla Tetrapanacis), 4.5-9g
Chuan Lian Zi (Fructus Toosendan), 6-9g
Lou Lu (Radix Rhapontici/Echinopsis), 9g
Gan Cao (Radix Glycyrrhizae), 3-9g

Tong Gan Shen Ru Tang
(Free the Flow of the Liver & Extend the Breast [Milk] Decoction)
Bai Shao (Radix Albus Paeoniae Lactiflorae), 9g
Dang Gui (Radix Angelicae Sinensis), 9g
Bai Zhu (Rhizoma Atractylodis Macrocephalae), 9g
Shu Di (cooked Radix Rehmanniae), 9-15g
Mai Men Dong (Tuber Ophiopogonis), 9-12g
Tong Cao (Medulla Tetrapanacis), 4.5-9g
Chai Hu (Radix Bupleuri), 9g
Yuan Zhi (Radix Polygalae), 6-9g

This formula treats liver depression complicated by qi and blood insufficiency.

Tong Ru Tang (Free the Flow of the Breast [Milk] Decoction)
Dang Gui (Radix Angelicae Sinensis), 9g
Sheng Di (uncooked Radix Rehmanniae), 12-15g
Mai Men Dong (Tuber Ophiopogonis), 9-12g
Tian Hua Fen (Radix Trichosanthis), 9g
Bai Shao (Radix Albus Paeoniae Lactiflorae), 9g

Wang Bu Liu Xing (Semen Vaccariae), 9g
Shan Jia (Squama Manitis), 9-15g
Sheng Ma (Rhizoma Cimicifugae), 3-4.5g
Chuan Xiong (Radix Ligustici Wallichii), 6-9g
Jie Geng (Radix Platycodi), 6-9g

Lou Lu San (Rhaponticus Powder)
Lou Lu (Radix Rhapontici/Echinopsis), 9g
Chi Shao (Radix Rubrus Paeoniae Lactiflorae), 9g
Jie Geng (Radix Platycodi), 6-9g
Bai Zhi (Radix Angelicae Dahuricae), 9-15g
Gan Cao (Radix Glycyrrhizae), 3-9g
Zao Jiao Ci (Spina Gleditschiae Chinensis), 6-9g
Dang Gui (Radix Angelicae Sinensis), 9g
Chuan Xiong (Radix Ligustici Wallichii), 9g
Zhi Ke (Fructus Aurantii), 6-9g
Mu Xiang (Radix Auklandiae), 6-9g

This formula is for swelling and lumps with the beginnings of inflammation and abscess.

Acupuncture & moxibustion: *Ru Gen* (St 18), *Shan Zhong* (CV 17), *Shao Ze* (SI 1), *Gan Shu* (Bl 18), *Qi Men* (Liv 14)

Ear points: Chest, Liver, Gallbladder, Brain, Subcortex, Sympathetic

Wind cold external contraction

Main symptoms: Rapid onset agalactia with a palpable swelling or lump in the breast that is painful upon pressure, aversion to cold, fever, a pale tongue with white fur, and a floating, fine, bowstring pulse

Treatment principles: Dispel wind and nourish the blood, quicken the network vessels and transform stasis

Guiding formula:

Shu Feng Huo Luo Tong Ru Yin (Course Wind, Quicken the Network Vessels & Free the Flow of the Breast [Milk] Drink)
Fang Feng (Radix Sapshnikoviae), 9g
Hai Tong Pi (Cortex Erythrinae Variegatae), 9g
Xi Xian Cao (Herba Siegesbeckiae Orientalis), 9g
Wei Ling Xian (Radix Clematidis), 9g
Xu Duan (Radix Dipsaci), 9g
Dang Gui (Radix Angelicae Sinensis), 9g
Bai Shao (Radix Albus Paeoniae Lactiflorae), 9g
Bai Wei (Radix Cynanchi Atrati), 9g
Liu Ji Nu (Radix Angelicae Anomalae), 9g
Wang Bu Liu Xing (Semen Vaccariae), 9g

Lou Lu (Radix Rhapontici/Echinopsis), 9g
Chuan Shan Jia (Squama Manitis), 9-15g
Qing Pi (stir-fried Pericarpium Citri Reticulatae Viride), 6-9g
Xi Xin (Herba Asari), 1-3g

Acupuncture & moxibustion: *Ru Gen* (St 18), *Shan Zhong* (CV 17), *Shao Ze* (SI 1), *He Gu* (LI 4), *Qu Chi* (LI 11), *Wai Guan* (TB 5)

Abstracts of representative Chinese research

From "The Treatment of 64 Cases of Postpartum Insufficient Lactation with *Chi Xiao Dang Qi Tang* (Aduki Bean, Dang Gui & Astragalus Decoction)" by Zhao Rui-fen & Wang Hong-zhao, *Xin Zhong Yi (New Chinese Medicine)*, #12, 2001, p. 53-54

Cohort description:

The 64 women in this study were 24-32 years old and all were 4-28 days postpartum. Forty-two had given birth normally, while 22 had had cesarean deliveries. Twenty-six patients were able to discharge less than 10ml of milk, 16 were able to discharge less than 20ml of milk, and 22 cases had no milk. In addition, 21 cases had anemia.

Treatment method:

The basic formula consisted of: *Chi Xiao Dou* (Semen Phaseoli), 30g, *Huang Qi* (Radix Astragali), 30-40g, *Dang Gui* (Radix Angelicae Sinensis), 10g, blast-fried *Chuan Shan Jia* (Squama Manitis), 6g, *Lu Lu Tong* (Fructus Liquidambaris Taiwaniae), 10g, *Tong Cao* (Medulla Tetrapanacis), 5g, and *Chai Hu* (Radix Bupleuri), 3g. If the breasts were soft and flaccid and there was lack of strength, *Dang Shen* (Radix Codonopsitis) was added. If the breasts were distended and painful, *Chuan Lian Zi* (Fructus Toosendan) was added. If there was low back pain, *Xu Duan* (Radix Dipsaci) and *Tu Si Zi* (Semen Cuscutae) were added. One packet was decocted in water and administered orally per day in two divided doses, and this treatment was continued 3-5 days.

Treatment outcomes:

Thirty-two cases got a marked effect. This meant that their milk increased to 50ml each time within 3-5 days. Twenty-two cases were judged improved. This meant that their milk production increased but still did not reach 30ml. No result meant that, after five days of treatment, there was still not secretion of milk, and 10 cases were judged not to have gotten any effect. Thus the total amelioration rate was 84.3%. Seven of the 10 women who did not get any effect had had c-sections.

From "The Treatment of 104 Cases of Postpartum Insufficient Lactation with *Sheng Yu Zeng Ru Yin* (Sagely Curing & Increasing Breast [Milk] Drink)" by Chen Li-fu & Xie Lin, *Ji Lin Zhong Yi Yao (Jilin Chinese Medicine & Medicinals)*, #4, 1999, p. 27

Cohort description:

Seventy-two of the 104 patients in this study were 23-26 years old, and 32 were 27 or older, with the oldest patient being 38. Fifty-two patients had lack of milk beginning immediately after delivery, 30 had developed insufficient milk 4-14 days postpartum, and 22 had developed this condition more than 14 days postpartum, with the longest time to onset being 40 days after delivery. Sixty-eight patients had soft, atonic breasts and clear, thin milk, while 22 had accompanying chest and rib-side distention and oppression with slightly distended breasts due to psychoemotional stress. Seventy-five women had lusterless facial complexions, lassitude of the spirit, lack of strength, and other such qi and blood dual depletion symptoms. Twenty-four patients had accompanying constipation.

Treatment method:

The basic formula consisted of: *Huang Qi* (Radix Astragali), 30-50g, *Dang Shen* (Radix Codonopsitis) and *Wang Bu Liu Xing* (Semen Vaccariae), 30g each, *Shu Di* (cooked Radix Rehmanniae), *Dang Gui* (Radix Angelicae Sinensis), *Bai Shao* (Radix Albus Paeoniae Lactiflorae), *Chuan Shan Jia* (Squama Manitis), and *Lou Lu* (Radix Rhapontici/Echinposis), 15g each, and *Chuan Xiong* (Radix Ligustici Wallichii), *Tong Cao* (Medulla Tetrapanacis), and *Gan Cao* (Radix Glycyrrhizae), 6g each. If there was emotional discomfort with breast, chest, and rib-side distention, 12 grams each of *Qing Pi* (Pericarpium Citri Reticulatae Viride) and *Chai Hu* (Radix Bupleuri) were added. If there was yin vacuity and blood depletion with dry stools, 15 grams each of *Mai Men Dong* (Tuber Ophiopogonis) and processed *He Shou Wu* (Radix Polygoni Multiflori) were added. One packet of these medicinals was decocted in water and administered internally per day.

Treatment outcomes:

Cure was defined as sufficient breast milk with the ability to breastfeed the baby for six months without eating additional food. Improvement was defined as a marked increase in breast milk. However, breastfeeding could not be maintained for six months without eating more food. No effect meant that, after six packets, there was no marked increase in breast milk. Based on these criteria, 84 women (80.8%) were judged cured. Among these, 50 cases responded in 2-4 packets, 25 cases responded in 5-6 packets, and nine cases required seven or more packets. Fifteen cases (14.4%) were judged improved, and five cases (4.8%) got no effect. Thus the total amelioration rate was 95.2%.

From "A Clinical Audit of the Treatment of 78 Cases of Postpartum Insufficient Lactation with *Zeng Ru Tang* (Increase Breast [Milk] Decoction)" by Wang Jin-quan & Liu Xiao-ying, *Shan Xi Zhong Yi (Shanxi Chinese Medicine)*, #4, 1993, p. 27

Cohort description:

All 78 women in this study were 22-38 years of age. Fifty-two women were primiparas and 26 were multiparas. Fifty-six women had given birth at full term, nine had given birth prematurely, and 13 had been past due. Sixty-three women had given birth normally, and 15 had had c-sections. Forty-seven women had developed insufficient lactation within 10 days postpartum, 18 cases had developed insufficient lactation 11-30 days postpartum, 13 cases had developed this condition 31-60 days postpartum, and three cases had developed it more than 60 days postpartum. In 32 cases, there was either dribbling and dripping or no milk at all, while in 28 cases, there was accompanying breast swelling and distention.

Treatment method:

The basic formula consisted of: *Dang Gui* (Radix Angelicae Sinensis), 20g, uncooked *Huang Qi* (Radix Astragali), 20g, *Dang Shen* (Radix Codonopsitis), 20g, *Bai Zhi* (Radix Angelicae Dahuricae), 5g, *Mu Tong* (Caulis Akebiae), 4g, *Tong Cao* (Medulla Tetrapanacis), 4g, *Lu Lu Tong* (Fructus Liquidambaris Taiwaniae), 5g, *Jie Geng* (Radix Platycodi), 5g, blast-fried *Chuan Shan Jia* (Squama Manitis), 5g, *Si Gua Luo* (Fasciulus Luffae Cylindricae), 6g, *Wang Bu Liu Xing* (Semen Vaccariae), 9g, *Mai Men Dong* (Tuber Ophiopogonis), 10g, *Tian Hua Fen* (Radix Trichosanthis), 10g, *Hei Zhi Ma* (Semen Sesami Indici), 15g, *Gua Lou* (Fructus Trichosanthis), 12g, uncooked *Gan Cao* (Radix Glycyrrhizae), 3g, *Tao Ren* (Semen Persicae), 5 pieces. If there was no breast distention but rather marked qi and blood vacuity, *Dang Gui, Huang Qi,* and *Dang Shen* were increased to 30 grams each and *Tian Hua Fen* was increased to 15 grams. If there was breast distention and hardness with lumps, 12 grams each of *Qing Pi* (Pericarpium Citri Reticulatae Viride), *Ju He* (Semen Citri Reticulatae), and *Zao Jiao Ci* (Spina Gleditschiae Chinensis) were added. If the breasts were distended, painful, and burning hot, 10 grams each of *Pu Gong Ying* (Herba Taraxaci) and *Lian Qiao* (Fructus Forsythiae) were added. If there was marked anger damaging the liver, six grams each of *Chai Hu* (Radix Bupleuri) and *Xiang Fu* (Rhizoma Cyperi) were added. One packet of these medicinals was decocted in water per day and administered internally in two divided doses, morning and evening.

Treatment outcomes:

Cure was defined as an increase in milk secretion after taking the above medicinals to the point where the child could gather all his or her nutrition from the breast milk alone. Some effect was defined as a marked increase in breast milk secretion, and no effect meant that there was no improvement in breast milk secretion after taking these medicinals. Based on these criteria, 49 cases were judged cured and 21 cases got some effect. Four cases got no effect. Thus the total amelioration rate was 89.7%. The smallest number of packets taken was one and the largest was nine, with an average of 4.3 packets. There were no observable side effects with this protocol.

From "The Treatment of 58 Cases of Insufficient Lactation with Self-composed *Cui Ru Yin* (Promote Breast [Milk] Drink)" by Yang Su-e, *Si Chuan Zhong Yi (Sichuan Chinese Medicine)*, #12, 2001, p. 51

Cohort description:

Of the 58 patients in this study, the oldest was 37 and the youngest was 20 years old. the shortest period of insufficient lactation was two months and the longest was six months. Forty-eight women were primiparas, eight women were second-time mothers, and two women were third-time mothers. All the women had soft, atonic breasts, and none had lumps or pressure pain.

Treatment method:

The basic formula consisted of: *Dang Shen* (Radix Codonopsitis), 20g, *Dang Gui* (Radix Angelicae Sinensis), 9g, *Mu Tong* (Caulis Akebiae), 5g, *Lou Lu* (Radix Rhapontici/Echinopsis), *Wang Bu Liu Xing* (Semen Vaccariae), *Gan Cao* (Radix Glycyrrhizae), and *Tian Hua Fen* (Radix Trichosanthis), 6g each. If qi and blood vacuity was severe, 10 grams of *Huang Qi* (Radix Astragali) and five grams of *Jie Geng* (Radix Platycodi) were added. If liver depression qi stagnation was severe, nine grams of *Bai Shao* (Radix Albus Paeoniae Lactiflorae) and six grams each of *Chuan Xiong* (Radix Ligustici Wallichii), *Qing Pi* (Pericarpium Citri Reticulatae Viride), *Chai Hu* (Radix Bupleuri), and *Tong Cao* (Medulla Tetrapanacis) were added. If there was poor appetite, nine grams of *Shen Qu* (Massa Medica Fermentata) and six grams of *Mai Ya* (Fructus Germinatus Hordei) were added. If liver depression had transformed heat, six grams each of *Huang Qin* (Radix Scutellariae) and *Jin Yin Hua* (Flos Lonicerae) or *Lian Qiao* (Fructus Forsythiae) were added. One packet was decocted in water and administered per day, with 10 days equaling one course of treatment.

Treatment outcomes:

Marked effect meant that, after one course of treatment, women had enough milk to feed a 4-6 month-old child. Some effect meant that the women got the same effect after two courses. No effect meant that this result was not achieved after three or more courses of treatment. Based on these criteria, 30 cases (51.7%) got a marked effect, 26 cases (44.8%) got some effect, and two cases (3.4%) got no effect, for a total amelioration rate of 96.6%.

Representative case histories

Case 1: The patient was a 28 year-old female medical teacher who was one half month postpartum and whose breast milk was extremely scanty. The breasts did not feel distended, and they had a soft-looking appearance. The breast milk itself was clear and thin like water. The patient's lochia had recently ceased, however, she had lack of strength and poor appetite, and stirring caused her to become dizzy with blurred vision. The patient's tongue was pale and moist, and her pulse was fine and forceless. When pressed it was deep and faint. In addition, this patient had a habitually weak body. Therefore, her pattern was categorized as qi and blood vacuity weakness scanty lactation, and she was prescribed the following medicinals in order to supplement the qi to engender the blood: mix-fried *Huang Qi* (Radix Astragali), 15g, *Dang Shen* (Radix Codonopsitis), 12g, *Chuan Xiong* (Radix Angelicae Sinensis), 9g, *Dang Gui* (Radix Ligustici Wallichii), 6g, *Bai Zhu* (Rhizoma Atractylodis Macrocephalae), 9g, *Shu Di* (cooked Radix Rehmanniae), 9g, *Sha Ren* (Fructus Amomi), 3g, *Tong Cao* (Medulla Tetrapanacis), 4.5g, and *Wang Bu Liu Xing* (Semen Vaccariae), 6g. In addition, the patient was instructed to make a soup from ham hocks and to drink this.

At the second examination, after having taken four packets of the above medicinals, the patient's milk had descended. However, its amount was still scanty and its consistency was still thin. The woman now had a distended feeling in her breasts, but her breasts were still soft. This suggested that her qi and blood were still both vacuous. Therefore, she was prescribed three packets of the following medicinals: *Huang Qi* (Radix Astragali), 21g, *Dang Shen* (Radix Codonopsitis), 15g, *Dang Gui* (Radix Angelicae Sinensis), 15g, *Chuan Shan Jia* (Squama Manitis), 3g, plus the same amounts of the other same medicinals in the first formula. After taking these three packets, the patient reported that her strength was back, her breasts were full, and her milk had significantly increased.

Case 2: The patient was a 26 year-old female agricultural worker who was newly delivered and first seen on June 24, 1988. This patient habitually ate acrid, peppery foods. After giving birth, her stools were dry and bound and hemafecia was profuse. Six days postpartum, the woman's milk would not move. When examined, both breasts were swollen and distended, her tongue had slimy, yellow fur, and her pulse was fine and rapid. Based on these signs and symptoms, the woman's pattern was categorized as damp heat brewing and binding. This had caused the hemafecia below and the nonmoving breast milk above. Therefore, the treatment principles were to clear heat and disinhibit dampness, harmonize the blood and moisten dryness. For this, *Chi Xiao Dou Dang Gui San* (Aduki Bean & Dang Gui Powder) was prescribed: *Dang Gui* (Radix Angelicae Sinensis), 60g, and *Chi Xiao Dou* (Semen Phaseoli), 90g. One packet of these medicinals was decocted in water and administered orally per day. After four days, the patient's stools were regulated and moist and her breast milk was freely and easily moving.

Case 3: The patient was a 31 year-old female cadre who was first seen on Nov. 6, 1989. The patient had recently delivered. The woman had a habitually weak body and had had a miscarriage four years before. At this birth, she had lost a lot of blood, and, afterwards, her breast milk was scanty, providing her baby with only half of what it needed to eat. The patient self-administered *Cui Ru Pian* (Promote Breast [Milk] Tablets), but, after taking these for seven days, there was no effect. She also had taken three packets of *Tong Ru Dan* (Free the Flow of the Breast [Milk] Elixir), also without effect. When examined, the patient's breasts were soft and atonic. Her tongue was dark but pale with scanty fur, and her pulse was deep, fine, and choppy. Therefore, she was prescribed *Dang Gui Si Ni Tang Jia Wei* (Dang Gui Four Counterflows Decoction with Added Flavors): *Dang Gui* (Radix Angelicae Sinensis), 30g, *Chi Shao* (Radix Rubrus Paeoniae Lactiflorae), 15g, *Gui Zhi* (Ramulus Cinnamomi), 15g, *Xi Xin* (Herba Asari), 3g, *Tong Cao* (Medulla Tetrapanacis), 10g, mix-fried *Gan Cao* (Radix Glycyrrhizae), 5g, and *Da Zao* (Fructus Jujubae), 10 pieces. One packet was decocted in water and administered per day, and, after taking three packets the patient's hands and feet had become warm, her breasts felt more distended, and her breast milk increased. After taking six more packets of this formula, the woman's hands and feet were warm and comfortable and her breast milk was full.

Case 4: The patient was a 36 year-old female teacher who was first seen on Jul. 20, 1990. After the patient's second birth, this patient suffered the bitterness of no breast milk. Each day she had to feed her new baby daughter with cow's milk. The patient self-administered two bottles of *Cui Ru Pian* (Promote Breast [Milk] Tablets) but without effect. She had also received four acupuncture treatments and had been prescribed six packets of Chinese medicinals, all also without effect. Now the patient was 40 days postpartum. Both breasts were slightly distended, breast milk was extremely scanty, there was a severely dry mouth with thirst and a liking for hot drinks. Urination was inhibited, and the patient's lower limbs were cold and chilly. She wore several pairs of socks to try to keep her feet warm. Her tongue was pale, tender, and had scanty fluids, while her pulse was deep, fine, and forceless.

Based on the above signs and symptoms, this case was categorized as yang vacuity with qi not transforming fluids. Instead, water had collected and obstructed the network vessels, thus the scanty lactation, cold lower limbs, and dryness above. The patient was prescribed three packets of the following medicinals: *Tian Hua Fen* (Radix Trichosanthis), 20g, *Qu Mai* (Herba Dianthi), 15g, *Shan Yao* (Radix Dioscoreae), 15g, *Fu Ling* (Poria), 30g, *Zhi Fu Zi* (Radix Lateralis Praeparatus Aconiti Carmichaeli), 10g, and *Tong Cao* (Medulla Tetrapanacis), 10g, one packet per day. After taking these medicinals, the patient reported that her thrist had decreased and her lower limbs had become warm. In addition, her urination had increased and so, markedly, had her breast milk. After taking another three packets, the inhibited urination, chilled lower extremities, and thirst were all basically cured and her breast milk had greatly increased. Therefore, she was told to take nine grams each time of the same formula made into pills, two times per day. After another 15 days, the patient's breast milk was full.

Remarks

1. While Western medical texts suggest that insufficient milk is a relatively rare phenomenon, I have had numerous occasions to treat this condition over the last 22 years of practice. Perhaps this is because, when it does occur, Western medicine has no treatment to offer. Therefore, women are forced to seek out alternatives. In any case, my experience is that Chinese medicine treats this condition extremely well.

2. Song and Yu say that eight out of 10 cases of postpartum insufficient lactation in China are due to insufficiency. My experience in America is that most cases of insufficient lactation are due to a combination of vacuity and repletion. This is because of the relationship between the liver and spleen. In real-life Western women, it is rare for liver depression not to cause simultaneous spleen vacuity. However, because the spleen is the latter heaven root of the engenderment and transformation of qi and blood, most cases of spleen vacuity, especially in women, are complicated by blood vacuity, and milk is made out of blood. Therefore, in my experi-

ence, most women with insufficient lactation have a liver-spleen disharmony with a qi and blood vacuity. Then, depending on their age and body type, they may also have a yin vacuity as well.

3. Certain Chinese medicinals have a special tropism for the breasts and, empirically, free the flow of the breast milk by freeing the flow of the qi and blood within the breasts. These specical medicinals include *Wang Bu Liu Xing* (Semen Vaccariae), *Chuan Shan Jia* (Squama Manitis), *Mu Tong* (Caulis Akebiae), *Lu Lu Tong* (Fructus Liquidambaris Taiwaniae), *Tong Cao* (Medulla Tetrapanacis), *Lou Lu* (Radix Rhapontici/Echinopsis), and *Gua Lou* (Fructus Trichosanthis) to name the most important of these. As the reader will see, one or more of these medicinals is found in almost every one of the above formulas.

Endnotes:

[1] www.breastfeedingbasics.com/html/why_breastfeed.htm

[2] www.parentsplace.com/expert/lactation/qas/0,10338,239801_108781,00.html

[3] http://classes.aces.uiuc.edu/AnSci308/HumanLact.html

[4] http://mammary.nih.gov/reviews/lactation/Hartmann001/

[5] http://classes.aces.uiuc.edu, *op. cit.*

[6] www.parentsplace.com, *op. cit.*

28

Postpartum Areolar Eczema

Some breastfeeding women experience cracking, chapping, pain, and itching of their nipples. The most common Western medical diagnosis of this is areolar eczema. Most often this occurs in primiparas. Because, cracked nipples may allow entry of *Staphylococcus* bacteria from the baby's mouth and throat to enter the breast causing mastitis, this condition may not only cause its own discomfort but lead to more serious conditions. Western medicine treats areolar eczema by internally administered corticosteroids and externally administered moisturizing creams. Breast-feeding mothers are recommended to suspend breastfeeding until the lesions have healed.[1]

Chinese medical disease categorization

In Chinese, this condition is most commonly referred to as *ru tou po sui*. *Ru tou* means the nipple (literally, breast head), and *po sui* means tattered and cracked. In premodern texts, this condition is also referred to as *ru tou feng*, nipple wind.

Disease causes & disease mechanisms

As discussed above, the liver channel homes to the nipple, and the breast itself is traversed by the foot *yang ming*. Depressive anger may damage the liver with qi depression transforming fire. At the same time, since liver wood disease often affects spleen earth, spleen-stomach movement and transformation may lose their normalcy. In that case, clear and turbid are not separated, and damp heat may be engenderd internally. This fire and damp heat may then bind together causing inflammation, dryness, bleeding, and exudation of the nipples.

Classical Chinese texts say this condition is due to wind from the suckling baby's mouth. If wind here means an unseeable, microscopic pathogen, then this description is not wrong since most commonly this condition occurs in women whose babies suffer from oral thrush. In this case, the microbial pathogen is the commensal saprophyte, Candida albicans. However, before such a commensal microbe can cause a pathological response, there must be a resonant imbalance in the mother establishing a terrain for the microbe to flourish inappropriately.

Treatment based on pattern discrimination

Mutual binding of fire & damp heat

Main symptoms: Dry, itchy, chapped, and/or cracked nipples in a breastfeeding mother causing cutting or lancinating pain when the baby suckles, possible bleeding and/or discharge of a thick, watery fluid or a greasy yellow exudate, yellow tongue fur, and a bowstring, rapid pulse

Treatment principles: Clear heat, eliminate dampness, and resolve depression

Guiding formulas:

Long Dan Xie Gan Tang (Gentiana Drain the Liver Decoction)
Long Dan Cao (Radix Gentianae), 6-9g
Huang Qin (Radix Scutellariae), 9-12g
Zhi Zi (Fructus Gardeniae), 6-9g
Ze Xie (Rhizoma Alismatis), 6-9g
Che Qian Zi (Semen Plantaginis), 6-9g
Mu Tong (Caulis Akebiae), 6-9g
Sheng Di (uncooked Radix Rehmanniae), 12-15g
Dang Gui Wei (Extremitas Radicis Angelicae Sinensis), 6-9g
Chai Hu (Radix Bupleuri), 6-9g
Gan Cao (Radix Glycyrrhizae), 3-9g

If there is constipation, add *Da Huang* (Radix Et Rhizoma Rhei). This formula is for prominent damp heat. In this case, there will be thick, yellow fur and a slippery, rapid pulse with yellowish exudation from the nipples.

Qing Re Chu Shi Tang (Clear Heat & Eliminate Dampness Decoction)
Jin Yin Hua (Flos Lonicerae), 9-15g
Bai Xian Pi (Cortex Dictamni), 9-15g
Hua Shi (Talcum), 9-15g
Yi Yi Ren (Semen Coicis), 15-30g
Huang Bai (Cortex Phellodendri), 9g
Huang Qin (Radix Scutellariae), 9-12g
Yin Chen Hao (Herba Capillaris), 9g
Che Qian Zi (Semen Plantaginis), 6-9g
Cang Zhu (Rhizoma Atractylodis), 9g
Ku Shen (Radix Sophorae Flavescentis), 9-15g
Mu Tong (Caulis Akebiae), 6-9g
Gan Cao (Radix Glycyrrhizae), 3-9g

Likewise, this formula is for marked damp heat.

Dan Zhi Xiao Yao San Jia Jian
(Moutan & Gardenia Rambling Powder with Additions & Subtractions)
Dan Pi (Cortex Moutan), 6-9g
Zhi Zi (Fructus Gardeniae), 6-9g
Chai Hu (Radix Bupleuri), 9g
Bai Shao (Radix Albus Paeoniae Lactiflorae), 9g
Dang Gui (Radix Angelicae Sinensis), 9g
Bai Zhu (Rhizoma Atractylodis Macrocephalae), 9g
Fu Ling (Poria), 9-12g
Gan Cao (Radix Glycyrrhizae), 3-9g
Xia Ku Cao (Spica Prunellae), 9-15g
Bai Zhi (Radix Angelicae Dahuricae), 9-15g

This formula is for more prominent depressive liver fire and less dampness. This patient's condition is reactive to stress, and the nipples are more chapped, cracked, and inflamed but present no particular exudation. Rather they are more apt to bleed.

External treatments:

Ku Shen Tang (Sophora Decoction)
Ku Shen (Radix Sophorae Flavescentis), 9-15g
Ye Ju Hua (Flos Chrysanthemi Indici), 9-15g
She Chuang Zi (Semen Cnidii Monnieri), 9-15g
Jin Yin Hua (Flos Lonicerae), 9-15g
Bai Zhi (Radix Angelicae Dahuricae), 9-15g
Huang Bai (Cortex Phellodendri), 9g
Di Fu Zi (Fructus Kochiae), 9-15g
Shi Chang Pu (Rhizoma Acori Tatarinowii), 6-9g

It is also possible to add *Da Qing Ye* (Folium Daqingye) and *Ban Lan Gen* (Radix Istadis/Baphicacanthi). These ingredients should be decocted in water and the breast washed repeatedly with this liquid. This formula is suitable if there is exudation, in which case one should not apply an oil-based ointment.

Bai Zhi San (Angelica Dahurica Powder)
Bai Zhi (Radix Angelicae Dahuricae)

Grind this into a fine powder and dust the affected area. This may be used after washing the nipple with the above formula and is useful when there is exudation from the affected area.

Qing Dai San (Indigo Powder)
Qing Dai (Indigo Naturalis)
Huang Bai (Cortex Phellodendri)
Shi Gao (Gypsum Fibrosum)
Hua Shi (Talcum)

Grind equal amounts of the above ingredients into a fine powder and mix with cold water. Apply to the affected area if there is serous exudation, inflammation, and itching. If there is no exudation, this powder may be mixed with an ointment base and applied as an ointment. This is called *Qing Dai Gao* (Indigo Ointment) and moistens dryness as it clears heat and kills microbes. This ointment is available from Blue Poppy Herbs under the name "Antifungal Ointment."

Si Huang San (Four Yellows Powder)
Da Huang (Radix Et Rhizoma Rhei)
Huang Qin (Radix Scutellariae)
Huang Lian (Rhizoma Coptidis)
Huang Bai (Cortex Phellodendri)

Grind equal amounts of the above ingredients into a fine powder and mix with cold water. Apply to the affected area if there is serous exudation. Like *Qing Dai San* above, this powder may also be mixed with an ointment base if there is no exudation. Then it is called *Si Huang Gao* (Four Yellows Ointment). It is also available from Blue Poppy Herbs under the name "Clear Heat Ointment."

For chapping, dryness, and parching, use *Gui Ban* (mix-fried Plastrum Testudinis) and *Zhang Nao* (Camphora). Grind into a fine powder, mix with roasted sesame seed oil, and apply.

For damp, suppurating ulcers, use *Huang Bai* (Cortex Phellodendri), *Zi Cao* (Radix Lithospermi/Arnebiae), *Ku Fan* (Alum), and *Mang Xiao* (Mirabilitum). Decoct in water and apply as a wet compress.

Abstracts of representative Chinese research

From "Ophiopogon in the Treatment of Cracked Nipple" by Song Shu-qing & Xu Shao-hua, *Shan Dong Zhong Yi Za Zhi (Shandong Journal of Chinese Medicine)*, #1, 1995, p. 34

Cohort description:

Over a number of years, the author has used *Mai Men Dong* (Tuber Ophiopogonis) as an external application in the treatment of 31 cases of cracked nipples. Twenty-two of the women were primiparas and nine were multiparas. The duration of the disease ranged from 5-20 days. Eight women were cured after one course of treatment, 16 were cured after two courses, and seven were cured after three courses of treatment.

Treatment method:

Fifty grams of *Mai Men Dong* were ground and placed in a bottle to be stored for use. At the time of treatment, the affected area was first washed with physiologic salt water. Then a suitable amount of the ground *Mai Men Dong* was mixed with vinegar and made into a plaster. This was applied to the affected area and changed once every five hours. Three days equaled one course of treatment. While being treated with these medicinals, patients were forbidden to eat acrid, peppery foods and were instructed to temporarily suspend breastfeeding.

Treatment outcomes:

Eight women were cured after one course of treatment, 16 were cured after two courses, and seven were cured after three courses of treatment.

From "The Treatment of 34 Cases of Cracked Nipples with *Bai Jin Tang* (Alum & Lonicera Decoction)" by Niu Wu-qun, *Zhe Jiang Zhong Yi Za Zhi (Zhejiang Journal of Chinese Medicine)*, #11, 1995, p. 518

Cohort description:

From 1988-1992, the author of this clinical audit treated 34 cases of cracked nipples with the external application of *Bai Jin Tang* with very good results.

Treatment method:

Bai Jin Tang consisted of: *Ku Fan* (Alum) and *Bai Ji* (Rhizoma Bletillae), 30g each, and *Jin Yin Hua* (Flos Lonicerae), 20g. These medicinals were decocted in water two times in order to achieve 100ml of medicinal liquid. This was then used to wash the affected area 10 times each day. During the time these medicinals were used, the number of times of breastfeeding was reduced as much as possible in order to allow the wound to heal. Ten days equaled one course of treatment.

Treatment outcomes:

Thirteen cases were cured in one course, and 14 cases in two courses. Three cases saw their aching and pain diminish and the wounds shrink after being treated for two courses, while four cases got no effect after two courses of treatment.

Remarks

1. Western women with this condition typically present with a combination of repletion and vacuity. In that case, *Long Dan Xie Gan Tang* (Gentiana Drain the Liver Decoction) is too harsh and attacking, even for short-term use, and should be modified by appropriate additions and subtractions so that it does not further damage the spleen.

2. In my experience, most patients with this condition have a history of candidiasis or intestinal dysbiosis associated with atopic dermatitis and other allergic or even autoimmune conditions. In such cases, a clear, bland diet is extremely important for the overall effectiveness of Chinese medical treatment.

Endnote:

[1] www.totalskincare.com/library/totalskincare_n_nipple-eczema.html

29

Postpartum Mastitis

Postpartum mastitis refers to infection of a mammary duct or gland leading to inflammation of the affected breast during the puerperium. Along with postpartum urinary tract infections, mastitis is one of the two most common postpartum infections.[1] This condition is most likely during the first three months postpartum, and usually occurs during the first 3-4 weeks postpartum.[2] The most common organism implicated in this infection is *Staphylococcus aureus* which usually comes from the breast-feeding infant's mouth or throat.[3] Predisposing factors include fatigue, stress, plugged duct, abrupt change in feeding pattern, engorgement, oversupply, tight or under-wire bra, and cracked nipple. The signs and symptoms of this condition include sudden onset of fever, chills, and flu-like symptoms accompanied by a red, hot, swollen breast (often in the upper outer quadrant).[4] The Western medical treatment of this condition mainly consists of the administration of dicloxacillin, penicillinase-resistant penicillin, or clindamycin, the continuation of breast-feeding, the use of analgesics for pain control, possible ice packs over the affected area, and support of the breast. If an abscess forms, this may need to be drained surgically.

Chinese medical disease categorization

In Chinese, *chan hou ru yong* means postpartum breast welling abscess, while *chan hou ru yan* means postpartum breast rock. The first condition corresponds to non-purulent mastitis, while the second corresponds to a breast abscess. Typically, breast rock refers to the latter stages of a breast abscess which has either not been or not successfully treated.

Disease causes & disease mechanisms

In Chinese medicine, mastitis is most often due to emotional agitation and excessive anger. This gives rise to depressive fire within the liver channel. The liver homes to the nipple via an internal branch. In addition, liver heat often gives rise to stomach heat since both participate in the larger vision of lifegate fire. When one becomes pathologically hot, so often does the other. This is called mutual engenderment.

Since the foot *yang ming* stomach channel also traverses the breast, this combination of liver and stomach heat may stagnate in the breast and impede the free flow of qi and blood in that area. Stomach heat can be further aggravated by over-eating hot, greasy, spicy food or by postpartum food stagnation.

It is also possible that external wind cold evils may take advantage of postpartum vacuity and weakness to invade the body in the region of the breast. These external evils block the free flow of qi and blood and this accumulation can transform into heat according to Liu Wan-su's theory of similar transformation.

Yet another potential cause of postpartum breast abscess is simple amassment of breast milk due to changes in feeding schedule and subsequent engorgement. Because the breast milk is transformed and engendered from the blood and it is moved upward to and through the breasts by the qi, if breast milk amasses and does not flow, the qi associated with it becomes stagnant and depressed and may transform heat.

If a woman's qi and blood are both vacuous and depleted, her body may not be able to out-thrust heat toxins which have been engendered. In that case, there may be swollen lumps which are only slightly or not painful, or there may be ulceration followed by unending suppuration and nonhealing.

Patterns common to this condition

Evil toxins externally assailing
Liver qi depression & binding
Breast milk amassment & accumulation
Qi & blood dual vacuity

Treatment based on pattern discrimination

Evil toxins externally assailing

Main symptoms: Postpartum breast swelling and pain, difficulty breast-feeding, cracked nipple, localized burning, heat, and possible redness, possible nodular lumps, generalized aversion to cold, fever, headache, muscular soreness and pain, thin, white or thin, yellow tongue fur, and a floating, rapid pulse

Treatment principles: Emit the exterior and scatter evils, course the liver and clear the stomach

Guiding formulas:

***Jing Fang Niu Bang Tang Jia Jian* (Schizonepeta, Ledebouriella & Arctium Decoction with Additions & Subtractions)**
Jing Jie (Herba Schizonepetae), 9g
Fang Feng (Radix Sapshnikoviae), 9g
Huang Qin (Radix Scutellariae), 9-12g
Niu Bang Zi (Fructus Arctii), 9g

Jin Yin Hua (Flos Lonicerae), 9-15g
Tian Hua Fen (Radix Trichosanthis), 9g
Lian Qiao (Fructus Forsythiae), 9-15g
Xiang Fu (Rhizoma Cyperi), 9g
Pu Gong Ying (Herba Taraxaci), 9-30g
Chai Hu (Radix Bupleuri), 9g
uncooked *Gan Cao* (Radix Glycyrrhizae), 3-6g
Zao Jiao Ci (Spina Gleditschiae Chinensis), 6-9g

If the breast milk is not free-flowing, add mix-fried *Chuan Shan Jia* (Squama Manitis), *Wang Bu Liu Xing* (Semen Vaccariae), and *Mu Tong* (Caulis Akebiae). If there is rib-side pain and distention, add *Yu Jin* (Tuber Curcumae) and *Chuan Lian Zi* (Fructus Toosendan). If there is severe swelling and pain, add processed *Ru Xiang* (Resina Olibani) and processed *Mo Yao* (Resina Myrrhae). If interior heat is severe, add *Shi Gao* (Gypsum Fibrosum) and *Zhi Mu* (Rhizoma Anemarrhenae).

Xian Fang Huo Ming Yin Jia Jian
(Immortal Formula Rescue Life Drink with Additions & Subtractions)
Jin Yin Hua (Flos Lonicerae), 9-15g
Lian Qiao (Fructus Forsythiae), 9-15g
Bai Zhi (Radix Angelicae Dahuricae), 9-15g
Fang Feng (Radix Sapshnikoviae), 9g
Dang Gui (Radix Angelicae Sinensis), 9g
Chen Pi (Pericarpium Citri Reticulatae), 6g
Gan Cao (Radix Glycyrrhizae), 3-9g
Zhe Bei Mu (Bulbus Fritillariae Thunbergii), 6-9g
Tian Hua Fen (Radix Trichosanthis), 9g
Mo Yao (Resina Myrrhae), 3-6g
Ru Xiang (Resina Olibani), 3-6g
Zao Jiao Ci (Spina Gleditschiae Chinensis), 6-9g

Gua Lou Niu Bang Tang Jia Jian
(Trichosanthes & Arctium Decoction with Additions & Subtractions)
Quan Gua Lou (Fructus Trichosanthis), 9g
Niu Bang Zi (Fructus Arctii), 9g
Pu Gong Ying (Herba Taraxaci), 9-30g
Jing Jie (Herba Schizonepetae), 9g
Fang Feng (Radix Sapshnikoviae), 9g
Ju Ye (Folium Citri Reticulatae), 9g
Huang Qin (Radix Scutellariae), 9-12g
Chai Hu (Radix Bupleuri), 9g
Wang Bu Liu Xing (Semen Vaccariae), 9-15g
Lu Lu Tong (Fructus Liquidambaris Taiwaniae), 9g

This formula is for the initial stage of a breast abscess before any pus has been brewed.

Qing Chuang Yin Jia Jian
(Clear Sores Drink with Additions & Subtractions)
Pu Gong Ying (Herba Taraxaci), 9-30g
Jin Yin Hua (Flos Lonicerae), 9-15g
Lian Qiao (Fructus Forsythiae), 9-15g
Gan Cao (Radix Glycyrrhizae), 3-9g
Tian Hua Fen (Radix Trichosanthis), 9g
Zhe Bei Mu (Bulbus Fritillariae Thunbergii), 9g
Chuan Shan Jia (Squama Manitis), 9-15g
Dang Gui (Radix Angelicae Sinensis), 9g
Zao Jiao Ci (Spina Gleditschiae Chinensis), 6-9g
Chi Shao (Radix Rubrus Paeoniae Lactiflorae), 9g
Ru Xiang (Resina Olibani), 3-6g
Mo Yao (Resina Myrrhae), 3-6g
Chen Pi (Pericarpium Citri Reticulatae), 6g

This formula is for the second stage of a breast abscess, referred to as brewing pus stage, when the breast is more severely red, swollen, hot, and painful. The fever does not recede, while the swollen lumps gradually soften. If pressed, there is a wavelike sensation. The tongue fur is slimy, yellow, and the pulse is bow-string, slippery, and rapid.

Acupuncture & moxibustion: *Qi Men* (Liv 14), *Jian Jing* (GB 21), *Nei Guan* (Per 6)

Liver qi depression & binding

Main symptoms: Postpartum breast distention and pain, obvious nodular lumps which are hard in substance, no change in the skin color, chest and rib-side distention and fullness, diminished appetite, thin, possibly slimy tongue fur, and a bowstring pulse

Treatment principles: Course the liver and resolve depression, move the qi, quicken the blood, and scatter nodulation

Guiding formulas:

Xiao Yao San Jia Wei (Rambling Powder with Added Flavors)
Chai Hu (Radix Bupleuri), 9g
Dang Gui (Radix Angelicae Sinensis), 9g
Bai Shao (Radix Albus Paeoniae Lactiflorae), 9g
Bai Zhu (Rhizoma Atractylodis Macrocephalae), 9g
Fu Ling (Poria), 9-12g
mix-fried *Gan Cao* (Radix Glycyrrhizae), 6-9g
Bo He (Herba Menthae Haplocalycis), 3-6g
Sheng Jiang (uncooked Rhizoma Zingiberis), 6g
Qing Pi (Pericarpium Citri Reticulatae Viride), 6-9g
Gua Lou (Fructus Trichosanthis), 9g
Yu Jin (Tuber Curcumae), 9g

Chuan Lian (Fructus Toosendan), 6-9g
Dan Shen (Radix Salviae Miltiorrhizae), 9-15g

If the breast milk is not smoothly flowing, add mix-fried *Chuan Shan Jia* (Squama Manitis), *Zao Jiao Ci* (Spina Gleditschiae Chinensis), and *Lu Lu Tong* (Fructus Liquidambaris Taiwaniae). If pain is severe, add *Lian Qiao* (Fructus Forsythiae), *Pu Gong Ying* (Herba Taraxaci), and *Ju He* (Semen Citri Reticulatae). If there is simultaneous aversion to cold and fever, add *Jin Yin Hua* (Flos Lonicerae) and *Huang Qin* (Radix Scutellariae) to resolve both the exterior and interior.

Chai Pu He Ji (Bupleurum & Dandelion Harmonizing Prescription)
Chai Hu (Radix Bupleuri), 9g
Pu Gong Ying (Herba Taraxaci), 9-30g
Hong Hua (Flos Carthami), 9g
Chi Shao (Radix Rubrus Paeoniae Lactiflorae), 9g
processed *Xiang Fu* (Rhizoma Cyperi), 9g

If there is swelling and a lump, add *Shan Zha* (Fructus Crataegi). If there is distention and pain, add *Wang Bu Liu Xing* (Semen Vaccariae). If there is pain in the chest and rib-sides with fever, add *Dan Shen* (Radix Salviae Miltiorrhizae). And if qi and blood are vacuous, add *Dang Shen* (Radix Codonopsitis), *Huang Qi* (Radix Astragali), *Dang Gui* (Radix Angelicae Sinensis), and *Shu Di* (cooked Radix Rehmanniae).

Xiao Chai Hu Tang Jia Wei
(Minor Bupleurum Decoction with Added Flavors)
Chai Hu (Radix Bupleuri), 9g
Dang Shen (Radix Codonopsitis), 9g
Ban Xia (Rhizoma Pinelliae), 9g
Huang Qin (Radix Scutellariae), 9-12g
mix-fried *Gan Cao* (Radix Glycyrrhizae), 6-9g
Da Zao (Fructus Jujubae), 3 pieces
Sheng Jiang (uncooked Rhizoma Zingiberis), 6g
Pu Gong Ying (Herba Taraxaci), 9-30g
Chuan Shan Jia (Squama Manitis), 9-15g
Mu Tong (Caulis Akebiae), 6-9g

This formula is for mastitis in a patient with a liver-spleen-stomach disharmony with or without alternating fever and chills. If fever is high and local inflammation is pronounced, add *Jin Yin Hua* (Flos Lonicerae) and *Lian Qiao* (Fructus Forsythiae). If nodulations are present, add *Zhe Bei Mu* (Bulbus Fritillariae Thunbergii) and *Xia Ku Cao* (Spica Prunellae). If there is accompanying thirst, add *Tian Hua Fen* (Radix Trichisanthis) and *Xuan Shen* (Radix Scrophulariae).

Acupuncture & moxibustion: *Qi Men* (Liv 14), *Liang Qiu* (St 34), *Nei Guan* (Per 6), *Gan Shu* (Bl 18)

Breast milk amassment & accumulation

Main symptoms: Postpartum swollen lumps in the breast which begin soft and gradually harden, nonfreely flowing breast milk, local distention and pain, chest oppression, vexation and agitation, slimy tongue fur, and a deep, bowstring pulse

Treatment principles: Move the qi, open the breasts, and scatter nodulation

Guiding formulas:

Xia Ru Yong Quan San (Precipitate Milk Gushing Spring Powder)
Dang Gui (Radix Angelicae Sinensis), 9g
Chuan Xiong (Radix Ligustici Wallichii), 9g
Bai Shao (Radix Albus Paeoniae Lactiflorae), 9g
Sheng Di (uncooked Radix Rehmanniae), 12-15g
Chai Hu (Radix Bupleuri), 9g
Tian Hua Fen (Radix Trichosanthis), 9g
Lou Lu (Radix Rhapontici/Echinopsis), 9g
Qing Pi (Pericarpium Citri Reticulatae Viride), 6-9g
Jie Geng (Radix Platycodi), 6-9g
Tong Cao (Medulla Tetrapanacis), 4.5-9g
Bai Zhi (Radix Angelicae Dahuricae), 9-15g
Chuan Shan Jia (Squama Manitis), 9-15g
Gan Cao (Radix Glycyrrhizae), 3-9g
Wang Bu Liu Xing (Semen Vaccariae), 9g
Mu Tong (Caulis Akebiae), 6-9g

If there is localized redness, swelling, aching and pain with fever, oral thirst, reddish urination, and dry stools, these are the manifestations of many days enduring transformation of heat brewing pus. In that case, it is OK to use *Ru Yong Yan Fang Jia Jian* (Breast Welling Abscess Experiential Formula with Additions & Subtractions): *Pu Gong Ying* (Herba Taraxaci), *Qing Pi* (Pericarpium Citri Reticulatae Viride), *Chen Pi* (Pericarpium Citri Reticulatae), *Chuan Shan Jia* (Squama Manitis), *Chuan Bei Mu* (Bulbus Fritillariae Cirrhosae), *Chai Hu* (Radix Bupleuri), *Gan Cao* (Radix Glycyrrhizae), *Gua Lou* (Fructus Trichosanthis), *Xiang Fu* (Rhizoma Cyperi), *Jie Ye* (Folium Platycodi), *Dang Gui* (Radix Angelicae Sinensis), *Lou Lu* (Radix Rhapontici/Echinopsis), *Wang Bu Liu Xing* (Semen Vaccariae).

Experiential formula #1
Gua Lou (Fructus Trichosanthis), 9g
Xia Ku Cao (Spica Prunellae), 9-15g
Zhe Bei Mu (Bulbus Fritillariae Thunbergii), 9g
mix-fried *Chuan Shan Jia* (Squama Manitis), 9-15g
Mu Tong (Caulis Akebiae), 6-9g
Lou Lu (Radix Rhapontici/Echinopsis), 9g
stir-fried *Mai Ya* (Fructus Germinatus Hordei), 15g
Niu Xi (Radix Achyranthis Bidentatae), 9-12g
uncooked *Gan Cao* (Radix Glycyrrhizae), 3-6g

Experiential formula #2
Ren Dong Teng (Caulis Lonicerae), 15g
Li Zhi He (Semen Litchi), 9g
Jin Yin Hua (Flos Lonicerae), 9-15g
mix-fried *Chuan Shan Jia* (Squama Manitis), 9-15g
Wang Bu Liu Xing (Semen Vaccariae), 9g
Lou Lu (Radix Rhapontici/Echinopsis), 9g

Acupuncture & moxibustion: *Tai Chong* (Liv 3), *Zu San Li* (St 36), *Shan Zhong* (CV 17), *Wei Shu* (Bl 21)

Qi & blood dual vacuity

Main symptoms: This pattern is mostly seen after breast abscesses have ruptured. There is pussy water which is clear and dilute. The opening of the sore is slow to close or endures for days without healing. There is also lassitude of the spirit, lack of strength, shortness of breath, disinclination to speak, insomnia, profuse dreams, a lusterless facial complexion, a pale tongue with thin, white fur, and a fine, forceless pulse

Treatment principles: Greatly supplement the qi and blood

Guiding formulas:

Ren Shen Yang Rong Tang (Ginseng Nourish the Constructive Decoction)
Bai Shao (Radix Albus Paeoniae Lactiflorae), 9g
Dang Gui (Radix Angelicae Sinensis), 9g
Chen Pi (Pericarpium Citri Reticulatae), 6g
Huang Qi (Radix Astragali), 9-18g
Rou Gui (Cortex Cinnamomi), 3-9g
Ren Shen (Radix Ginseng), 3-9g
Bai Zhu (Rhizoma Atractylodis Macrocephalae), 9g
mix-fried *Gan Cao* (Radix Glycyrrhizae), 6-9g
Shu Di (cooked Radix Rehmanniae), 12-15g
Wu Wei Zi (Fructus Schisandrae), 9g
Fu Ling (Poria), 9-12g
Yuan Zhi (Radix Polygalae), 6-9g

Tuo Li Xiao Du San Jia Wei
(Expel the Interior & Disperse Toxins Powder with Added Flavors)
Ren Shen (Radix Ginseng), 3-9g
Huang Qi (Radix Astragali), 9-18g
Zao Jiao Ci (Spina Gleditschiae Chinensis), 6-9g
Jie Geng (Radix Platycodi), 6-9g
Chuan Shan Jia (Squama Manitis), 9-15g

Acupuncture & moxibustion: Moxa *Zu San Li* (St 36) and *San Yin Jiao* (Sp 6)

Externally applied therapies:

In the early and middle stages when there is obvious localized burning heat, redness, swelling, aching and pain, use *Jin Huang San* (Golden Yellow Powder) or *Qing Fu Yao* (Green Application Medicine) applied externally. One can also use equal amounts of fresh *Pu Gong Ying* (Herba Taraxaci) and *Mang Xiao* (Mirabilitum) ground in a mortar and applied externally. Or one can put 250 grams of *Mang Xiao* in a cotton gauze bag and apply this externally. Keep the *Mang Xiao* over the nodular lumps and presently they will change.

Jin Huang San: *Da Huang* (Radix Et Rhizoma Rhei), *Huang Bai* (Cortex Phellodendri), *Jiang Huang* (Rhizoma Curcumae Longae), *Bai Zhi* (Radix Angelicae Dahuricae), 2500g each, *Nan Xing* (Rhizoma Arisaematis), *Chen Pi* (Pericarpium Citri Reticulatae), *Cang Zhu* (Rhizoma Atractylodis), *Hou Po* (Cortex Magnoliae Officinalis), *Gan Cao* (Radix Glycyrrhizae), 1000g each, *Tian Hua Fen* (Radix Trichosanthis), 5000g. Grind into a fine powder and apply externally.

Qing Fu Yao: *Da Huang* (Radix Et Rhizoma Rhei), *Jiang Huang* (Rhizoma Curcumae Longae), *Huang Bai* (Cortex Phellodendri), 240g each, *Bai Ji* (Rhizoma Bletillae), 180g, *Bai Zhi* (Radix Angelicae Dahuricae), *Chi Shao* (Radix Rubrus Paeoniae Lactiflorae), *Tian Hua Fen* (Radix Trichosanthis), *Qing Dai* (Pulvis Indigonis), *Gan Cao* (Radix Glycyrrhizae), 120g each. Grind into a fine powder. Use malt sugar or honey to mix into a paste.

Cong Yun Fa (Scallion Ironing Method)
Apply mashed *Cong Bai* (Bulbus Allii Fistulosi, scallion bulbs) to the affected area. Place a piece of smoldering charcoal over this and cover with a jar. Leave in place until the patient begins to perspire profusely. The swelling should be alleviated when the jar is withdrawn.

Xiang Fu Bing (Cyperus Pancake)
Xiang Fu (Rhizoma Cyperi)
She Xiang (Secretio Moschi Moschiferi)
Pu Gong Ying (Herba Taraxaci)
Jiu (alcohal)

Grind equal amounts of the first two ingredients into a fine powder. Decoct the *Pu Gong Ying* in wine and remove the dregs. Mix the remaining alcohol with the powdered medicinals and form into a flat cake. Apply warm over the affected area. *Mo Yao* (Resina Myrrhae) and/or *Ru Xiang* (Resina Olibani) may be substituted for *She Xiang*.

Unnamed formula from the Yi Zong Jin Jian (Golden Mirror of Ancestral Medicine)
Nan Xing (Rhizoma Arisaematis)
Ban Xia (Rhizoma Pinelliae)
Jiang Can (Bombyx Batryticatus)
Bai Zhi (Radix Angelicae Dahuricae)
Zao Jiao Ci (Spina Gleditschiae Chinensis)

Cao Wu (Radix Aconiti Kusnezoffii)

Grind the above ingredients and mix with onion juice and honey. Form into a flat cake and apply to the affected area.

Abstract of representative Chinese research:

From "The Treatment of 120 Cases of Mastitis with Self-composed *Ru Yong San* (Breast Abscess Powder)" by Chen Ti–zhang, *Zhe jiang Zhong Yi Za Zhi (Zhejiang Journal of Chinese Medicine)*, #11, 1994, p. 513

Cohort description:

Of the 120 women in this study, 104 were primiparas and 16 were multiparas. All were postpartum. The youngest primipara was 19 and the oldest was 26 years old. The multiparas were aged 23-37 years. The majority of these patients had been ill for 2-8 days, with 87 cases having been sick for three days or less. Twenty-two cases had been sick for 4-8 days, seven cases had been ill for nine days or more, and four cases had been ill for more than 15 days. Those who had been sick for nine days or more had all taken antibiotics which had been ineffective. All exhibited aversion to cold, fever, redness, swelling, pain of and lumps in the breast.

Treatment method:

The basic formula consisted of: *Ma Huang* (Herba Ephedrae), *Lian Qiao* (Fructus Forsythiae), and *Gan Cao* (Radix Glycyrrhizae), 20-25g each. If heat was exuberant, 12 grams each of *Pu Gong Ying* (Herba Taraxaci), *Zi Hua Di Ding* (Herba Violae), *Jin Yin Hua* (Flos Lonicerae), and *Ye Ju Hua* (Flos Chrysanthemi Indici) were added. If there was a tendency to cold, 15-20 grams of *Lu Jiao Shuang* (Cornu Degelatinum Cervi) and 10-15 grams of *Dang Gui* (Radix Angelicae Sinensis) were added. If the milk was not freely flowing or purulence was not being discharged easily, 12 grams of *Wang Bu Liu Xing* (Semen Vaccariae) were added. These medicinals were decocted in water and administered orally in divided doses.

Treatment outcomes:

All 120 patients were cured by this protocol. Forty-eight cases were cured with one packet of the above medicinals, 54 were cured with two packets, and 18 were cured after taking three packets.

Representative case histories

Case 1: The patient was a 30 year-old female worker. The woman had been breast-feeding for two months when some emotional upset caused her to develop pain in her right breast which was hard to palpation. There was a lump as big as a chicken egg, and pressure pain was marked. There was no change in color of the overlying skin. However, there was a dry cough, chest pain, vexation and agitation, easy anger, a bitter taste in the mouth, reduced appetite, generalized lack of strength, and a deep, bowstring, slippery pulse.

Based on these signs and symptoms, the patient's pattern was discriminated as liver depression transforming fire with obstruction and stagnation of the vessels and network vessels. Therefore, she was prescribed six packets of the following medicinals: *Wu Yao* (Radix Linderae), *Sha Shen* (Radix Glehniae), *Qing Pi* (Pericarpium Citri Reticulatae Viride), and *Chi Shao* (Radix Rubrus Paeoniae Lactiflorae), 10g each, *Pu Gong Ying* (Herba Taraxaci), 50g, *Jie Geng* (Radix Platycodi), 9g, *Chen Xiang* (Lignum Aquilariae), 6g, and *Bai Hua She She Cao* (Herba Hedyotis Diffusae), 15g. After taking these medicinals, the patient was cured.

Case 2: The patient was a 26 year-old female who had had postpartum swelling, hardness, distention, and pain in her right breast for five days. Initially, there had been fever and aversion to cold. After treatment, her fever had receded, but her breast swelling, pain, and hardness had not. On examination, it was found that both breasts were distended and full and that the patient's breast milk was thick. The patient's tongue was red with yellow fur, and her pulse was slippery and slightly rapid. In order to clear heat and resolve toxins, free the flow of the network vessels and move the milk, she was prescribed two packets of the following medicinals: *Pu Gong Ying* (Herba Taraxaci), 120g, *Jin Yin Hua* (Flos Lonicerae), *Zao Jiao Ci* (Spina Gleditschiae Chinensis), and *Gua Lou* (Fructus Trichosanthis), 60g each, *Sheng Ma* (Rhizoma Cimicifugae) and *Tian Hua Fen* (Radix Trichosanthis), 30g each. These were decocted in water and administered internally. In addition, 100 grams of *Mang Xiao* (Mirabilitum) and 50 grams of mashed *Sheng Ma* (Rhizoma Cimicifugae) were placed in a cotton bag which was soaked in alcohol and then placed over the affected area for 60-90 minutes. Using this protocol, the patient was healed after two days.

Case 3: The patient was a 22 year-old postpartum female who had lumps in both breasts which were red, swollen, and painful and from which the milk flowed uneasily. This had been going on for six days and was accompanied by aversion to cold and fever. The woman had already used externally applied poultices of fresh medicinals but without effect. Likewise, Western medical treatment had also been ineffective. At the time of examination, the patient's fever was 39∞ C. There was aversion to cold, and both breasts had lumps with marked pressure pain but no sensation of wavelike movement. The woman's tongue was pale red with thin fur, and her pulse was slippery and rapid. The patient's pattern was categorized as blood stasis obstructing the network vessels and was administered two packets of the following medicinals: *Dang Gui* (Radix Angelicae Sinensis), *Chuan Xiong* (Radix Ligustici Wallichii), *Yi Mu Cao* (Herba Leonuri), *Ze Lan* (Herba Lycopi), and *Cang Er Zi* (Fructus Xanthii), 12g each. These medicinals were boiled in a combination of water and rice wine.

After taking the above medicinals, the patient's breast swelling and pain decreased and her fever and aversion to cold disappeared. She was given another five packets of the same formula, all her symptoms disappeared, and her disease was considered cured.

Remarks

1. In my experience, Chinese medicine treats mastitis extremely well. However, great care should be taken and possible referral to Western medical services may be made if there has been fever and breast pain for more than 48 hours, if there is a high temperature, if there is a painful lump in the breast, and/or if there are swollen, tender glands in the arm pit.

2. Patients with mastitis should be fed a clear, bland diet. They should use hot ginger compresses over the site of inflammation during breast-feeding, and they should be encouraged to breast-feed from the affected breast.

3. Certain Chinese medicinals have a special tropism for the breasts. These include *Pu Gong Ying* (Herba Taraxaci), *Wang Bu Liu Xing* (Semen Vaccariae), *Chuan Shan Jia* (Squama Manitis), *Mu Tong* (Caulis Akebiae), *Lu Lu Tong* (Fructus Liquidambaris Taiwaniae), and *Tong Cao* (Medulla Tetrapanacis) to name some of the most important of these. In addition, all of the Citrus medicinals, such as *Ju He* (Semen Citri Reticulatae), *Ju Ye* (Folium Citri Reticulatae), *Chen Pi* (Pericarpium Citri Reticulatae), *Qing Pi* (Pericarpium Citri Reticulatae Viride), *Zhi Ke* (Fructus Aurantii), and *Zhi Shi* (Fructus Immaturus Aurantii) also have special tropism for the breasts. When using *Pu Gong Ying*, it is usually best to use large dosages, starting at not less than 18-24 grams per day and going up to 60 grams per day. This medicinal does not achieve marked effects at lower doses. *Lou Lu* (Radix Rhapontici/Echinopsis) is another medicinal with a special tropism for the breasts, but I have had no good luck using it. It has always caused unwanted indigestion in any patients I have tried to use it with. Therefore, I no longer prescribe it.

Endnotes:

[1] www.cdc.gov/ncidod/eid/vol7no5/yokoe.htm

[2] www.wdxcyber.com/mbrfeed.htm#m01

[3] www.emedicine.com/emerg/topic482.htm

[4] www.parentsplace.com/features/primer/qas/0,10338,258693_113637,00.html

30

Postpartum Weeping Breasts

In modern Western medicine, galactorrhea refers to spontaneous lactation in a man or a nonpuerperal woman. In Western medicine, there is no category of galactorrhea in a postpartum, breastfeeding mother. However, in Chinese medicine, we do recognize a situation where a puerperal, breastfeeding woman has unwanted leakage or spilling over from her breasts. If the postpartum woman has a strong constitution and her qi and blood are effulgent and flourishing, even if her breasts are distended and the breast milk is overflowing, this is considered normal and should not be treated with medicinal prescriptions. On the other hand, if the woman is either feverish with painful, distended breasts or presents signs and symptoms of qi vacuity and has spontaneously weeping or leaking breasts, this is considered pathological and should be treated.

Chinese medical disease categorization

Ru ye zi chu means spontaneous exiting of breast milk. Traditionally, this is also called *lou ru*, leaking breasts, *ru qi*, weeping breasts, and *ru ye zi tong*, breast milk spontaneously free-flowing.

Disease causes & disease mechanisms

There are two basic mechanisms involved in pathological postpartum weeping of the breasts. Either the qi and blood are vacuous and weak, leading to the qi being unable to secure and astringe body fluids, or there is depressive heat in the liver channel. In the latter case, coursing and discharge lose their normalcy and depressive heat forces the milk to overflow and spill outside.

Patterns common to this condition

Qi vacuity not securing
Liver channel depressive heat

Treatment based on pattern discrimination

Qi vacuity not securing

Main symptoms: Postpartum spontaneous weeping of the breasts, no distention or pain in the breasts, the amount of spillage not large, clear, thin, watery milk, dizziness, heart palpitations, shortness of breath, spontaneous perspiration, diminished intake of food and drink, a sallow yellow facial complexion, a pale, moist tongue, and a vacuous, big, moderate (*i.e.*, relaxed or slightly slow), or fine and forceless pulse

Treatment principles: Boost the qi and nourish the blood assisted by securing and astringing

Guiding formulas:

Ba Zhen Tang Jia Jian
(Eight Pearls Decoction with Additions & Subtractions)
Dang Gui (Radix Angelicae Sinensis), 9g
Shu Di (cooked Radix Rehmanniae), 9-15g
Bai Shao (Radix Albus Paeoniae Lactiflorae), 9g
Ren Shen (Radix Ginseng), 3-9g
mix-fried *Gan Cao* (Radix Glycyrrhizae), 6-9g
Bai Zhu (Rhizoma Atractylodis Macrocephalae), 9g
Fu Ling (Poria), 9-12g
Huang Qi (Radix Astragali), 9-18g
Wu Wei Zi (Fructus Schisandrae), 9g
Qian Shi (Semen Euryalis), 9g

Shi Quan Da Bu Tang Jia Wei (Ten [Ingredients] Completely & Greatly
Supplementing Decoction with Added Flavors)
Dang Gui (Radix Angelicae Sinensis), 9g
Bai Shao (Radix Albus Paeoniae Lactiflorae), 9g
Shu Di (cooked Radix Rehmanniae), 9-15g
Chuan Xiong (Radix Ligustici Wallichii), 6-9g
Ren Shen (Radix Ginseng), 3-9g
mix-fried *Gan Cao* (Radix Glycyrrhizae), 6-9g
Bai Zhu (Rhizoma Atractylodis Macrocephalae), 9g
Fu Ling (Poria), 9-12g
Rou Gui (Cortex Cinnamomi), 3-9g
Huang Qi (Radix Astragali), 9-18g
Mu Li (Concha Ostreae), 9-18g

Wu Wei Zi (Fructus Schisandrae), 9g

Acupuncture & moxibustion: *Zu San Li* (St 36), *San Yin Jiao* (Sp 6), *Pi Shu* (Bl 20), *Wei Shu* (Bl 21), *Shan Zhong* (CV 17)

If eating is diminished and the stools are loose, add *Zhong Wan* (CV 12) and *Tian Shu* (St 25). If there is lassitude of the spirit and shortness of breath, also moxa *Qi Hai* (CV 6) and *Guan Yuan* (CV 4).

Liver channel depressive heat

Main symptoms: Spontaneous postpartum discharge of breast milk accompanied by breast distention, fullness, and possible pain, a bitter taste in the mouth, dry mouth and parched throat, heart vexation, easy anger, emotional depression, heart palpitations or reduced sleep, constipation and dry stools, yellow or reddish urine, chest and rib-side pain and distention, yellow, thick breast milk or scanty milk mixed with bloody fluids, a red facial complexion, a red tongue with thin, dry, yellow fur, and a bowstring, rapid pulse

Treatment principles: Soothe the liver, resolve depression, and clear heat

Guiding formulas:

Han Bai-ling's Dan Zhi Xiao Yao San Jia Jian
(Moutan & Gardenia Rambling Powder with Additions & Subtractions)
Dan Pi (Cortex Moutan), 6-9g
Zhi Zi (Fructus Gardeniae), 6-9g
Dang Gui (Radix Angelicae Sinensis), 9g
Bai Shao (Radix Albus Paeoniae Lactiflorae), 9g
Chai Hu (Radix Bupleuri), 9g
Fu Ling (Poria), 9-12g
Bai Zhu (Rhizoma Atractylodis Macrocephalae), 9g
Bo He (Herba Menthae Haplocalycis), 3-6g
Gan Cao (Radix Glycyrrhizae), 3-9g
Huang Qin (Radix Scutellariae), 9-12g
Sheng Di (uncooked Radix Rehmanniae), 12-15g

If there is a bloody discharge from the nipples, add *Bai Mao Gen* (Rhizoma Imperatae) and *Xiao Ji* (Herba Cephalanoplos). If there is constipation, add a small amount of *Da Huang* (Radix Et Rhizoma Rhei).

Sun Jiu-ling's Dan Zhi Xiao Yao San Jia Jian
(Moutan & Gardenia Rambling Powder with Additions & Subtractions)
Dan Pi (Cortex Moutan), 6-9g
Zhi Zi (Fructus Gardeniae), 6-9g
Chai Hu (Radix Bupleuri), 9g
Bai Shao (Radix Albus Paeoniae Lactiflorae), 9g
Dang Gui (Radix Angelicae Sinensis), 9g
Gan Cao (Radix Glycyrrhizae), 3-9g

Bo He (Herba Menthae Haploclycis), 3-6g
Bai Zhu (Rhizoma Atractylodis Macrocephalae), 9g
Fu Ling (Poria), 9-12g
Sheng Di (uncooked Radix Rehmmaniae), 12-15g
Mai Men Dong (Tuber Ophiopogonis), 9-12g
uncooked *Mu Li* (Concha Ostreae), 9-18g

Luo Yuan-huang's Dan Zhi Xiao Yao San Jia Jian
(Moutan & Gardenia Rambling Powder with Additions & Subtractions)
Dan Pi (Cortex Moutan), 6-9g
Zhi Zi (Fructus Gardeniae), 6-9g
Chai Hu (Radix Bupleuri), 9g
Dang Gui (Radix Angelicae Sinensis), 9g
Bai Shao (Radix Albus Paeoniae Lactiflorae), 9g
Bai Zhu (Rhizoma Atractylodis Macrocephalae), 9g
Fu Ling (Poria), 9-12g
Gan Cao (Radix Glycyrrhizae), 3-9g
Bo He (Herba Menthae Haploclycis), 3-6g
Sheng Di (uncooked Radix Rehmanniae), 12-15g
Xia Ku Cao (Spica Prunellae), 9-15g
uncooked *Mu Li* (Concha Ostreae), 9-18g

Acupuncture & moxibustion: *Jian Jing* (GB 21), *Guang Ming* (GB 37), *Zu Lin Qi* (GB 41), *Tai Chong* (Liv 3), *Nei Guan* (Per 6)

If there is chest and rib-side distention and fullness, add *Qi Men* (Liv 14). If there is stomach duct distention and fullness, add *Zhong Wan* (CV 12) and *Zu San Li* (St 36).

Representative case history

The patient was a 29 year-old female who was initially examined on Jun. 20, 1979. This patient's milk was thin and watery and occasionally spontaneously spilled over. The patient was worried that this would lead to not enough milk for her baby, even though the child's urinary and fecal output was normal. The patient's tongue was pale and her pulse was fine. Therefore, her pattern was discriminated as postpartum qi and blood dual vacuity, with qi vacuity not able to secure and contain, and she was prescribed the following medicinals: *Huang Qi* (Radix Astragali), 30g, *Dang Gui* (Radix Angelicae Sinensis), 15g, *Lu Rong* (Cornum Parvum Cervi), 10g, *Bai Shao* (Radix Albus Paeoniae Lactiflorae), 10g, *Tian Hua Fen* (Radix Trichosanthis), 10g, *Wang Bu Liu Xing* (Semen Vaccariae), 8g, *Shu Di* (cooked Radix Rehmanniae), 15g, *Gou Qi Zi* (Fructus Lycii), 10g, *Chen Pi* (Pericarpium Citri Reticulatae), 10g. After taking three packets of these medicinals, the patient reported that her milk had gradually become thicker and that its amount had increased. Thus she was given another five packets, after which her milk no longer spilled over spontaneously.

Remarks

Chinese medicine is typically quite effective for stopping galactorrhea. A main ingredient for this purpose is large doses (30-60g) of stir-fried till fragrant *Mai Ya* (Fructus Germinatus Hordei). Another medicinal that has empirically verified milk-stopping properties is *Shan Zha* (Fructus Crataegi).

31

Postpartum Depression

Postpartum depression, also called "baby blues" refers to depression experienced in the postpartum period. Such depression may appear within 24 hours of delivery. It is usually limited in duration (36-48 hours) and is very common. This type of depression may require treatment if it lasts for more than 72 hours or is associated with lack of interest in the infant, suicidal or homicidal thoughts, hallucinations, or psychotic behavior. Contemporary Western psychiatry recognizes many syndromes that occur in the immediate postpartum time frame. However, in the current nosology, these symptom patterns are described as "specifiers" of broader categories of mood disorders or psychotic disorders. The *DSM-IV* mentions postpartum onset as a specifier in seven separate psychiatric disorders:

Major depressive disorder—single episode

Major depressive disorder—recurrent

Bipolar disorder I—single manic episode

Bipolar disorder I—most recent episode manic

Bipolar disorder I—most recent episode mixed

Bipolar disorder I—most recent episode depressed

Bipolar disorder II—depressed

Depressed mood with or without psychotic symptoms is the focus of clinical attention in four of these. Manic or mixed depressive-manic symptoms with or without psychotic symptoms are specified in the remaining three symptom patterns. According to *DSM-IV* criteria, postpartum onset means that symptoms begin sometime during the first four weeks after childbirth. Other Western mental health organizations define the postpartum period as lasting up to one year following childbirth. Definitional differences in the timeframe required for symptom onset significantly influence the number of cases diagnosed as postpartum disorders. The same general criteria required to diagnose an episode of major depression, mania, or mixed manic-depressive symptoms are also required to diagnose postpartum depression. In Western psychiatric nosology, psychotic symptoms sometimes occur together with a manic or depressive episode but are not necessary to diagnose either.

Epidemiologic surveys of Western populations indicate that prevalence rates of postpartum psychiatric disorders vary depending on the number of pregnancies. Postpartum psychosis occurs in first-time pregnancies at a rate of one in 500 (0.005%), and almost one-third of women who have had a postpartum psychotic episode experience similar symptoms in subsequent pregnancies.

Symptom patterns of several medical disorders that begin or worsen during or soon after pregnancy resemble postpartum psychiatric disorders. Ruling out delirium is the most important medical consideration in the differential diagnosis of postpartum depression or psychosis. Delirium in the postpartum period can be caused by medication side effects, infection, or blood loss. By definition, delirium is characterized by a change in level of consciousness, confusion, and disorientation. The delirious patient typically alternates between alert wakefulness and confused stupor. Specific medical disorders that may undergo exacerbation during or after pregnancy include multiple sclerosis (MS), systemic lupus erythematosus (SLE), hyperthyroidism, hypothyroidism, and other endocrinological disorders. It is difficult to distinguish postpartum mood or psychotic symptoms from neuropsychiatric sequelae of these or other medical disorders on the basis of clinical findings alone. Laboratory studies and brain-imaging usually clarify the differential diagnosis, verifying or excluding possible underlying medical causes.

Chronic abuse of alcohol or illicit substances during pregnancy or following delivery can result in persisting depressed mood. Use of certain prescription medications, including antihypertensives and steroids, can also result in depressive mood changes.

When primary medical disorders have been excluded, a thorough history clarifies the psychiatric differential diagnosis. The goal is to establish a pattern of mood or psychotic symptoms that occur predominantly in the weeks following childbirth. When this pattern cannot be established, other primary psychiatric disorders must be considered. For unclear reasons, transient worsening in schizophrenia, obsessive-compulsive disorder (OCD), and many anxiety disorders sometimes takes place in the postpartum time frame. According to the *DSM-IV* approach, the correct diagnosis depends on the long-term course and specific symptom pattern.

Many biological, psychological, and social theories have been advanced as putative explanations of postpartum psychiatric syndromes. Most of these derive from observations of the effects of specific neuroendocrinological changes on mood and behavior. This approach to understanding the pathogenesis of psychiatric disorders with postpartum onset can be traced to the discovery that anterior pituitary damage caused by a sudden transient drop in blood pressure during delivery manifests as symptom patterns that closely match diagnostic criteria for postpartum psychosis or depression. This disorder, called Sheehan's syndrome, is characterized by depression, agitation, confusion, and auditory or visual hallucinations. Further, hormonal replacement therapy with cortisone and thyroxine (two master hormones whose production declines in Sheehan's syndrome) typically results in normalization of postpartum psychiatric syndromes. Other evidence suggests that severe agitation or psychotic symptoms tend to occur in the first days following childbirth in contrast to depressed mood, which gradually evolves over a period of weeks. A neuroendocrinological basis for this pattern has not been clearly established. Independently from pituitary dysregulation in Sheehan's syndrome, maternal thyroid hormone serum levels typically change from high to low between the final trimester and the first postpartum days. The majority of women who experience this change in serum thyroid hormone levels report psychiatric symptoms that resemble postpartum depression. Treatment with thyroid hormones effectively reverses depressed mood and other psychiatric symptoms in approximately 50% of cases. In addition to pituitary-mediated hormonal influences, dysregulation in several neurotransmitters has been implicated as a possible cause of postpartum psychiatric syndromes. Studies investigating the role of serotonin, dopamine and norepinephrine have been inconclusive to date.

Although many studies have explored the potential contribution of psychological and social factors to the pathogenesis of postpartum psychiatric disorders, no causal relationships have been established.

In Western medicine, prompt treatment of identified medical etiologies (including hypothyroidism) usually leads to rapid clinical improvement in symptoms of agitation, psychosis, or depression. Aggressive treatment of postpartum psychotic states with high potency antipsychotics in the first days after symptom onset is usually more effective than starting treatment several weeks into the illness. Delaying the start of treatment can be a consequence of unreported or unrecognized psychotic symptoms. For unclear reasons, delayed treatment sometimes results in refractory psychotic states. The standard of care in contemporary Western psychiatry is to continue antipsychotic medications at least six weeks after a therapeutic response has been achieved and as long as one year after onset of postpartum psychotic symptoms. Antipsychotics may be safely continued during breast-feeding. Because of the very high risk of recurring psychosis following subsequent pregnancies, it is reasonable to start antipsychotics at childbirth in women with a history of postpartum psychosis.

In contrast to postpartum psychosis, which typically starts in the first days after childbirth, postpartum depressive or manic states tend to evolve gradually over several months. Most classes of antidepressants, including SSRIs, tricyclic agents, and atypical agents, have been used with some success. Several studies of nursing mothers have demonstrated that most antidepressants are secreted into the breast milk at concentrations that affect infants, resulting in significant behavioral side effects or discontinuation syndromes. As the long-term consequences of neonatal exposure to antidepressants have not been established, the recommended conservative approach is to avoid breast-feeding if severe postpartum psychiatric symptoms interfere with functioning, placing the mother's or infant's welfare at risk.

Progesterone therapy has been used to treat postpartum depression but with mixed results. When depressive symptoms are severe or refractory to trials of appropriate medications, electroconvulsive therapy (ECT) is considered to be the most reasonable alternative treatment available in contemporary Western medicine. Women who experience postpartum depression or mania are several times more likely to have clinically significant mood changes during or after future pregnancies. Because of the high probability of recurrence, prophylactic treatment is often started after subsequent births. Supportive psychotherapy often benefits mothers who are coping with the fatigue, anxiety, and stresses of caring for an infant while depressed. Perhaps the optimum treatment approach is combined medications and psychotherapy.[1]

Chinese medical disease categorization

Chan hou jing ji refers to postpartum fright and anxiety with heart palpitations. *Chan hou huang hu* literally means that one is abstracted from their surroundings as if in a trance postpartum. As a disease category, it includes impaired memory, restlessness and agitation, and confused, chaotic speech. *Chan hou xu fan* means postpartum vacuity vexation, agitation, lack of tranquility, restless fidgeting, and insomnia.

Disease causes & disease mechanisms

Most postpartum mental-emotional disorders are rooted in vacuity. Due to excessive blood and fluid loss during delivery and consumption of blood and fluids due to breast-feeding, heart qi and blood may become vacuous and weak. The heart treasures the spirit, and heart blood nourishes and secures the spirit. Therefore, if heart qi and blood become vacuous and weak, the spirit may become unsettled and nervous. This then may give rise to fright palpitations, impaired memory, and deranged speech. Since heart qi and blood are rooted in the spleen, heart vacuity is typically complicated by spleen vacuity, and spleen vacuity may give rise to fatigue, somnolence, lethargy, and lack of strength. Because the spleen qi and kidney yang are mutually rooted, spleen qi vacuity may also involve kidney yang vacuity.

However, a righteous postpartum vacuity is often complicated by various types of evil qi. For instance, postpartum blood vacuity may fail to nourish and moisten the liver sufficiently which then fails to control coursing and discharge. Hence the liver becomes depressed and the qi becomes stagnant, leading to irritability and easy anger. If liver depression transforms heat, this heat may ascend to harass the heart spirit. If it endures, it will also further consume yin and blood. If the liver invades the spleen, the spleen may become even more vacuous and weak. If the spleen fails to do its duty in controlling the movement and transformation of body fluids, dampness may be engendered which may further give rise to phlegm and turbidity misting and obstructing the clear orifices. Likewise, yin vacuity may engender internal heat. When this ascends and collects in the heart, it harasses the spirit, causing vexation and agitation, impaired memory, dizziness, insomnia, and heart palpitations. It is also possible for a righteous vacuity to allow for easy contraction of external wind evils which then cause heart palpitations, fearful throbbing, heart vexation, restlessness, insomnia, profuse dreams, and/or mental-emotional chaos and confusion.

In addition, it is possible to have completely replete postpartum disease mechanisms of essence spirit disorders. If spoilt blood (*i.e.*, static blood) is retained after delivery and penetrates upward, it may disturb the heart spirit causing heart palpitations, oppression, agitation, and insomnia. If severe, such spoilt or static blood may even result in mania, visual and auditory hallucinations, and deranged speech.

Patterns common to this condition

Heart qi vacuity weakness
Blood stasis penetrating the heart
Yin vacuity-fire effulgence
Righteous vacuity with contraction of evils

Treatment based on pattern discrimination

Heart qi vacuity weakness

Main symptoms: Postpartum heart palpitations, nervous anxiety, vertigo, dizziness, impaired memory, deranged speech, spontaneous perspiration, vexation and agitation, insomnia, a pale white or sallow yellow facial complexion, a pale, dry tongue, and a bowstring, fine pulse

Treatment principles: Boost the qi and nourish the blood, quiet the spirit and tranquilize palpitations

Guiding formula:

***Gui Pi Tang Jia Wei* (Restore the Spleen Decoction with Added Flavors)**
Ren Shen (Radix Ginseng), 3-9g
Bai Zhu (Rhizoma Atractylodis Macrocephalae),9g
Long Yan Rou (Arillus Euphoriae Longanae,9g)
Yuan Zhi (Radix Polygalae), 6-9g
Fu Shen (Sclerotium Pararadicis Poriae Cocos), 9-12g
Mu Xiang (Radix Auklandiae), 6-9g
Huang Qi (Radix Astragali), 9-18g
Dang Gui (Radix Angelicae Sinensis), 9g
mix-fried *Gan Cao* (Radix Glycyrrhizae), 6-9g
Suan Zao Ren (Semen Zizyphi Spinosae), 9-15g
Mai Men Dong (Tuber Ophiopogonis), 9-12g
Wu Wei Zi (Fructus Schisandrae), 9g
Mu Li (Concha Ostreae), 9-18g
Long Chi (Dens Draconis), 9-18g

Acupuncture & moxibustion: *Xin Shu* (Bl 15), *Ge Shu* (Bl 17), *Pi Shu* (Bl 20), *Shen Men* (Ht 7), *Zu San Li* (St 36), *Bai Hui* (GV 20), *Yin Tang* (M-HN-3)

Blood stasis penetrating the heart

Main symptoms: Postpartum heart palpitations, restlessness, nondescension of the lochia or a dark, purplish lochia which contains clots, possible lower abdominal pain which refuses pressure, possible mania, in extreme, possible visual and auditory hallucinations, deranged speech, and acting as if possessed, loss of sleep, a purple, dark facial complexion, deep red lips, static spots or macules on the tongue, and a bowstring, choppy, forceful pulse

Treatment principles: Free the flow of the channels and quicken the network vessels

Guiding formula:

Jia Wei Chuan Xiong San **(Added Flavors Ligusticum Powder)**
Chuan Xiong (Radix Ligustici Wallichii), 9-15g
Sheng Di (uncooked Radix Rehmanniae), 12-15g
Bai Shao (Radix Albus Paeoniae Lactiflorae), 9g
Niu Xi (Radix Achyranthis Bidentatae), 9-15g
Pu Huang (Pollen Typhae), 9g
Wu Ling Zhi (Feces Trogopterori Seu Pteromi), 9g

Acupuncture & moxibustion: *Xue Hai* (Sp 10), *San Yin Jiao* (Sp 6), *Tai Chong* (Liv 3), *He Gu* (LI 4), *Qi Hai* (CV 6), *Guan Yuan* (CV 4)

Yin vacuity-fire effulgence

Main symptoms: Postpartum heart vexation, restlessness, dizziness, tinnitus, impaired memory, insomnia, heart palpitations, night sweats, vexatious heat in the hands and feet, tidal heat, flushed red cheeks, a dry mouth but no particular thirst, low back and knee soreness and limpness, a red tongue with scanty, dry fur, and a bowstring, fine, rapid pulse

Treatment principles: Nourish yin and clear heat, quiet the spirit and tranquilize palpitations

Guiding formula:

Ren Shen Dang Gui Tang Jia Wei
(Ginseng & Dang Gui Decoction with Added Flavors)
Ren Shen (Radix Ginseng), 3-9g
Dang Gui (Radix Angelicae Sinensis), 9g
Shu Di (cooked Radix Rehmanniae), 12-15g
Tian Men Dong (Tuber Asparagi), 9-12g
Rou Gui (Cortex Cinnamomi), 3-9g
Bai Shao (Radix Albus Paeoniae Lactiflorae), 9g
Mai Men Dong (Tuber Ophiopogonis), 9-12g
Zhu Ru (Caulis Bambusae In Taeniis), 6-9g
Zhi Mu (Rhizoma Anemarrhenae), 9g

If yin vacuity causes internal engenderment of the heat which damages stomach and intestinal fluids with constipation and marked thirst, then use *Zeng Ye Cheng Qi Tang Jia Wei* (Increase Fluids Order the Qi Decoction with Added Flavors): *Xuan Shen* (Radix Scrophulariae), *Long Gu* (Os Draconis), *Mu Li* (Concha Ostreae), *Mai Men Dong* (Tuber Ophiopogonis), *Sheng Di* (uncooked Radix Rehmanniae), *Da Huang* (Radix Et Rhizoma Rhei), *Mang Xiao* (Mirabilitum)

Acupuncture & moxibustion: *Xin Shu* (Bl 15), *Shen Shu* (Bl 23), *Shen Men* (Ht 7), *Yin Xi* (Ht 6), *Da Ling* (Per 7), *Tai Xi* (Ki 3), *San Yin Jiao* (Sp 6), *Bai Hui* (GV 20), *Yin Tang* (M-HN-3)

Righteous vacuity with contraction of evils

Main symptoms: Postpartum dizziness, headache, agitation and restlessness, heart palpitations, fearful throbbing, heart vexation, insomnia, profuse dreams, if severe, chaotic and confused thinking, possible tics and spasms or convulsions, alternating fever and chills, a pale, possibly enlarged tongue with white fur, and a faint, forceless pulse

Treatment principles: Course wind and dispel evils, harmonize the qi and blood and quiet the spirit

Guiding formula:

Xiao Chai Hu Tang He Si Wu Tang Jia Wei **(Minor Bupleurum Decoction plus Four Materials Decoction with Added Flavors)**
Long Gu (Os Draconis), 9-18g
Mu Li (Concha Ostreae), 9-18g
Chai Hu (Radix Bupleuri), 9g
Dang Shen (Radix Codonopsitis), 9g
Huang Qin (Radix Scutellariae), 9-15g
Ban Xia (Rhizoma Pinelliae), 9g
Dang Gui (Radix Angelicae Sinensis), 9g
Bai Shao (Radix Albus Paeoniae Lactiflorae), 9g
Shu Di (cooked Radix Rehmanniae), 12-15g
Chuan Xiong (Radix Ligustici Wallichii), 9-15g
mix-fried *Gan Cao* (Radix Glycyrrhizae), 6-9g
Sheng Jiang (uncooked Rhizoma Zingiberis), 2-3 slices
Da Zao (Fructus Jujubae), 3-5 pieces

Acupuncture & moxibustion: *Feng Chi* (GB 20), *Feng Fu* (GV 16), *Feng Men* (Bl 12), *Bai Hui* (GV 20), *Yin Tang* (M-HN-3), *Wai Guan* (TB 5), *He Gu* (LI 4)

Representative case history

Neither the patient's age, marital status, occupation, or date of first examination are given in this case history. The patient had given birth twice before without problem. However, after her third delivery, she developed a number of psychological complaints, including insomnia, anxiety, and vexation and agitation. These were accompanied by heart fluster (*i.e.*, fright palpitations), shortness of breath, sweating, disinclination to speak, headache, lack of strength, and generalized soreness and pain. Her heart rate was 100 BPM, her respiratory rate was 24 times per minute, her temperature was 36.6° C, and her blood pressure was 13.3/8.0kPa. Her abdomen was level and soft, neither her liver or spleen were enlarged, and her uterus had shrunk to 3.0 *cun* below her navel. There was a slight degree of pressure pain over the uterus, her lochia was slightly profuse in amount, fresh red in color, and had a fishy odor. Her two excretions were normal. The patient's tongue was pale with thin, white fur, and her pulse was fine, rapid, and forceless. Her throat was slightly hyperemic, but neither her tonsils or submaxillary glands were enlarged.

Based on the above signs and symptoms, the patient was diagnosed as suffering from postpartum insomnia and her pattern was categorized as great postpartum damage to the true source or origin. Therefore, her qi and blood were both debilitated and unable to enrich and nourish the heart spirit. Therefore, the treatment principles were to supplement the qi, nourish the blood, and quiet the spirit. The medicinals she was given consisted of: *Ren Shen* (Radix Ginseng), 15g, *Huang Qi* (Radix Astragali), 25g, *Bai Zhu* (Rhizoma Atractylodis Macrocephalae), 15g, *Dang Gui* (Radix Angelicae Sinensis), 15g, *Fu Shen* (Sclerotium Pararadicis Poriae Cocos), 30g, *Yuan Zhi* (Radix Polygalae), 25g, *Suan Zao Ren* (Semen Zizyphi Spinosae), 25g, *He Huan Pi* (Cortex Albizziae), 15g, *Mu Xiang* (Radix Auklandiae), 15g, *Long Yan Rou* (Arillus Euphoriae Longanae), 25g, *Wu Wei Zi* (Fructus Schisandrae), 15g, *Shu Di (*cooked Radix Rehmanniae), 30g, mix-fried *Gan Cao* (Radix Glycyrrhizae), 5g, *Da Zao* (Fructus Jujubae), 5 pieces, *Sheng Jiang* (uncooked Rhizoma Zingiberis), 3 slices, and *E Jiao* (Gelatinum Corii Asini), 20g. One packet was administered per day, decocted in water, and given in two divided doses, morning and evening.

Remarks

In most women with postpartum depression, postpartum vacuity of qi, blood, and/or yin plays a large part. However, this postpartum vacuity is always complicated in real-life by liver depression qi stagnation, and this qi stagnation may be further complicated by blood stasis. Although the Chinese literature does not say anything about phlegm turbidity, if the patient over-eats fatty, greasy, so-called nutritious food postpartum and their spleen is vacuous and weak, there may also be complications from phlegm misting the orifices. Righteous vacuity with external contraction of evils mostly describes postpartum deranged speech, clouded spirit, and convulsions due to high fever associated with acute postpartum endomyometritis. This is not so commonly seen in developed countries.

Endnote:

[1] This Western medical introduction has mostly been written by Dr. James Lake and is taken from Bob Flaws and Dr. Lake's *Chinese Medical Psychiatry* also available from Blue Poppy Press.

General Index

Formula Index

OTHER BOOKS ON CHINESE MEDICINE AVAILABLE FROM:
BLUE POPPY PRESS

1990 North 57th Court, Unit A, Boulder, CO 80301
For ordering 1-800-487-9296 PH. 303\447-8372 FAX 303\245-8362
Email: info@bluepoppy.com Website: www.bluepoppy.com

ACUPOINT POCKET REFERENCE
by Bob Flaws
ISBN 0-936185-93-7
ISBN 978-0-936185-93-4

ACUPUNCTURE & IVF
by Lifang Liang
ISBN 0-891845-24-1
ISBN 978-0-891845-24-6

ACUPUNCTURE, CHINESE MEDICINE &
HEALTHY WEIGHT LOSS   Revised Edition
by Juliette Aiyana, L. Ac.
ISBN 1-891845-61-6
ISBN 978-1-891845-61-1

ACUPUNCTURE FOR STROKE REHABILITATION
Three Decades of Information from China
by Hoy Ping Yee Chan, et al.
ISBN 1-891845-35-7
ISBN 978-1-891845-35-2

ACUPUNCTURE PHYSICAL MEDICINE:
An Acupuncture Touchpoint Approach to the
Treatment of Chronic Pain, Fatigue, and Stress
Disorders
by Mark Seem
ISBN 1-891845-13-6
ISBN 978-1-891845-13-0

AGING & BLOOD STASIS:
A New Approach to TCM Geriatrics
by Yan De-xin
ISBN 0-936185-63-6
ISBN 978-0-936185-63-7

AN ACUPUNCTURISTS GUIDE TO MEDICAL RED
FLAGS & REFERRALS
by Dr. David Anzaldua, MD
ISBN 1-891845-54-3
ISBN 978-1-891845-54-3

BETTER BREAST HEALTH NATURALLY
with CHINESE MEDICINE
by Honora Lee Wolfe & Bob Flaws
ISBN 0-936185-90-2
ISBN 978-0-936185-90-3

BIOMEDICINE: A TEXTBOOK FOR PRACTITIONERS
OF ACUPUNCTURE AND ORIENTAL MEDICINE
by Bruce H. Robinson, MD
ISBN 1-891845-38-1
ISBN 978-1-891845-38-3

THE BOOK OF JOOK: Chinese Medicinal Porridges
by Bob Flaws
ISBN 0-936185-60-6
ISBN 978-0-936185-60-0

CHANNEL DIVERGENCES Deeper Pathways of the
Web
by Miki Shima and Charles Chase
ISBN 1-891845-15-2
ISBN 978-1-891845-15-4

CHINESE MEDICAL OBSTETRICS
by Bob Flaws
ISBN 1-891845-30-6
ISBN 978-1-891845-30-7

CHINESE MEDICAL PALMISTRY:
Your Health in Your Hand
by Zong Xiao-fan & Gary Liscum
ISBN 0-936185-64-3
ISBN 978-0-936185-64-4

CHINESE MEDICAL PSYCHIATRY
A Textbook and Clinical Manual
by Bob Flaws and James Lake, MD
ISBN 1-845891-17-9
ISBN 978-1-845891-17-8

CHINESE MEDICINAL TEAS: Simple, Proven, Folk
Formulas for Common Diseases & Promoting Health
by Zong Xiao-fan & Gary Liscum
ISBN 0-936185-76-7
ISBN 978-0-936185-76-7

CHINESE MEDICINAL WINES & ELIXIRS
by Bob Flaws   Revised Edition
ISBN 0-936185-58-9
ISBN 978-0-936185-58-3

CHINESE PEDIATRIC MASSAGE THERAPY: A
Parent's & Practitioner's Guide to the Prevention &
Treatment of Childhood Illness
by Fan Ya-li
ISBN 0-936185-54-6
ISBN 978-0-936185-54-5

CHINESE SCALP ACUPUNCTURE
by Jason Jishun Hao & Linda Lingzhi Hao
ISBN 1-891845-60-8
ISBN 978-1-891845-60-4

CHINESE SELF-MASSAGE THERAPY:
The Easy Way to Health
by Fan Ya-li
ISBN 0-936185-74-0
ISBN 978-0-936185-74-3

THE CLASSIC OF DIFFICULTIES:
A Translation of the *Nan Jing*
translation by Bob Flaws
ISBN 1-891845-07-1
ISBN 978-1-891845-07-9

A CLINICIAN'S GUIDE TO USING GRANULE
EXTRACTS
by Eric Brand
ISBN 1-891845-51-9
ISBN 978-1-891845-51-2

A COMPENDIUM OF CHINESE MEDICAL
MENSTRUAL DISEASES
by Bob Flaws
ISBN 1-891845-31-4
ISBN 978-1-891845-31-4

CONCISE CHINESE MATERIA MEDICA
by Eric Brand and Nigel Wiseman
ISBN 0-912111-82-8
ISBN 978-0-912111-82-7

CONTEMPORARY GYNECOLOGY: An Integrated
Chinese-Western Approach
by Lifang Liang
ISBN 1-891845-50-0
ISBN 978-1-891845-50-5

CONTROLLING DIABETES NATURALLY WITH
CHINESE MEDICINE
by Lynn Kuchinski
ISBN 0-936185-06-3
ISBN 978-0-936185-06-2

CURING ARTHRITIS NATURALLY WITH
CHINESE MEDICINE
by Douglas Frank & Bob Flaws
ISBN 0-936185-87-2
ISBN 978-0-936185-87-3

CURING DEPRESSION NATURALLY WITH
CHINESE MEDICINE
by Rosa Schnyer & Bob Flaws
ISBN 0-936185-94-5
ISBN 978-0-936185-94-1

CURING FIBROMYALGIA NATURALLY WITH
CHINESE MEDICINE
by Bob Flaws
ISBN 1-891845-09-8
ISBN 978-1-891845-09-3

CURING HAY FEVER NATURALLY WITH
CHINESE MEDICINE
by Bob Flaws
ISBN 0-936185-91-0
ISBN 978-0-936185-91-0

CURING HEADACHES NATURALLY WITH
CHINESE MEDICINE
by Bob Flaws
ISBN 0-936185-95-3
ISBN 978-0-936185-95-8

CURING IBS NATURALLY WITH CHINESE
MEDICINE
by Jane Bean Oberski
ISBN 1-891845-11-X
ISBN 978-1-891845-11-6

CURING INSOMNIA NATURALLY WITH
CHINESE MEDICINE
by Bob Flaws
ISBN 0-936185-86-4
ISBN 978-0-936185-86-6

CURING PMS NATURALLY WITH CHINESE
MEDICINE
by Bob Flaws
ISBN 0-936185-85-6
ISBN 978-0-936185-85-9

DISEASES OF THE KIDNEY & BLADDER
by Hoy Ping Yee Chan, *et al.*
ISBN 1-891845-37-3
ISBN 978-1-891845-35-6

THE DIVINE FARMER'S MATERIA MEDICA
A Translation of the Shen Nong Ben Cao
translation by Yang Shouz-zhong
ISBN 0-936185-96-1
ISBN 978-0-936185-96-5

DUI YAO: THE ART OF COMBINING
CHINESE HERBAL MEDICINALS
by Philippe Sionneau
ISBN 0-936185-81-3
ISBN 978-0-936185-81-1

ENDOMETRIOSIS, INFERTILITY AND
TRADITIONAL CHINESE MEDICINE:
A Layperson's Guide
by Bob Flaws
ISBN 0-936185-14-7
ISBN 978-0-936185-14-9

THE ESSENCE OF LIU FENG-WU'S GYNECOLOGY
by Liu Feng-wu, translated by Yang Shou-zhong
ISBN 0-936185-88-0
ISBN 978-0-936185-88-0

EXTRA TREATISES BASED ON INVESTIGATION &
INQUIRY: A Translation of Zhu Dan-xi's Ge Zhi Yu
Lun
translation by Yang Shou-zhong
ISBN 0-936185-53-8
ISBN 978-0-936185-53-8

FIRE IN THE VALLEY: TCM Diagnosis & Treatment
of Vaginal Diseases
by Bob Flaws
ISBN 0-936185-25-2
ISBN 978-0-936185-25-5

FULFILLING THE ESSENCE:
A Handbook of Traditional & Contemporary
Treatments for Female Infertility
by Bob Flaws
ISBN 0-936185-48-1
ISBN 978-0-936185-48-4

FU QING-ZHU'S GYNECOLOGY
trans. by Yang Shou-zhong and Liu Da-wei
ISBN 0-936185-35-X
ISBN 978-0-936185-35-4

GOLDEN NEEDLE WANG LE-TING: A 20th Century
Master's Approach to Acupuncture
by Yu Hui-chan and Han Fu-ru, trans. by Shuai Xue-zhong
ISBN 0-936185-78-3
ISBN 978-0-936185-78-1

A HANDBOOK OF CHINESE HEMATOLOGY
by Simon Becker
ISBN 1-891845-16-0
ISBN 978-1-891845-16-1

A HANDBOOK OF TCM PATTERNS
& THEIR TREATMENTS   Second Edition
by Bob Flaws & Daniel Finney
ISBN 0-936185-70-8
ISBN 978-0-936185-70-5

A HANDBOOK OF TRADITIONAL
CHINESE DERMATOLOGY
by Liang Jian-hui, trans. by Zhang Ting-liang
& Bob Flaws
ISBN 0-936185-46-5
ISBN 978-0-936185-46-0

A HANDBOOK OF TRADITIONAL
CHINESE GYNECOLOGY
by Zhejiang College of TCM, trans. by Zhang Ting-liang
& Bob Flaws
ISBN 0-936185-06-6 (4th edit.)
ISBN 978-0-936185-06-4

A HANDBOOK of TCM PEDIATRICS
by Bob Flaws
ISBN 0-936185-72-4
ISBN 978-0-936185-72-9

THE HEART & ESSENCE OF DAN-XI'S
METHODS OF TREATMENT
by Xu Dan-xi, trans. by Yang Shou-zhong
ISBN 0-926185-50-3
ISBN 978-0-936185-50-7

HERB TOXICITIES & DRUG INTERACTIONS:
A Formula Approach
by Fred Jennes with Bob Flaws
ISBN 1-891845-26-8
ISBN 978-1-891845-26-0

IMPERIAL SECRETS OF HEALTH & LONGEVITY
by Bob Flaws
ISBN 0-936185-51-1
ISBN 978-0-936185-51-4

INSIGHTS OF A SENIOR ACUPUNCTURIST
by Miriam Lee
ISBN 0-936185-33-3
ISBN 978-0-936185-33-0

INTEGRATED PHARMACOLOGY: Combining Modern Pharmacology with Chinese Medicine
by Dr. Greg Sperber with Bob Flaws
ISBN 1-891845-41-1
ISBN 978-0-936185-41-3

INTRODUCTION TO THE USE OF PROCESSED CHINESE MEDICINALS
by Philippe Sionneau
ISBN 0-936185-62-7
ISBN 978-0-936185-62-0

KEEPING YOUR CHILD HEALTHY WITH CHINESE MEDICINE
by Bob Flaws
ISBN 0-936185-71-6
ISBN 978-0-936185-71-2

THE LAKESIDE MASTER'S STUDY OF THE PULSE
by Li Shi-zhen, trans. by Bob Flaws
ISBN 1-891845-01-2
ISBN 978-1-891845-01-7

MANAGING MENOPAUSE NATURALLY WITH CHINESE MEDICINE
by Honora Lee Wolfe
ISBN 0-936185-98-8
ISBN 978-0-936185-98-9

MASTER HUA'S CLASSIC OF THE CENTRAL VISCERA
by Hua Tuo, trans. by Yang Shou-zhong
ISBN 0-936185-43-0
ISBN 978-0-936185-43-9

THE MEDICAL I CHING: Oracle of the Healer Within
by Miki Shima
ISBN 0-936185-38-4
ISBN 978-0-936185-38-5

MENOPAIUSE & CHINESE MEDICINE
by Bob Flaws
ISBN 1-891845-40-3
ISBN 978-1-891845-40-6

MOXIBUSTION: A MODERN CLINICAL HANDBOOK
by Lorraine Wilcox
ISBN 1-891845-49-7
ISBN 978-1-891845-49-9

MOXIBUSTION: THE POWER OF MUGWORT FIRE
by Lorraine Wilcox
ISBN 1-891845-46-2
ISBN 978-1-891845-46-8

A NEW AMERICAN ACUPUNTURE By Mark Seem
ISBN 0-936185-44-9
ISBN 978-0-936185-44-6

PLAYING THE GAME: A Step-by-Step Approach to Accepting Insurance as an Acupuncturist
by Greg Sperber & Tiffany Anderson-Hefner
ISBN 3-131416-11-7
ISBN 978-3-131416-11-7

POCKET ATLAS OF CHINESE MEDICINE
Edited by Marne and Kevin Ergil
ISBN 1-891-845-59-4
ISBN 978-1-891845-59-8

POINTS FOR PROFIT: The Essential Guide to Practice Success for Acupuncturists 4rd Edition
by Honora Wolfe, Eric Strand & Marilyn Allen
ISBN 1-891845-25-X
ISBN 978-1-891845-25-3

PRINCIPLES OF CHINESE MEDICAL ANDROLOGY: An Integrated Approach to Male Reproductive and Urological Health by Bob Damone
ISBN 1-891845-45-4
ISBN 978-1-891845-45-1

PRINCE WEN HUI's COOK: Chinese Dietary Therapy
By Bob Flaws & Honora Wolfe
ISBN 0-912111-05-4
ISBN 978-0-912111-05-6

THE PULSE CLASSIC:
A Translation of the Mai Jing
by Wang Shu-he, trans. by Yang Shou-zhong
ISBN 0-936185-75-9
ISBN 978-0-936185-75-0

THE SECRET OF CHINESE PULSE DIAGNOSIS
by Bob Flaws
ISBN 0-936185-67-8
ISBN 978-0-936185-67-5

SECRET SHAOLIN FORMULAS FOR THE TREATMENT OF EXTERNAL INJURY
by De Chan, trans. by Zhang Ting-liang & Bob Flaws
ISBN 0-936185-08-2
ISBN 978-0-936185-08-8

STATEMENTS OF FACT IN TRADITIONAL CHINESE MEDICINE   Revised & Expanded
by Bob Flaws
ISBN 0-936185-52-X
ISBN 978-0-936185-52-1

STICKING TO THE POINT: A Step-by-Step Approach to TCM Acupuncture Therapy
by Bob Flaws & Honora Wolfe   2 Condensed Books
ISBN 1-891845-47-0
ISBN 978-1-891845-47-5

A STUDY OF DAOIST ACUPUNCTURE
by Liu Zheng-cai
ISBN 1-891845-08-X
ISBN 978-1-891845-08-6

THE SUCCESSFUL CHINESE HERBALIST
by Bob Flaws and Honora Lee Wolfe
ISBN 1-891845-29-2
ISBN 978-1-891845-29-1

THE SYSTEMATIC CLASSIC OF ACUPUNCTURE & MOXIBUSTION
A translation of the Jia Yi Jing
by Huang-fu Mi, trans. by Yang Shou-zhong & Charles Chace
ISBN 0-936185-29-5
ISBN 978-0-936185-29-3

THE TAO OF HEALTHY EATING: DIETARY WISDOM ACCORDING TO CHINESE MEDICINE
by Bob Flaws   Second Edition
ISBN 0-936185-92-9
ISBN 978-0-936185-92-7

TEACH YOURSELF TO READ MODERN MEDICAL CHINESE
by Bob Flaws
ISBN 0-936185-99-6
ISBN 978-0-936185-99-6

TEST PREP WORKBOOK FOR BASIC TCM THEORY
by Zhong Bai-song
ISBN 1-891845-43-8
ISBN 978-1-891845-43-7

TEST PREP WORKBOOK FOR THE NCCAOM BIO-MEDICINE MODULE: Exam Preparation & Study Guide
by Zhong Bai-song
ISBN 1-891845-34-9
ISBN 978-1-891845-34-5

TREATING PEDIATRIC BED-WETTING WITH ACUPUNCTURE & CHINESE MEDICINE
by Robert Helmer
ISBN 1-891845-33-0
ISBN 978-1-891845-33-8

TREATISE on the SPLEEN & STOMACH: A
Translation and annotation of Li Dong-yuan's
Pi Wei Lun
by Bob Flaws
ISBN 0-936185-41-4
ISBN 978-0-936185-41-5

THE TREATMENT OF CARDIOVASCULAR DIS-
EASES WITH CHINESE MEDICINE
by Simon Becker, Bob Flaws &
Robert Casañas, MD
ISBN 1-891845-27-6
ISBN 978-1-891845-27-7

THE TREATMENT OF DIABETES MELLITUS WITH
CHINESE MEDICINE
by Bob Flaws, Lynn Kuchinski &
Robert Casañas, M.D.
ISBN 1-891845-21-7
ISBN 978-1-891845-21-5

THE TREATMENT OF DISEASE IN TCM, Vol. 1:
Diseases of the Head & Face, Including Mental &
Emotional Disorders   New Edition
by Philippe Sionneau & Lü Gang
ISBN 0-936185-69-4
ISBN 978-0-936185-69-9

THE TREATMENT OF DISEASE IN TCM, Vol. II:
Diseases of the Eyes, Ears, Nose, & Throat
by Sionneau & Lü
ISBN 0-936185-73-2
ISBN 978-0-936185-73-6

THE TREATMENT OF DISEASE IN TCM, Vol. III:
Diseases of the Mouth, Lips, Tongue, Teeth & Gums
by Sionneau & Lü
ISBN 0-936185-79-1
ISBN 978-0-936185-79-8

THE TREATMENT OF DISEASE IN TCM, Vol IV:
Diseases of the Neck, Shoulders, Back, & Limbs
by Philippe Sionneau & Lü Gang
ISBN 0-936185-89-9
ISBN 978-0-936185-89-7

THE TREATMENT OF DISEASE IN TCM, Vol V:
Diseases of the Chest & Abdomen
by Philippe Sionneau & Lü Gang
ISBN 1-891845-02-0
ISBN 978-1-891845-02-4

THE TREATMENT OF DISEASE IN TCM, Vol VI:
Diseases of the Urogential System & Proctology
by Philippe Sionneau & Lü Gang
ISBN 1-891845-05-5
ISBN 978-1-891845-05-5

THE TREATMENT OF DISEASE IN TCM, Vol VII:
General Symptoms
by Philippe Sionneau & Lü Gang
ISBN 1-891845-14-4
ISBN 978-1-891845-14-7

THE TREATMENT OF EXTERNAL DISEASES WITH
ACUPUNCTURE & MOXIBUSTION
by Yan Cui-lan and Zhu Yun-long, trans. by Yang Shou-zhong
ISBN 0-936185-80-5
ISBN 978-0-936185-80-4

THE TREATMENT OF MODERN WESTERN
MEDICAL DISEASES WITH CHINESE MEDICINE
by Bob Flaws & Philippe Sionneau
ISBN 1-891845-20-9
ISBN 978-1-891845-20-8

UNDERSTANDING THE DIFFICULT PATIENT: A
Guide for Practitioners of Oriental Medicine
by Nancy Bilello, RN, L.ac.
ISBN 1-891845-32-2
ISBN 978-1-891845-32-1

WESTERN PHYSICAL EXAM SKILLS FOR
PRACTITIONERS OF ASIAN MEDICINE
by Bruce H. Robinson & Honora Lee Wolfe
ISBN 1-891845-48-9
ISBN 978-1-891845-48-2

YI LIN GAI CUO (Correcting the Errors in the Forest
of Medicine)
by Wang Qing-ren
ISBN 1-891845-39-X
ISBN 978-1-891845-39-0

70 ESSENTIAL CHINESE HERBAL FORMULAS
by Bob Flaws
ISBN 0-936185-59-7
ISBN 978-0-936185-59-0

160 ESSENTIAL CHINESE READY-MADE
MEDICINES
by Bob Flaws
ISBN 1-891945-12-8
ISBN 978-1-891945-12-3

630 QUESTIONS & ANSWERS ABOUT CHINESE
HERBAL MEDICINE:
A Workbook & Study Guide
by Bob Flaws
ISBN 1-891845-04-7
ISBN 978-1-891845-04-8

260 ESSENTIAL CHINESE MEDICINALS
by Bob Flaws
ISBN 1-891845-03-9
ISBN 978-1-891845-03-1

750 QUESTIONS & ANSWERS ABOUT
ACUPUNCTURE
Exam Preparation & Study Guide
by Fred Jennes
ISBN 1-891845-22-5
ISBN 978-1-891845-22-2